African Studies
History, Politics, Economics, and Culture

Edited by
Molefi Asante
Temple University

A Routledge Series

African Studies

History, Politics, Economics, and Culture

Molefi Asante, *General Editor*

The Human Cost of African Migrations

Toyin Falola and
Niyi Afolabi

Routledge
New York & London

Routledge
Taylor & Francis Group
270 Madison Avenue
New York, NY 10016

Routledge
Taylor & Francis Group
2 Park Square
Milton Park, Abingdon
Oxon OX14 4RN

Routledge is an imprint of Taylor & Francis Group, an Informa business

Transferred to Digital Printing 2009

International Standard Book Number-13: 978-0-415-95837-0 (Hardcover)

Library of Congress Cataloging-in-Publication Data

The human cost of African migrations / edited by Toyin Falola and Niyi Afolabi.
p. cm.
Includes bibliographical references and index.
ISBN 0-415-95837-7 (alk. paper)
1. Africa--Emigration and immigration. 2. Migration, Internal--Africa. 3. Medical personnel--Africa. 4. Medical care--Africa. I. Falola, Toyin. II. Afolabi, Niyi.

JV8790.H86 2007
304.8096--dc22 2007006125

ISBN10: 0-415-95837-7 (hbk)
ISBN10: 0-415-80239-3 (pbk)

ISBN13: 978-0-415-95837-0 (hbk)
ISBN13: 978-0-415-80239-0 (pbk)

Visit the Taylor & Francis Web site at
http://www.taylorandfrancis.com

and the Routledge Web site at
http://www.routledge.com

To
Dennis Cordell, scholar, humanist and world citizen
&
Isidore Okpewho, scholar and able navigator of our global Odyssey

Contents

PART IV: REFUGEES, DISPLACEMENT, AND RE-SETTLEMENT

List of Tables

TABLES

List of Abbreviations, Acronyms, Language Clusters

ABBREVIATIONS & ACRONYMS

AESM	All Ethiopian Socialist Movement
AIDB	Agricultural and Industrial Development Bank
AIDS	Acquired Immune Deficiency Syndrome
ANDM	Amhara National Democratic Movement
ANC	African National Congress
BBC	British Broadcasting Corporation
CEDAW	Convention on the Elimination of All Forms of Discrimination Against Women
CODESA	Convention for a Democratic South Africa
COLTS	Culture of Teaching and Learning Services
COR	Commission of Refugees (Sudan)
CSWs	Commercial Sex Workers
DfEE	Department for Education and Development
DfES	Department for Education and Skills
DOE	Department of Education
DRC	Democratic Republic of Congo
ECOMOG	Economic Community of West African States Monitoring Group
ECOWAS	Economic Community of West African States
EDU	Ehiopian Democratic Union

ELF	Eritrean Liberation Front
EPID	Extension and Project Implementation Department
EPLF	Eritrean People's Liberation Front
EPRDF	Ethiopian People's Revolutionary Democratic Forces
EPRP	Ethiopian People's Revolutionary party
ERA	Eritrean Relief Association
GAATW	Global Alliance Against Trafficking in Women
FEDSAW	Federation of South African Women
GATS	General Agreement in Trade and Services
GATT	General Agreement on Tariffs and Trade
GDP	Gross Domestic Product
GEAR	Growth Employment and Redistribution
HIV	Human Immunodeficiency Virus
ICJ	International Court of Justice
ICM	International Committee for Migration
ICMC	International Catholic Migration Committee
ICRC	International Committee of the Red Cross
IDPs	Internally Displaced Persons
IMF	International Monetary Fund
IRC	International Rescue Committee
JSS	Junior Secondary School
MONUC	UN Mission in the Democratic Republic of Congo
MRA	Manpower Requirement Approach
NAPTIP	National Agency for the Prohibition of Traffic in Persons and Other Related Matters
NFD	Northern Frontier District
NGO	Non-Governmental Organization
NHIS	National Health Interview Surveys
OAU	Organization of African Unity
OCHA	UN Office for the Coordination of Humanitarian Affairs

OFSTED	Office for Standards in Education
OLF	Oromo Liberation Front
OPDO	Oromo People's Democratic Organization
ORA	Oromo Relief Association
PCIJ	Permanent Court of International Justice
PED	Papers in Education and Development
PSA	Prostate Specific Antigen
RDP	Reconstruction and Development Program
REST	Relief Society of Tigray (Sudan)
RNC	Revised National Curriculum
RST	Relief Society of Tigray
SABC	South African Broadcasting Co-operation
SACTU	South African Congress of Trade Unions
SANA	South African Nursing Association
SANC	South African Nursing Council
SANDF	South African National Defense Force
SAP	Structural Adjustment Program
SEM	Senior Education Managers
SGBs	School Governing Bodies
SPLA	Sudanese People's Liberation Army
SSA	Sub-Saharan Africa
SSS	Senior Secondary School
STD	Sexually Transmitted Disease
TANU	Tangayika African National Union
TB	Tuberculosis
TPLF	Tigrian People's Liberation Front (Now EPRDF)
UNICEF	United Nations International Children's Emergency Fund
UNIFEM	United Nations Development Fund for Women
UNHCHR	United Nations High Commission for Human Rights
UNHCR	United Nations High Commission for Refugees

UK	United Kingdom
UN	United Nations
UNCTAD	United Nations Conference on Trade and Development
UNN	University of Nigeria
UNODC	United Nations Office on Drugs and Crime
UNSC	United Nations Security Council
UPE	Universal Primary Education
US	United States
USSR	Union of Soviet Socialist Republics
WHO	World Health Organization
WOTCLEF	Women Trafficking and Child Labor Eradication Foundation
WTO	World Trade Organization

LINGUISTIC CLUSTERS

African Languages

Edo: An African language of southwestern Nigeria.

Obiemwen:	Wife of the earth.
Ogiuwu:	Deity of death.
Osanobua:	The highest God.

Ge'ez: An ancient southwest Semitic language that is the ancestor to Amharic, Tigrinya and Gurage languages. Spoken in Ethiopia.

Timkitgena:	Chauvinist
Neftegna:	Colonizer

Yoruba: An African language of southwestern Nigeria.

ObiemwenOgun:	Deity of iron or metals.
Olokun:	Great god of the sea.
Orunmila:	God of divination.
Osanyin:	Deity of medicine.

Zulu

European Languages

ENGLISH

Contract: An agreement recognized by the law as stipulating the legal rights and duties of the parties involved.

Habitus: Refers to the physical characteristics and condition of an individual, especially with regards to the potential to develop a certain disease.

House Girls: Domestics.

FRENCH

'Au pair': Means "at the peer level." Refers to someone who boards temporarily in someone else's home as a "live in" domestic.

SPECIALIZED TERMS

DERG (Dergue): Refers to the military junta that came to power in Ethiopia (1974) after Haile Selassie was outsted. An abbreviated name for the Coordinating Committee of the Armed Forces, Police, and Territorial Army. The word *derg* means a committee or council in Ge'ez language.

EBOLA: A deadly virus that causes high fever and massive internal bleeding.

GTZ: A German organization in East Africa.

UMKHONTO WE SIZWE: Military wing of the African National Congress

MK Cadres: Militant combatants (men and women) trained by the African National Congress.

OROMO: The largest indigenous African ethnic group found in Ethiopia and to some extent, in Kenya.

SOMAFCO: The African National Congress school in Tanzania, 1978 to 1992. Has the reputation of being a good school in exile that produces tough and adaptable students.

Preface

The Human Cost of African Migrations contributes to the discourse on the beneficiaries, benefactors, and casualties of African displacement, whether as part of forced migrations or voluntary labor-related exigencies, in the perpetual search for the metaphorical greener pastures. Conceptually, the volume is motivated by the absence of a cohesive body of work addressing the human cost of African migrations, specifically. Human cost implies a number of consequential sacrifices that include health, social and financial well-being, psychological and physical violation, and in some instances, the toleration of abuse in its varied manifestations.

Echoing the spirit of "Suffering and Smiling," a 1978 record album ("Shuffering and Schmiling") by the deceased world-class Afro-Beat musician, Fela Anikulapo-Kuti, this book captures the essential paradox inherent in African migration. On the one hand, the migrant's hopes and aspirations call for some celebrative "smiling," but on the other, the harsh realities of adjustment in a new but enchanting setting turns "smiling" into a necessary mask, a disguise or even therapy to cope with the nightmarish "suffering" engendered by displacement.

Drawn from an international conference on "Movements, Migrations, and Displacements," held at the University of Texas-Austin in March 2006, this volume brings together fifteen prominent and emerging scholars who share their expertise on the subject. Divided into four main parts, namely, "Migration and Health Issues," "Human Trafficking and Exploitation," "Migration and Education," and "Refugees, Displacement, and Re-Settlement," these thematic clusters summarize issues that are not only intellectually provocative but also emotionally draining. These cogent chapters appeal to the intellect as well as to the spirit of all concerned with the human investment and sacrifices inherent in migration.

Other issues covered by the book range from the stereotypes and discrimination faced by new African immigrants to the international political economy of prostitution and health care economics, as trade agreements between Africa and the New World, and between naïve girls and women co-opted into prostitution, figuratively and technically replace the traditional trans-Atlantic human cargo of ages past. Given this extensive scope, the timing of the conference could not have been more appropriate, as it sets out to theorize the human cost of African migration as an aspect that has received the least attention in emerging African migration studies in the age of economic globalization.

We want to thank all the contributors who, despite security and financial concerns, traveled long distances to be with us in Texas. Presenters and participants engaged in lively discussion throughout the three-day period. Such an undertaking does not come without copious debts. We are grateful to a host of graduate students (Roy Doron, Tyler Fleming, Matthew Heaton, Ann Genova, and Saheed Aderinto); the technical personnel (Sam Saverance); and many staff at the University of Texas (Gail Davis, Laura Flack and Martha Gail Moore). The organizations and departments that supported us financially include the Departments of History, Government, and English, the Center for African and African American Studies, the Office of the Vice President, College of Liberal Arts, Office of the Dean of Students, the Texas Cowboys Fund, The Louann and Larry Temple Fund, The Frances Higgenbotham Nalle Fund, and Dedman College, Southern Methodist University, Dallas. We are also grateful to Dr. Vik Bahl of Green River Community College in Auburn, Ms. Ronke Obadina of Austin, and Dr. Segun Fayemi of New York for their commitment to the conference.

Toyin Falola, University of Texas at Austin

Niyi Afolabi, University of Massachusetts at Amherst

Chapter One

Introduction: Migration Fantasies, Nightmarish Realities

Toyin Falola and Niyi Afolabi

OVERVIEW

In the age of globalization, one of the major challenges faced by the international community, as well as local governments, lies in the pervasive rise in migration patterns and the determination of migrants to pay any price necessary to better their lives. From the perilous clandestine trips across borders, to the deadly confrontation with Atlantic currents, to questionable exploitative arrangements made with dubious migration tycoons, migration has indeed become for many, what international trade was in the mid twentieth century.[1] Despite the human rights protections accorded to international migrants through the UN International Convention on the Protection of the Rights of all Migrant Workers and Members of their Families, the gap between policy and implementation is staggering, due to the economic cost for the receiving countries. It is against this background that a Conference on "Movements, Migrations, and Displacements," is plausible, since in addition to examining the economic cost, it has focused on the human cost–especially in this volume.

Let us cite extensively from the welcome address of the convener, Professor Toyin Falola, whose laconic vision of the conference has generated an edited volume of compelling breadth—a timely venture that sets out to explore major topical issues facing Africa and the World, especially regarding the issues of African migrations:

> Africans have always been on the move, ever since the time they created civilization and scattered it around the continent and elsewhere. . . . We are ready to listen to fresh ideas on new cultural, historical, sociological, methodological, and theoretical questions that will address relevant, recurring and urgent issues or raise neglected

> topics. . . . The richness is reflected in the wide variety of issues that are represented . . . : migration and shifting identity; hybridity and transculturation, the impact of Western and Asian settlers in Africa, trans-national struggles and ideas, and the African diaspora in other continents. Other major issues include those with regard to refugees, the representations of migrations in literature, films, and media, exile and homecoming narratives, sociological issues such as crime, juvenile delinquency, unemployment, family structures, gender and generational disparities, and memoirs of migrancy.[2]

Given this extensive scope, the timing of the conference could not have been more appropriate, as it sets out to theorize on the human cost of African migration as an aspect that has received the least attention in emerging studies of African migration in the age of economic globalization.

THEORIZING THE HUMAN COST

Going by the multidisciplinary thrust of this book, any discussion of African migration, whether internal or external, must be conceived as only one aspect of a more complex, organic, and global patterning of "flux and reflux,"[3] necessitated by constantly shifting dynamics of world socio-economic, cultural, and political order. While existing scholarly studies by Adepoju,[4] Akpraku,[5] Gordon,[6] Arthur,[7] Okafor,[8] and Schulman[9] among others, have emphasized economic motivation as the primary factor triggering African migration, this volume promotes multivalent perspectives that are reflected in the diversity of the issues covered by the four sections that range in their thematic foci from the medical, the economic, the socio-political, the pedagogical, to the developmental. This volume extends the debate by challenging assumptions and proposing novel frameworks and new methodological vistas for understanding the complexity of African migrations.

In theorizing on the human cost of African migrations, the following premises provide the fundamental determinants for its attraction, persistence, and contradictions: (i) The push-pull dynamics seem to favor, respectively, both the beneficiaries and the benefactors, depending on the perspective from which the "benefits" are defined and processed—as well as who is defining and processing. (ii) Internal economic, political, and socio-religious crises have made migration very alluring to African migrants seeking economic or political refuge in the West. (iii) Displacement caused by the foregoing crises, especially those of African refugees, has made migration or immigration a humanitarian policy issue for developed countries such as the United States, Canada, and the European Union. (iv) Issues relating to labor shortages in the West, especially in the healthcare profession, make the migration of health care professionals from Africa beneficial to Euro-America. (v) Questionable elements, including unsuspecting parents in Africa, take undue advantage of young, naïve African girls, as well as older women, by selling them into prostitution and servitude in Europe and America through organized, criminally entrepreneurial middlemen and women. (vi) African migration is not only external but internal, as witnessed in the pattern of job-seeking Africans settling in South Africa, Kenya, Ghana, and other countries. (vii) African migration, while beneficial in some instances, has a developmental cost for Africa, since the education of some of the highly trained professionals who are migrating to the West was financed by local, state, and federal governments in Africa.

In the final analysis, the benefit of migration is ultimately in the eye of the beholder, for some scholars argue that African migrants are developing Africa if they are able to send capital accumulated in the West back to Africa. Other scholars argue in favor of those few professionals who return home to impart their knowledge and skills in Africa. Ironically, this group of voluntary returnees is in the minority. Essentially, the human cost of migration is expected to rise proportionately to the capital gain which, often times, is the arena of only a select few who are usually ashamed to confess the nightmarish sacrifices and compromises they are often compelled to make, in order to achieve and sustain the ever glorified Western dream.

MIGRATIONS AND HEALTH ISSUES

This section addresses the implications of migration for African health professionals, as well as the relative quality of health care on both sides of the Atlantic. Good health is considered one of the fundamental human rights, but for the migrant, nothing can be farther from the truth, especially during the long journey toward integration and citizenship. In fact, the Yoruba say that *eni to ba ti ni alafia, oun gbogbo lo ni*—that is, one's health is the best of all riches. Ironically, global migration patterns of African professionals, especially health-care providers, have complicated the quality of health care in African countries. Essentially, Africa is being abandoned for better opportunities in the West and in the Caribbean, as well as in the Gulf States, particularly Saudi Arabia, to mention but a few locations of migration for African medical professionals. In their unity and diversity, the five chapters in this section engage the conditioning roles of migration and health care in Africa and the African Diaspora. From the human cost to Africa, to the market driven opportunities for Africans in the West, to the global gain for the rest of the world, this section complicates the idea of health, access and equality, forcing us to revisit and rethink our notions of the relationship between World Health Organization (WHO) and World Trade Organization (WTO). In this corrupt and corrupting partnership, health care ceases to be a fundamental human right, but becomes a fundamental human business with serious consequences for those naïve casualties caught in its web of apparent "philanthropy," indifference, and capitalist calculation. Unfortunately, the African migrant is the silent participant in this global quagmire of supply-demand dynamics that care less about human capital and more about economic exigency and expediency.

In Chapter Two, "Migration and Health in Africa and the African Diaspora," Kathryn H. Jacobsen argues, in a quadripartite approach, that there is a direct relationship between migration and the health of African immigrants, whether in the era of forced migration (slavery) or during voluntary migrations in search of a better life. First, Jacobsen posits that migration (whether intra or inter) significantly impacts the health of Africans. Second, migration often improves or deteriorates the health of Africans depending on where they go, and their relative status upon entry (refugee or voluntary migrant). Third, African migrants are often comparatively in better health, as compared to the African descendants. Fourth, African migrants' combined level of infectious diseases are higher, their mortality rates are lower, their susceptibilities to chronic disease are lower, while infant mortality rate is higher in Africa in comparison to their African descendants and Euro-American counterparts. In sum, the study reveals that Africans have a relatively sound health condition that may gradually deteriorate due to migration patterns of health professionals from Africa to the West. Consequently, in terms of African health condition, the ratio of at-risk populations left behind in Africa increases proportionately to the ratio of health practitioners pursuing better opportunities outside of Africa. The implications of this study are several: on the one hand it demystifies the stereotypes associated with images of Africans in the Western media, as sickly and dying of malnutrition; on the other hand, it educates us regarding the medical cost of migration in human and financial terms, in Africa as well as in the African Diaspora.

Along the lines of the stereotypical images of Africans in Western media, Charles Adeyanju, in Chapter Three, "Discourse of Health Risks and Anti-Racial Diversity in the Media Coverage of the Non-Ebola Panic," documents and analyzes the relationship between immigration policies, race/racism, and the media in Canada. Through the pretext of the case study of a sick visitor to Canada, incidentally from the Congo (Zaire/Africa), the study unmasks the subtleties and ambiguities of racism especially in the media, and how such racism becomes pervasive and political. Using four newspapers' coverage of this event in Ontario, Canada, the study concludes that through the media's appeal to the emotions and feelings of the Canadian people, they are able to sensationalize the debate on anti-racial diversity in Canada. The implications of this study imply that Canadians are urging their government to reform immigration policies in the name of their well being (health) and national security. As the author's title indicates ("Non-Ebola Panic"), the irony of the case-study is that the so called "health-risk" associated with the visitor's misdiagnosis as "Ebola," actually turned out not to be Ebola related at all. However, through the negative media coverage, the panic had already done the intended damage by mobilizing Canadians to speak against racial diversity, since every African visitor or resident is now a potential health risk to Canadians.

While anti-diversity campaign is highlighted in Canada with the foregoing case-study, Obijiofor Aginam, in Chapter Four, "'Predatory Globalization'?: The World Trade Organization, General Agreement on Trade in services, and Migration of African Health Professionals to the West," revisits the contradiction of portraying Africans as carriers of infectious diseases on the one hand, while on the other hand, recruiting their health professionals to work in the health care profession. In this compelling study, Aginam exposes the double-edged nature of trade agreements (WTO, GATS, etc) between developed and developing nations under the guise of economic globalization. As the author convincingly argues, the agreements are, indeed, pretexts to justify labor migration (and exploitation) from the developing world to the West. The author lays out the serious and precarious implications of such non-reciprocal migration for the African continent. In essence, Aginam sees Africa as ultimately receiving the short end of the bargain, as further accentuated in his conclusion: "GATS must be situated in a broader global social policy context, and globalization needs to be humane. Managed migration ought to bring benefits to source countries without crippling their health and other sectors. Some of the proposals made on ethical recruitment of doctors and nurses from developing countries will most likely be trumped by the intrusive provisions of GATS and the WTO trade regime." Such an incisive conclusion is unmistakable in its direct indictment of questionable economic globalization in the health care sector.

In a curious case-study of three graduating classes of a Nigerian medical school, Ike Anya, Chikwe Ihekweazu, and Enyi Anosike, in Chapter Five, "Searching the World: Following Three Graduating Classes of a Nigerian Medical School," painstakingly provide a brief and exploratory study, suggesting that about 40% of trained medical professionals from the University of Nigeria medical school have left Nigeria within ten years of their graduation. While their destination countries of choice are listed as USA, UK, Ireland, and South Africa, the authors conclude by projecting that the next stage of the study will include an email questionnaire, examining the motivation, career paths, and future plans for those medical graduates who are living abroad. Complementing this case-study is Sifiso M. Ndlovu's Chapter Six, "A Group of Twenty Nurses and the Pan African Struggle for Liberation," a rather extensive and compelling analysis of the specific experiences of intra-African migration (from South Africa to Tanzania) and their return (post-Apartheid). Drawing on the experiences of twenty South African nurses who volunteered to go and help alleviate staff shortages in the medical field in Tanzania, the chapter offers a provocative insider view of the contradictions of medical aid, especially coming from a neighboring African country to another African country. The significance of this chapter lies in its combination of issues of migration on both sides of the spectrum—workforce gain and workforce exploitation—ironically within Africa. The experiences narrated are melancholic and informative—providing first hand narratives of exploitation, double standards, frustration, and anxiety even for those nurses who had good intentions in going to help a neighboring country, only to be maltreated. These chapters provide two opposing views of migration for health care providers, whether they are looking forward to practicing in the West, or within Africa.

HUMAN TRAFFICKING AND EXPLOITATION

This section deals with the often silenced narratives of young African women sold into domestic labor and prostitution within Africa and in the West. Despite their melancholic exposition, the three chapters call our attention to the dark side of migration as it affects the most vulnerable and naïve in African society: women and children. By uncovering the pretexts, myths, motivations and disappointing realities, the chapters sum up one of the ugliest human ventures after slavery—human trafficking. In fact, it is arguable that sexual exploitation, regardless of the financial "gain" promised to the unsuspecting victims of this offensive trade, is a modern form of slavery. In Chapter Seven, "Trafficking of Young Women and Girls: A Case of "Au Pair" and Domestic Laborers in Tanzania," Elinami Veraeli Swai contends that due to the general unequal treatment of women in Tanzanian society, traffickers take advantage of young women who see domestic work as their only alternative to poverty and oppression. Drawing upon Bourdieu's theory of habitus in the construction of womanhood, Swai takes on the negative portrayal of African women as victims of male partners, relatives or neighbors, suggesting that such construction is part of societal historical and political process that must be challenged and redressed. In a very informative comparative analysis of the narratives of two women working as domestics in Tanzania and in the United States, respectively, Swai argues that despite the panicky nature of illegal trafficking of women for domestic work, lack of access to resources and unequal treatment of women in society is partly responsible for the oppression and exploitation of women. The author sees herself as part of the movement to change the status quo despite what she calls the "criminalization and demonization" of women's agency in a global economy.

Both chapters by Victor Nnamdi Opara deal with human trafficking and sexual exploitation. Chapter Eight, "Emerging Issues in the Trafficking of African Women for Prostitution," provides the cultural, social, economic, political and psychological causative factors for the success of traffickers in luring unsuspecting and naïve young girls into the clandestine industry of prostitution abroad. The chapter queries both local and international organizations for their passivity in the face of an urgent and perplexing moral pandemic. Conclusively, the chapter argues that fighting the trafficking of women "on the surface" only postpones the inevitable while the lasting approach is to return to the table, to compose a long-term plan of action that will erase the internal factors promoting the trafficking of African women such as political and economic inequalities, lack of equal access to education, and social mobility. In Chapter Nine, "Trafficking Contracts: Myth or Reality?: A Re-Examination of *Consent* in Human Trafficking," Opara demystifies the "consent" argument as an excuse usually deployed to justify the trafficking of African women. He posits that there is a "hidden matrix of inequality, domination, exploitation, oppression, dehumanization, threat, and lack of liberty and freedom," that makes any contractual agreements issued under such conditions not only invalid but analogous to contracts of slavery which must be banned. Swai and Opara are quite right that educational opportunities will go a long way in bringing about equality and empowerment for African women—as a point of departure to a full expression of their humanity, citizenship, and rejection of the debasement inherent in sexual exploitation and human trafficking.

MIGRATION AND EDUCATION

This section addresses the impact of education on women's subjugation, as well as the disparities in education for blacks and whites in South Africa. In order to gain access to a good education in this context, migration of students to a "white" school, if permitted and lawful, becomes inevitable. Education has always been regarded as the best weapon against ignorance, oppression, and servitude. If there is a direct relationship between education, the cultivation of the mind, and freedom, it stands to reason that every society should make this topmost on the priority list of policy issues. Given this knowledge, some societies have used lack of access to education as an instrument of social control. Indeed, in the case of South Africa under the Apartheid regime, inequality in educational access for blacks and whites was one of the issues that led to student protests, much violence, and death. In the absence of equal education, there is no social justice. Some traditional societies also saw fit to segregate education on the basis of gender; that is, certain basic educational opportunities are provided up to a certain level, and higher education favored males. In fact, having a higher education was considered to be the arena of the elite, the rich, and the fortunate. European colonization of Africa did not help matters, as Europeans targeted a select few for training and educational opportunities in order to facilitate their colonial objectives of divide and conquer, exploitation, and ease for the administrative burdens of the ruling class.

Both chapters in this section engage the "push-pull" dynamics of education and its relationship with migration in order to gain better access to social opportunities and mobility. In Chapter Ten, "School Migration: A Major Concern in Historically Disadvantaged Schools in South Africa," Myra Maboya presents an interesting study of the factors responsible for school migration from black or historically disadvantaged schools to more "committed" schools. In addition to enumerating the factors (financial/budgetary issues, insufficient training for teachers, low morale due to need to survive economically, etc.), the chapter calls for alternative developmental measures to improve black schools and discourage school migration. The individual narratives are particularly compelling and convincing while the methodology (focus group) seems unscientific. The conclusions reached provide a starting point for redressing the imbalances between "black" and disadvantaged schools in comparison to white or "committed" schools in South Africa. Jamaine Abidogun, in Chapter Eleven, "Pushing and Pulling: Western Education's Impact on Women's Subjugation in Ghana," complements the previous study on unequal access to education, but within the specificity of gender roles. This chapter showcases the unequal treatment of women in life and education. In essence, it argues for the need to establish role changes for women as opposed to the unequal and oppressive roles assigned to them due to cultural and traditional values. Taking the premise that the combination of Islamic and Christian/European influences on indigenous societies, such as the Ghanaian, has brought about detrimental gender role assignments that are now being challenged through education, the chapter hopes for a future where social and economic democracy will apply to both women and men.

REFUGEES, DISPLACEMENT, AND RE-SETTLEMENT

Beyond a broad survey of displacement as a security issue in Africa, this section focuses on the reality of displacement, refugee crisis, and resettlement efforts, using as case-studies the refugee crises in Democratic Republic of Congo, Nigeria, Ethiopia and Sudan. Home and homelessness, exile, civil wars, political repression, ethnic cleansing, violence, relocation, repatriation, and resettlement are some of the issues affecting refugees in their "suspended" predicament. Constantly on the move until they reach the proverbial "safe haven," refugees are doubly displaced in the sense that they long for the home they had to leave while at the same time they are not fully integrated in the temporary "camp" giving them a new lease on life. It is saddening to know that one out of two refugees in the entire world comes from Africa. This makes the situation dire and urgent. Beyond the trauma of displacement, refugees often receive inadequate assistance from international organizations, generally live in permanent fear of the oppressive governments from whom they fled, and are usually at the mercy of aid, developmental and relief organizations for their immediate survival and possibility of return to their homelands. While this section cannot claim to have exhausted the many issues relative to refugee crisis on the African continent and its implications for the rest of the world, it does draw attention to its seriousness and the need to fashion a long-term strategy to confront this dilemma.

Bukola Adeyemi Oyeniyi, in Chapter Twelve, "Peoples without Homes: Displacement and Security Situation in Africa," identifies two pertinent variables in the study of displacement, namely, refugees and internally displaced persons (IDPs). Using the Democratic Republic of the Congo to analyze the countries-in-conflict model, and Nigeria as a model for countries out-of-conflict, Oyeniyi argues that "DR Congo is but a representation of nations wrecked by many years of conflicts and war, while Nigeria represents nations that have experienced limited or relative peace over the years." In this cogent and well-documented chapter, the author conceptualizes refugee crisis and displacement as formidable factors in continental security and as an aspect that is yet to be diagnosed as a contributing variable to the underdevelopment of Africa. The author concludes by arguing for the direct relationship between displacement and sustainable development in Africa. While Oyeniyi focuses comparatively on the variables of displacement, Solomon A. Getahun, in Chapter Thirteen, "Determinants of Ethiopian Refugee Flow in the Horn of Africa, 1970–2000," seeks to understand why Sudan is the favorite destination of refugees from Ethiopia. In addition to a historical background, the chapter highlights the fact that some African refugees or displaced laborers are deciding to remain in Africa (i.e. South Africa, Kenya, Ghana, etc.) instead of going to the West. The author concludes that while Kenya emerged as a preferred location of refuge, especially between 2001 and 2005 (see Table 2 of chapter), Sudan remained the main destination for Ethiopian refugees. The study gives a positive dimension to the refugee crisis in Africa, by turning to internal measures and solutions as opposed to the external.

Getahun's positive spin on the refugee crisis notwithstanding, the dilemma of displacement and estrangement in a new setting is real. In this regard, Terence Ranger raises a series of questions geared towards theorizing repatriation as part of African social historiography: "How do returned refugees perceive 'home'? How do they define their 'identity'?" The answer to these questions is critical to understanding mechanisms of 'integration.'"[10] In an effort to reach for that answer, Ranger goes on to note: "Yet this is precisely what is at stake in many contexts which generate refugees and returnees—in the Southern Sudan, in northern Uganda, and so on. Even in effectively operating nation-states, where the idea of return to one's 'country' is a national as well as a local sentiment, that idea co-exists and sometimes conflicts with many other senses of identity and entitlement," (289). Against this background may be understood the degree of estrangement and identitarian crises for the refugees while they are adapting, whether temporarily or permanently, in the host country. In a sense, it is a case of migrants giving up what they hold so dearly for something that is less compelling, at least in the initial stages of integration and negotiation of their shifting identities.

NOTES

1. Since labor has become another "exportable commodity," the arguments for and against it are heated; but those who argue for protection of international migrants suggest that it is in the interest of developed nations to protect the "goods" they need to keep their economies going, while those who argue against suggest that the uncontrolled flow of international migrants may actually complicate rising national unemployment. While industrialized countries do need migrants in areas in which they face shortages, such as highly skilled jobs in information technology, health services, or even manual jobs such as agriculture and construction, the UN International Convention on the Protection of the Rights of all Migrant Workers and Members of their Families, enacted in 2003, may thus be seen as a

contingency protection that may not be expressly enforceable in reality although it is highly desirable.

2. See Toyin Falola, "Welcome," Conference Program, *Movements, Migrations, and Displacements in Africa*, Africa Conference 2006, The University of Texas at Austin, March 25–27, 2006), 1.
3. We use this expression within the context of Pierre Verger's seminal work on the forced migrations of slaves from the West African coasts from the 17th to 19th centuries. See Pierre Verger, *Fluxo e Refluxo do Tráfico de Escravos entre o Golfo do Benin e a Bahia de Todos os Santos, dos Séculos XVII a IXX* (Nova Edição). Salvador: Corrupio, 1987. [1966-original French edition].
4. See for example, Aderanti Adepoju, "Linkages between Internal and International Migration: The African Situation," *International Social Science Journal* 23 (1984): 145–155 and Aderanti Adepoju, "Issues and Recent Trends in International Migration in Sub-Saharan Africa," *International Social Science Journal* 52.3 (2000): 383–389.
5. Akpraku provides the argument that African migration is costing Africa in terms of "uprooted" and displaced skilled labor, hence the "missing" link in African development in the post-independence era. See Kofi K. Akpraku, *African Émigrés in the United States: A Missing Link in Africa's Social and Economic Development*. New York: Praeger, 1991.
6. The notion of a "new" Diaspora is a welcome perspective to a global complication of ethnicity, diversity, population growth patterns, citizenship and the exigencies of labor migration. For a detailed case-study of the African experience, see April Gordon, "The New Diaspora: African Immigration to the United States," *Journal of Third World Studies* 15 (1998): 79–110.
7. Arthur's book constitutes the first in a series of recently published book-length studies on the plight and pleasures of Africans in the United States. Despite its timely and significant contribution, and with the exception of the author's discussion of the African refugee/resettlement situation in Minnesota, one limitation might be the fact that the author focused on "success" narratives as opposed to constructive perspectives that also point out the pitfalls of African migration. For a detailed study, see John Arthur, *Invisible Sojourners: African Immigrant Diaspora in the United States,* Westport: Praeger, 2000.
8. In addition to providing a historical background to voluntary African migration, the achievements and contributions to the USA and Africa, Okafor goes on to highlight the challenges of the stereotypical images of Africa in the American media as one of the hindrances to full integration of Africans in the USA, and their efforts to reach out to other ethnic minorities. See Lawrence A. Okafor, *Recent African Immigrants to the USA: Their Concerns and How Everyone Can Succeed in the USA*, New York: Rosedog Press, 2003.
9. In an innovative twist on African migration, Schulman's volume addresses the positive and negative effects of immigration on Americans. In focusing on how immigration affects African Americans specifically, the author raises issues of concern for African Americans in terms of low-level labor that is now being "taken over" or occupied by Mexicans, Africans, and other immigrants

who are deemed "hardworking and uncomplaining," as well as professional positions for which new professional minorities from Asia, Africa, and the Caribbean are now competing. From the viewpoint of building networks and political coalitions, such an unspoken conflict and invisible resentment towards Africans (often accused by African Americans to have collaborated in their enslavement, as well as for "taking over" the jobs they fought for through the Civil Rights movement) cannot be said to be an asset for Africans but a liability, hence another human cost of African migration. For further details, see Steven Schulman, ed., *The Impact of Immigration on African Americans*, New Brunswick: Transaction, 2005.

10. For a detailed discussion, see Terence Ranger, "Studying Repatriation as Part of African Social History," *When Refugees Go Home*, Tim Allen and Hubert Morsink, eds., (Trenton, NJ: Africa World Press/United Nations Research Institute, 1994), 279–294.

REFERENCES

Achanfuo-Yeboah, David. "Grounding a Theory of African Migration in Recent Data on Ghana." *International Sociology* 8.2 (1993): 215–226.

Adepoju, Aderanti. "Linkages between Internal and International Migration: The African Situation." *International Social Science Journal* 23 (1984): 145–155.

———."Issues and Recent Trends in International Migration in Sub-Saharan Africa." *International Social Science Journal* 52.3 (2000): 383–389.

Akpraku, Kofi K. *African Émigrés in the United States: A Missing Link in Africa's Social and Economic Development*. New York: Praeger, 1991.

Allen, Tim and Hubert Morsink, eds. *When Refugees Go Home: African Experiences*. Trenton, NJ: Africa World Press, 1994.

Allen, Tim, ed. *In Search of a Cool Ground: War, Flight & Homecoming in Northeast Africa*. Trenton, NJ: Africa World Press, 1996.

Arthur, John A. *Invisible Sojourners: African Immigrant Diaspora in the United States*. Westport: Praeger, 2000.

Bailey, Samuel L and Eduardo José Míguez, eds. *Mass Migration to Modern Latin America*. Wilmington, DE: Scholarly Resources, 2003.

Bloch, Alice. "Emigration from Zimbabwe: Migrant Perspectives." *Social Policy and Administration* 40.1(2006): 67–87.

Brettell, Caroline and James Hollifield, eds. *Migration Theory: Talking Across Disciplines* (New York: Routledge, 2000.

Castles, Stephen and Mark J. Miller. *The Age of Migration: International Population Movements in the Modern World*. New York: Guilford Press, 1993.

Clark, Kamari Maxine. *Mapping Yoruba Networks: Power and Agency in the Making of Transnational Communities*. Durham: Duke University Press, 2004.

Cohen, Lucy M. *Culture, Disease, and Stress among Latino Immigrants*. Washington: Smithsonian Institute, 1979.

Crush, Jonathan and Clarence Tshitereke. "Contesting Migrancy: The Foreign Labor Debate in Post-1994 South Africa." *Africa Today* 48.3 (2001): 49–70.

Daniel, Yvonne. *Dancing Wisdom: Embodied Knowledge in Haitian Vodou, Cuban Yoruba, and Bahian Candomblé*. Urbana: University of Illinois Press, 2005.

El-Khawas, Mohamed A. "Brain Drain: Putting Africa between a Rock and a Hard Place." *Mediterranean Quarterly* 15.4 (2004): 37–56.

Fabre, Geneviève and Klaus Benesch. *African Diasporas in the New and Old Worlds: Consciousness and Imagination*. Amsterdam/New York: Rodopi, 2004.

Falola, Toyin. "Nigeria in the Global Context of Refugees: Historical and Comparative Perspectives." Paul Lovejoy and Pat Williams, eds. *Displacement and The Politics of Violence in Nigeria*. Leiden and New York: Brill, 1997, 5–21.

———."Intellectuals and Africa in a Changing World Order." *Nationalism and African Intellectuals*. New York: University of Rochester Press, 2001. 262–293.

Falola, Toyin and Matt D. Childs, eds. *Yoruba Diaspora in the Atlantic World*. Bloomington, IN: Indiana University Press, 2005.

Gordon, April. "The New Diaspora: African Immigration to the United States." *Journal of Third World Studies* 15 (1998): 79–110.

Hagopian, A. et al., eds. "The Flight of Physicians from West Africa: Views of African Physicians and Implications for Policy." *Social Science and Medicine* 61.8 (2005): 1750–1760.

Hammar, Thomas et al., eds. *International Migration, Immobility and Development: Multidisciplinary Perspectives*. New York: Berg, 1997.

Hear, Nicholas Van. *New Diasporas: The Mass Exodus, Dispersal and Regrouping of Migrant Communities*. Seattle: University of Washington Press, 1998.

Henderson, George and Martha Primeaux. *Transcultural Health Care*. Menio Park, CA: Addison-Wesley, 1981.

Kibreab, Gaim. *African Refugees: Reflections on the African Refugee Problem*. Trenton, NJ: Africa World Press, 1985.

Kiluva-Ndunda, Mutindi Mumbua. "The Impact of Development on Women's Health and the Environment." *African Women & Globalization: Dawn of the 21st Century*. Jepkorir Rose Chepyator-Thompson, ed. Trenton, NJ: Africa World Press, 2005. 215–224.

Kiple, Kenneth F. *Another Dimension to the Black Diaspora*. Cambridge: Cambridge University Press, 1981.

Kramer, Elizabeth J. et al. eds. *Immigrant Women's Health: Problems and Solutions*. San Francisco: Jossey-Bass, 1999.

Lanza, Robert. *The Health and Survival of the Human Species in the 21st Century*. Santa Fe, NM: Health Press, 1996.

Lesser, Jeffrey, ed. *Welcoming the Undesirables: Brazil and the Jewish Question*. Berkeley: University of California Press, 1994.

———. *Negotiating National Identity: Immigrants, Minorities, and the Struggle for Ethnicity in Brazil*. Durham: Duke University Press, 1999.

Lindsay, Beverly, ed. *African Migration and National Development*. University Park: Pennsylvania State University Press, 1985.

Macklin, Audrey. "Our Sisters from Stable Countries": War, Globalization, and Accountability." *Social Politics: International Studies in Gender, State and Society* 10.2 (2003): 256–283.

Makoni, Sinfree, et al. eds. *Black Linguistics: Language, Society, and Politics in Africa and the Americas*. Foreward by Ngugi wa Thiong'o. London/New York: Routledge, 2003.

Martin, Philip L. and J. Edward Taylor. "Managing Migration: The Role of Economic Policies." *Global Migrants, Global Refugees: Problems and Solutions.* Aristide R. Zolberg and Peter M. Benda eds. New York: Berghahm Books, 2001. 95–120.

Meissner, Doris et al., eds. *International Migration: Challenges in a New Era.* New York: The Trilateral Commission, 1993.

Mobasher, Mohsen M and Mahmoud Sadri. *Migration, Globalization, and Ethnic Relations: An Interdisciplinary Approach.* Upper Saddle River, NJ: Pearson Prentice Hall, 2004.

Muller, Gilbert H. *New Strangers in Paradise.* Lexington KY: University Press of Kentucky, 1999.

Nelson, Lise and Joni Seager eds. *A Companion to Feminist Geography.* Malden, MA: Blackwell Publishers, 2005.

Okafor, Lawrence A. *Recent African Immigrants to the USA: Their Concerns and How Everyone Can Succeed in the USA.* New York: Rosedog Press, 2003.

Patterson, Andrew and Glenda Kruss. "Educational Migration and Its Effect on Access to Schooling in South Africa." *South African Journal of Education* 18.3 (1998): 149–156.

Pond, B. and B. McPake. "The Health Migration Crisis: The Role of Four Organizations for Economic Cooperation and Development Countries." *Lancet* 367 (2006): 1448–1455.

Ranger, Terence. "Studying Repatriation as Part of African Social History." *When Refugees Go Home.* Tim Allen and Hubert Morsink, eds. Trenton, NJ: Africa World Press/United Nations Research Institute, 1994, 279–294.

Reimers, David M. *Other Immigrants: The Global Origins of the American People.* New York: New York University Press, 2005.

Scott, Frankilin D. Ed. *World Migration in Modern Times.* New Jersey: Prentice Hall, 1968.

Sheldon, Kathleen, ed. *Courtyards, Markets, City Streets: Urban Women in Africa.* Boulder, CO: Westview Press, 1996.

Schulman, Steven, ed. *The Impact of Immigration on African Americans.* New Brunswick: Transaction, 2005.

Simelane, H.S. "The State, Chiefs and the Control of Female Migration in Colonial Swaziland, c. 1930–1950s." *Journal of African History* 45.1 (2004): 103–124.

Stilwell, B. et al. "Migration of Health-Care Workers from Developing Countries: Strategic Approaches to its Management." *Bulletin of the World Health Organization* 82.8 (2004): 595–600.

Sutlive, Vinson H. and Tomoko Hamada. *Physicians and Health Care in the Third World* (#55). Williamsburg: VA: Studies In Third World Societies/College of William & Mary, 1994.

United Nations. *Health and Mortality: Issues of Global Concern.* New York: United Nations, 1999.

Weiner, Myron. *The Global Migration Crisis: Challenge to States and to Human Rights.* New York: Harper Collins, 1995.

White, Evelyn C. *Black Women's Health Book: Speaking for Ourselves.* Seattle, WA: The Seal Press, 1990.

Zegeye, Abebe. *Forced Labour and Migration: Patterns of Movement within Africa*. London/NewYork: Zed Books, 1989.

Zeleza, Paul Tiyambe. "The African Academic Diaspora in the United States and Africa: The Challenges of Productive Engagement." *Comparative Studies of South Asia, Africa and the Middle East* 24.1 (2004): 261–275.

———."The Politics and Poetics of Exile: Edward Said in Africa." *Research in African Literatures* 36.3 (2005): 1–22.

Part I

Migrations and Health Issues

Chapter Two

Migration and Health in Africa and the African Diaspora

Kathryn H. Jacobsen

Thi s chapter uses published epidemiological reports to compare health status between various population groups in Africa and the African Diaspora. Health status can be measured by infant mortality rates, life expectancy, and the incidence and prevalence of selected communicable and non-communicable conditions, including heart disease and cancers, as well as a variety of other measures. Increases or decreases in the risk of both communicable diseases and non-communicable diseases may occur with migration. Infectious disease risk is associated with many types of population mobility, such as long-term migration to low-income or high-income countries, urbanization, and short-term travel.[1] Chronic disease risk is associated with changes in diet, lifestyle, and environmental exposures.

Migration has complex causes and diverse patterns. Migrants can be categorized by their reasons for migrating, intended length of stay in their host country, and other characteristics. Some are refugees and/or asylum seekers who have been forcibly displaced due to violence and/or persecution, or compelled to abandon their home region due to natural disasters. Some are economic migrants who, for instance, might move between rural and urban areas in search of economic opportunities. Others choose to emigrate for educational opportunities and higher paying jobs. Migrants in each category may be permanent settlers who intend to reside permanently in their host country, whereas others are expatriates or guest workers. Thus, it is impossible to speak generically of "migration and health," and data from studies of specific migrant groups must be used to assess health in various populations.

INTRA-AFRICAN MIGRATIONS

We begin with an assessment of the health impacts of population movement within Africa. The vast majority of migrants in West Africa[2] and, presumably, in other regions of Africa, move within-country and across national boundaries for employment purposes. Although some migrants have the economic means to secure healthcare for themselves and their families in new environs, most do not. Migrant laborers, truck drivers, itinerant traders, commercial sex workers (CSWs), and refugees have all been linked to the spread of sexually transmitted diseases in West Africa.[3] Analyses from other parts of sub-Saharan Africa, including South Africa,[4] report similar findings. However, while transportation and intra-African migration have long been viewed as a major cause for spread of infectious diseases like HIV/AIDS within sub-Saharan Africa, it may be more accurate to view migrants not as carriers of the virus to new areas, but as people whose living conditions facilitate the transmission of the virus, (Decosas, 826–828). New social situations, limited occupational options, possible language barriers, and lack of access to medical care and treatment all contribute to increased risk for acquiring HIV infection and other infections. This is exacerbated by the fact that limited treatment options may be available when illness occurs, (Decosas, 826–828).

Sub-Saharan Africa (SSA) is the world region with the highest urbanization rate; hence, rural-to-urban migration is a very common migration pattern. The World Bank estimates that the average annual percent increase in the urban population in SSA between 1990 and 2003 was 4.6%.[5] (By comparison, East Asia and the Pacific have a 3.6% urbanization rate and South Asia and the Middle East / North African regions have 2.8% rates.) There is a large difference in the current urbanized population between countries. Some countries are highly rural, like Rwanda (7% urban) and Burundi (10%), while others are highly urbanized, like Congo (67%) and Gabon (84%), (World Bank, 2005). In total, about 36% of sub-Saharan Africans now live in an urban area, and that percentage is rapidly increasing. For example, in 1975 about 23.4% of Nigerians lived in urban areas; by 2003 the proportion had increased to 46.6%, and the urban population is expected to reach 55.5% in 2015.[6] The experiences of rural-to-urban migrants may differ based on the presence or absence of urban structures, like sanitation facilities and transportation systems, to support their transition.

Rural residents often have reduced health status compared to urban residents even before moving. In general, rural residents have a higher incidence of infectious diseases and malnourishment than urban residents.

They may also have less access to health information. For example, urban Nigerian women are more aware of contraceptive options than women living in rural Nigeria.[7]

Brockerhoff et al. identified many pathways that link migrant status, and related household poverty, to negative health outcomes in urban areas.[8] Demographic, cultural, political, social, environmental, and economic consequences of movement may all be associated with increased exposure or susceptibility to disease or injury. For example, a household with limited resources upon entry into the city may require the employment of the main child caregiver, which may decrease the quality of child care and demand early weaning of breastfeeding babies, leading to a decrease in the nutritional status of the child. Economically challenged households may also lack consumer goods like mosquito nets and refrigerators that protect and enhance health; they may have inadequate caloric and micronutrient intake, and be unable to pay for health services. Furthermore, rural-urban migrants may be more likely than urban natives to live in residences without electricity, a flush toilet, or piped drinking water, and poor hygiene and sanitation are significant risk factors for the spread of infectious diseases. Not surprisingly, migrant women from rural areas have higher infant and child mortality risks after they settle in cities than lifelong city residents, (Child Survival, 1371–1383).

However, children born after their families have settled in urban areas have much better chance of survival than rural non-migrants.[9] Brockerhoff concludes, "many disadvantaged urban children would probably have been much worse off had their mothers remained in the village, and that millions of children's lives may have been saved in the 1980s as a result of mothers moving to urban areas," (Impact of Rural-Urban, 127–149). In general in Africa, urban women have lower fertility rates and infant mortality rates, higher rates of deliveries attended by a skilled birth attendant and use of modern contraceptives, and later age at first pregnancy.[10] Urban children are less likely to be underweight.

Rural-to-urban migrants may have unique health profiles that are intermediate to rural residents and long-term urban residents, indicating that a gradual health transition occurs following urban migration. A study conducted in Cameroon found higher prevalence of overweight, hypertension, and impaired fasting glycemia or diabetes in people who had lived in an urban environment for more than 10 years as compared to life-long rural residents. Recent urban migrants—those who had lived in an urban environment for 1 to 10 years—had intermediate prevalence of overweight and diabetes, but a reduced rate of hypertension to either of the other comparison groups.[11]

Some rural-to-urban migrants may make frequent visits to their rural homes, exposing themselves to the environmental health risks of both urban and rural residence. A study of movement patterns for residents of a medium-sized city in Zimbabwe found that 36% of urban migrants had originated in rural areas and 24% in smaller urban areas, and the vast majority had moved to the city for employment purposes. Of those migrants, less than one-tenth of respondents never made a rural home visit, two-thirds visited six times a year or less, and more than one-quarter visited their rural home at least seven times a year, indicating that many urban residents maintain close ties with their rural homes.[12] Maintaining family connections may be beneficial for health, but seasonal migration is also associated with some health risk. A study of adolescent females from rural Senegal found that those who migrated to the city to work (usually as maids) during the dry season weighed slightly more and had higher daily physical activity and less sleep, potential contributors to susceptibility to disease, than the non-migrants who stayed in the village year-round.[13] And short-term mobility (having left one's rural village for at least one day and one night in the past four weeks) is associated with increased HIV prevalence in both men and women in West Africa.[14]

While discussions of the risks of rural-to-urban migration are quite common, there are also risks with urban-to-rural and rural-to-rural migration. Studies of HIV risk and migration in Zimbabwe[15] and Ethiopia[16] have found an increased risk not just with rural-to-urban migration, but also with rural-to-rural migration. Both sending and receiving communities experience economic and environmental changes that might influence health.[17]

There are also health risks associated with urbanization and economic development. Urban residents have a higher risk of chronic non-communicable conditions such as hypertension[18] and diabetes[19] that are associated with over-nutrition and inactivity. Urban Nigerian men and women consume more calories daily than rural residents, have a significantly higher body mass index (BMI) and percentage of body fat, and generally have less healthy blood lipid profiles,[20] all of which are risk factors for cardiovascular disease. In southern Africa, urban residents have higher energy intake from fat, and decreased fiber intake, and higher obesity prevalence, especially in women.[21] It is not surprising that a study in Nigeria found that hypertension prevalence increased from 14% in rural farmers to 25% in the urban poor and 29% in railway workers.[22]

REFUGEE HEALTH

Refugees may move within a country or to neighboring or distant lands and have special health risks compared to other migrant groups. Refugee status is always caused by security concerns beyond the control of the refugee and is not voluntary—the destination is often unexpected and not determined before moving; hence, refugees often do not have the choice of returning to their countries of origin.[23] UNHCR estimates that there were more than 2.7 million African refugees in 2004.[24]

Refugees have special health concerns at different stages of the "cycle of displacement" that begins at the onset of a complex emergency and continues until a lasting solution is implemented. UNHCR has identified several conditions common to the refugee experience that increase the risk of health problems: "Many displaced people are exposed to insecurity and physical violence; lack adequate shelter and sanitation facilities; are packed into overcrowded camps or makeshift settlements; have insufficient access to appropriate food, clean water, and basic supplies for personal hygiene; have no immunity to the local diseases of their new environment; and suffer considerable emotional stress as a result of traumatic experiences and the uncertainty of their situation."[25] Increases in the incidence of malaria, diarrhea-related diseases, tuberculosis, measles, and acute respiratory infections are compounded by disruptions in agricultural production, food supplies, and health service provisions.[26] Refugee populations may also experience death, injury, disability, sexual assault, and psychological trauma as a result of violence.[27] Refugee children have a high risk of morbidity and mortality, especially when services related to food, water, environmental sanitation, shelter, and basic health services are interrupted or inadequate.[28] Furthermore, refugees are often exposed to environmental health problems. Thus, the health of refugees is often poor and must be addressed through both emergency relief efforts and long-term medical care.

MIGRATION OUT OF AFRICA

In this section we compare the health of Africans who voluntarily move to other continents to persons of African descent, and other population groups, who already reside in host countries. In general, health indicators from the United States, Europe, and other regions show a longer life expectancy, lower infant mortality, lower fertility rate, and better health status than those from any African nation. Table 2–1 shows some basic health statistics from selected countries. Although overall population health status in Europe, the United States, Canada, and many other nations is higher than that of African nations, the migrants to these countries from Africa often have better health than native-born residents.

African émigrés to destinations outside of Africa are often wealthy and educated. For example, a study of black immigrants to Houston, Texas, from more than twenty African nations found that a plurality moved to the United States for schooling,[29] an opportunity that would generally only be available to high-income households. "Brain drain," the emigration of highly educated Africans, especially health professionals, to other parts of the world, has become a considerable health concern for Africa. A study of medical graduates from sub-Saharan Africa estimates that about 10% of African-trained physicians live in the United States or Canada, and the proportion is much higher in some countries such as Liberia (43%), Ghana (30%), and Uganda (20%).[30] Hagopian et al. write: "There is now a well-developed culture of medical migration. This culture is firmly rooted, and does not simply fail to discourage medical migration but actually encourages it. Medical school faculty are role models for the benefits of migration (and subsequent return), and they are proud of their students who successfully emigrate."[31] The high socioeconomic status of many African emigrants is evident in the differences in health status between African emigrants and the residents of their host countries.

The contrast in health status is particularly obvious when comparing the health status of U.S.-born black and African-born blacks living in the United States. U.S. born blacks are significantly less healthy than immigrant blacks. The National Health Interview Surveys (NHIS) from 1992–1995 asked participants from the United States about their health status. More than 87% of the foreign-born black participants rated their health as excellent or very good compared to only 52% of U.S.-born black participants.[32] While 11% of foreign-born subjects reported being limited in some type of activity, 20% of U.S.-born subjects reported limitations, (Health Status of Non-Hispanic, 1–20). More recent NIHS surveys have consistently found that African-born black participants have better self-rated health, lower odds of activity limitation, and lower odds of limitation due to hypertension than U.S.-born black participants.[33] An analysis of the NHIS data from 2000 through 2002 found that when asked to rate health on a scale of 1 (poor) to 5 (excellent), the mean response for U.S.-born black respondents was 3.51, lower than foreign-born black respondents from any region of origin, including the West Indies (3.84), Europe (3.85), South America (4.00), and Africa (4.22).[34] U.S.-born respondents also reported more activity limitation, more hypertension, less education, lower incomes, and lower rates of health insurance, (Racial Context, 181–199).

Statistics reinforce the self-reporting of lower health status in African-Americans than African immigrants. A study of stroke mortality rates from 1979 through 1981 found a significantly lower mortality rate among black immigrants than U.S.-born blacks,[35] as did the National Longitudinal Mortality Study, which looked at all-cause mortality from 1979 through

1989.[36] A study in New York City found a significantly higher infant mortality rate in the children of native-born black women compared to foreign-born black women.[37] Breastfeeding is an important contributor to infant health, and in the United States foreign-born black women are significantly more likely to intend to breastfeed after delivery than continental U.S. born women.[38] There is even a notable difference in dental health. A study of the dental health of refugee children who were assessed within their first month in the United States found that African children were significantly less likely than African-American children to have caries (cavities) even though the African-born children were less likely to have ever seen a dentist.[39]

Health behaviors may differ by immigration status. Foreign-born blacks are less likely to smoke or use alcohol, (Health Status, Health Insurance, 1740–1777). Native-born African Americans are significantly more likely to be current smokers than foreign-born blacks,[40] and a study of childhood exposure to tobacco smoke found high rates for African-American children and low rates of exposure in Somali immigrant children.[41] Among college students in the United States, immigrants have less risky sexual behaviors and more physical activity, although they have less healthy diets.[42] First-generation African immigrants to the United States have lower body mass indexes than U.S.-born African Americans.[43]

It may be unfair to compare the health of immigrants only to black Americans since, although same-race comparisons may adjust for differences in genetic susceptibility, black American are generally less healthy than white Americans. However, an assessment that includes white Americans shows that the health status of African immigrants often exceeds the health status of both black and white Americans. An examination of death records in New York City from 1988 through 1992 found that while the death rate for blacks exceeded the death rate for whites, foreign-born blacks had a slightly lower death rate than whites.[44] While the contrast was greatest between U.S.-born and foreign-born blacks, and the study showed that U.S.-born black males were three times as likely and U.S.-born black females 2.5 times as likely to die as foreign-born blacks, (Nativity, Race, and Mortality, 689–701) the likelihood of death in a given year was lowest for foreign-born blacks, higher in white Americans, and highest in U.S.-born black Americans.

There are a few exceptions to this trend. Some ethnic and cultural immigrant groups may be high-risk populations for adverse birth outcomes. A study of Somali immigrants in Washington State found significantly elevated risk for numerous outcomes, including prolonged hospitalization, failed induction of labor, and gestational diabetes, compared to black American-born women.[45] A similar study in Sweden found that African immigrant women had higher risk of small-for-gestational-age babies, neonatal distress, and prenatal mortality compared to both Swedish-born women and foreign-born women from other parts of the world.[46] A comparison of female African-American residents of Rochester, Minnesota, to recent Somali immigrants found that the Somali women had significantly lower bone densities than the U.S.-born women.[47] Overall, cancer mortality among sub-Saharan African migrants in France is significantly lower than the native French population, although there is a higher risk of some specific cancers, such as liver cancer and bladder cancer in West Africans immigrants.[48] Similarly, immigrants from East Africa and the Caribbean to England and Wales have lower mortality than England and Wales-born populations, even though West African immigrants have a greater risk of cancer mortality due to high rates of liver cancer.[49] However, the general pattern is that immigrants from Africa have high health status.

AFRICA AND THE AFRICAN DIASPORA

The previous section looked at the difference in health status between recent immigrants and long-term black residents of host countries. This section looks at health disparities in the African Diaspora by comparing the health of long-term residents of African descent in different parts of the world. While recent immigrants may have a health status more similar to their country of origin than to their host country, over time a shift in risk profile occurs. Children of immigrants may have an intermediate risk profile, and their grandchildren may have a risk profile most similar to the host country (which is the birth country for this generation) or some unique risk profile.

Initially, migrants may have an increased risk for infectious disease due to differences in immunity and susceptibility due to lack of prior exposure or poor immune status. The risk of chronic diseases is likely to be similar to that of the home region. Acculturation and changes in health behavior, such as diet and activity level, gradually shift the risk profile from that of the home region to that of the host region. Finally, the health status of past migrants will be like long-term residents of the host country with similar genetic and socioeconomic profiles, even if health disparities may exist between population subgroups.

In general, the risk of infectious disease is higher in Africa than in Europe or the United States and the risk of chronic diseases is lower in Africa. This is partly due to increased life expectancy, since chronic conditions are often associated with age, and partly due to lifestyle differences. A meta-analysis of epidemiologic studies on hypertension, a symptom of cardiovascular disease, found that systolic blood pressure levels in both men and women are significantly higher in blacks from the northern Western hemisphere than in blacks from sub-Sahara Africa, (Systolic Blood Pressure, I87–91). A study comparing incidence of dementia in African Americans in Indianapolis, Indiana, to Yoruba in Ibadan, Nigeria, found a significantly lower rate of dementia and Alzheimer's disease in the Yoruba population.[50] Women from sub-Saharan Africa have a low incidence of breast cancer, largely due to protective reproductive histories that limit the number of ovular cycles over a lifetime, when compared to black women in the United States.[51] The risk profile of most for these population groups may currently be very similar to that of their region of origin, but the cancer prevalence will likely change with the adoption of new dietary practices and other lifestyle changes.

However, while the prevalence of cancer may be lower in Africa, the stage at diagnosis is often more advanced. A study of prostate cancer patients found that Senegalese men had a significantly worse tumor stage at diagnosis than patients from the United States.[52] Most Senegalese men were diagnosed after seeking treatment due to symptoms, but the vast majority of American men were diagnosed on the basis of an elevated PSA (Prostate Specific Antigen) screening test. Although the risk of developing a non-communicable condition is lower in low-income nations than high-income nations, the risk of dying from a chronic disease is greater.[53] In Tanzania, and presumably in many other African nations, the majority of deaths are now due to long-term illnesses rather than acute illness,[54] and other analyses have found that the majority of deaths from cardiovascular disease occur in developing countries.[55] Thus, while residence outside Africa is associated with increased incidence of some non-communicable conditions, increased access to health care may minimize the effects of the increased risk.

The health transition is perhaps most obvious in nutrition studies. Nutritionists refer to a nutrition transition, in which populations shift from a stage in which undernutrition and nutrient deficiencies are prevalent to an intermediate stage in which undernutrition and obesity are both problems in the population to a stage in which overweight and obesity are the dominant nutritional disorders.[56] West Africa is in the early stage and undernutrition is the most common nutritional problem. Descendents of Africans forced to other parts of the world by the slave trade represent populations at varying stages of the nutrition transition. Many Caribbean populations are in the middle stage of the transition whereas African-Americans and people of African descent living in the United Kingdom are in the later stage and suffer from many disorders of overnutrition including obesity, diabetes, hypertension, and heart disease (Luke, 47–71). The prevalence of obesity, diabetes, and hypertension among African Diaspora populations is lowest in African countries like Nigeria and Cameroon, higher in Caribbean nations like St. Lucia and Barbados, and highest in the United States and the United Kingdom.[57] An anthropometric study found 5% prevalence of obesity in Nigeria, 23% prevalence in Jamaica, and 39% prevalence among U.S. blacks.[58] Prevalence of type 2 diabetes increased from 2% in Nigeria to 9% in the Caribbean, and 11% in the United States and United Kingdom.[59] Hypertension increases from 16% in West Africa to 26% in the Caribbean and 33% in the United States.[60]

CONCLUSION

Table 2–2 summarizes the conclusions of this chapter. Intra-African migration often involves rural-to-urban movement that may, at least temporarily, increase risk of infectious disease and decrease access to health services. Over time, most urban residents in Africa become healthier than their rural counterparts. Maternal and child health may benefit most from the increased access to trained healthcare workers in cities. Refugees generally have poor health that results from violence, undernutrition, crowded living conditions, and poor environmental sanitation. Africans who voluntarily move to other parts of the world generally report better health than long-term residents of host nations. The health status of a given household several generations after emigration is related to socioeconomic status and the health status of their region of residence.

TABLE 2.1 Basic Health Statistics for Selected Countries [61]

Country	Total Fertility Rate, 2002	Life Expectancy at Birth (years), both sexes, 2002	Probability of Dying (per 1000) under age 5 years, 2002	
			Male	Female
Democratic Rep. of Congo	6.7	43.5	221	198
Ghana	4.2	57.6	106	99
Kenya	4.1	50.9	119	113
Nigeria	5.5	48.8	183	181
South Africa	2.6	50.7	86	81
Barbados	1.5	74.3	17	15
France	1.9	79.8	6	4
Jamaica	2.4	72.8	16	14
United Kingdom	1.6	78.2	7	6
United States	2.1	77.3	9	7

TABLE 2.2 Summary of Migration and Health

Migration Pattern	Health Trends Associated with Migration
Intra-African Migration	
Rural-to-Urban	Rural residents who move to an urban area may temporarily have an increased risk of infectious disease and decreased access to health services. Health status is usually higher than rural residents after several years, especially for women and children. Urban residents have higher risk of heart disease, diabetes, and obesity.
Urban-to-Urban / Rural-to-Rural /	
Urban-to-Rural	Movement to new locations is associated with increased infectious disease risk.
Short-term / Seasonal Migration	Short-term travel is associated with increased infectious disease risk.
Refugee Status (Refugeeism)	Refugees often experience poor health related to violence, undernutrition, crowded living conditions, and poor environmental sanitation.
Voluntary Migration Out of Africa	Migrants who voluntarily leave Africa generally have higher health status than both African non-migrants and long-term residents of their host country. Africans who voluntarily move to the United States, Canada, or Europe may have an increased risk of chronic diseases like cancer, but access to advanced health care technology may make earlier diagnosis and longer survival possible.

NOTES

1. Lance Saker, Kelley Lee, Barbara Cannito, Anna Gilmore, and Diarmid Campbell-Lendrum, "Globalization and Infectious Diseases: A Review of the Linkages" (TDR/STR/SEB/ST/04.2), Special Topics in Social, Economic and Behavioural Research (SEB) series, Geneva: Switzerland: WHO on

behalf of the UNICEF / UNDP / World Bank / WHO Special Programme for Research & Training in Tropical Diseases (TDR), 2004.

2. J. Decosas, F. Kane, J.K. Anarfi, K.D. Sodji, and H.U. Wagner, "Migration and AIDS," *Lancet* 346, no. 8978 (1995): 826–828.
3. Nathalie Lydié and Noah Jamie Robinson, "West and Central Africa," *International Migration* 36, no. 4 (1998): 469–512.
4. M. Colvin, S.S. Abdool Karim, and D. Wilkinson, "Migration and AIDS," *Lancet* 346, no. 8985 (1995): 1303–1304. Mark N. Lurie, Brian G. Williams, Khangelani Zuma, David Mkaya-Mwamburi, Geoff P. Garnett, Adriaan W. Sturm, Michael D. Sweat, Joel Gittelsohn, and Salim S. Abdool Karim, "The Impact of Migration on HIV-1 Transmission in South Africa," *Sexually Transmitted Diseases* 30, no. 2 (2003): 149–156. K. Zuma, E. Gouws, B. Williams, and M. Lurie, "Risk Factors for HIV Infection Among Women in Carletonville, South Africa: Migration, Demography, and Sexually Transmitted Diseases," *International Journal of STD & AIDS* 14, no. 12 (2003): 814–817. Brendan Girdler-Brown, "Eastern and Southern Africa," *International Migration* 36, no. 4 (1998): 513–552.
5. World Bank, *World Development Indicators 2005* (Washington, DC: World Bank, 2005); hereafter cited in text as World Bank, 2005.
6. United Nations Development Programme, *Human Development Report 2005* (New York: UNDP, 2006).
7. B.C. Ozumba, S.N. Obi, and N.N. Ijioma, "Knowledge, Attitude and Practice of Modern Contraception Among Single Women in a Rural and Urban Community in Southeast Nigeria," *Journal of Obstetrics and Gynaecology* 25, no. 3 (2005): 292–295.
8. Martin Brockerhoff, "Child Survival in Big Cities: The Disadvantages of Migrants," *Social Science and Medicine* 40, no. 10 (1995): 1371–1383; hereafter cited in text as Child Survival.
9. M. Brockerhoff, "The Impact of Rural-Urban Migration on Child Survival," *Health Transition Review* 4, no. 2 (1994): 127–149; hereafter cited as Impact of Rural-Urban.
10. UNFPA, *Country Profiles for Population and Reproductive Health: Policy Developments and Indicators 2005* (New York: United Nations Population Fund and the Population Reference Bureau, 2005).
11. Eugène Sobngwi, Jean-Claude Mbanya, Nigel C. Unwin, Raphael Porcher, André-Pascal Kengne, Léopold Fezeu, Etienne Magloire Minkoulou, Caroline Tournoux, Jean-Francois Gautie, Terence J. Aspray, and Kgmm Alberti, "Exposure Over the Life Course to an Urban Environment and Its Relation with Obesity, Diabetes, and Hypertension in Rural and Urban Cameroon," *International Journal of Epidemiology* 33, no. 4 (2004): 769–776.
12. Miriam Grant, "Movement Patterns and the Medium-Sized City: Tenants on the Move in Gweru, Zimbabwe," *Habitat International* 19, no. 3 (1995): 357–369.
13. D. Garnier and E. Bénéfice, "Habitual Physical Activity of Senegalese Adolescent Girls Under Different Working Conditions, As Assessed by a Questionnaire and Movement Registration," *Annals of Human Biology* 28, no. 1 (2001): 79–97.

14. E. Lagarde, M. Schim van der Loeff, C. Enel, B. Holmgren, R. Dray-Spira, G. Pison, J.P. Piau, V. Delaunay, S. M'Boup, M. Coeuret-Pellicer, H. Whittle, P. Aaby, and the MECORA Group, "Mobility and the Spread of Human Immunodeficiency Virus into Rural Areas of West Africa," *International Journal of Epidemiology* 32, no. 5 (2003): 744–752.
15. Megan P. Coffee, Geoffrey P. Garnett, Makalima Mlilo, Hélène A. Voeten, Stephen Chandiwana, and Simon Gregson, "Patterns of Movement and Risk of HIV Infection in Rural Zimbabwe," *The Journal of Infectious Diseases* 191, suppl. 1 (2005): S159–167.
16. I. Shabbir and C.P. Larson, "Urban to Rural Routes of HIV Infection Spread in Ethiopia," *Journal of Tropical Medicine and Hygiene* 98, no. 5 (1995): 338–342.
17. John A. Arthur, "Interregional Migration of Labor in Ghana, West Africa: Determinants, Consequences and Policy Intervention," Review of Black Political Economy 20, no. 2 (1991): 89–103.
18. T.W. Wilson, L.R. Hollifield, and C.E. Grim, "Systolic Blood Pressure Levels in Black Populations in Sub-Saharan Africa, the West Indies, and the United States: a Meta-Analysis," *Hypertension* 18, 3 suppl. (1991): I87–91; hereafter cited as Systolic Blood Pressure.

    Lionel H. Opie and Yackoob K. Seedat, "Hypertension in Sub-Saharan African Populations," *Circulation* 112, no. 23 (2005): 3562–3568. J. Mufunda, G. Mebrahtu, A. Usman, P. Nyarango, A. Kosia, Y. Ghebrat, A. Ogbamariam, M. Masjuan, and A. Gebremichael, "The Prevlance of Hypertension and Its Relationship with Obesity: Results from a National Blood Pressure Survey in Eritrea," *Journal of Human Hypertension* 20, no. 1 (2006): 59–65. K. Steyn, J.M. Kazenellenbogen, C.J. Lombard, and L.T. Bourne, "Urbanization and the Risk for Chronic Diseases of Lifestyle in the Black Population of the Cape Peninsula, South Africa," *Journal of Cardiovascular Risk* 4 (1997): 135–142.
19. Ayesha A. Motala, Mahomed A. Omar, and Fraser J. Pirie, "Diabetes in Africa. Epidemiology of Type 1 and Type 2 Diabetes in Africa," *Journal of Cardiovascular Risk* 10, no. 2 (2003): 77–83.
20. Robert H. Glew, Carole A. Conn, Thomas A. VanderJagt, Christine D. Calvin, Michael O. Obadofin, Michael Crossey, and Dorothy J. VanderJagt, "Risk factors for cardiovascular disease and diet of urban and rural dwellers in northern Nigeria," *Journal of Health, Population, and Nutrition* 22, no. 4 (2004): 357–369.
21. A.R. Walker, F. Adam, and B.F. Walker, "World Pandemic of Obesity: the Situation in Southern African Populations," *Public Health* 115, no. 6 (2001): 368–372.
22. J.S. Kaufman, E.E. Owoaje, S.A. James, C.N. Rotimi, and R.S. Cooper, "Determinants of Hypertension in West Africa: Contribution of Anthropometric and Dietary Factors to Urban-Rural and Socioeconomic Gradients," *American Journal of Epidemiology* 143, no. 12 (1996): 1203–1218.
23. John K. Akokpari, "The State, Refugees, and Migration in Sub-Saharan Africa," *International Migration* 36, no. 2 (1998): 211–234.

24. United Nations High Commissioner for Refugees (UNHCR), *2004 Global Refugee Trends: Overview of Refugee Populations, New Arrivals, Durable Solutions, Asylum-Seekers, Stateless and Other Persons of Concern to UNHCR*, Geneva, Switzerland: UNHCR, 20 June 2005.
25. UNHCR, *Improving Refugee Health Worldwide*, 30 November 2003; http://www.unhcr.ch/cgi-bin/texis/vtx/partners/opendoc.pdf?tbl=PARTNERS&id=3fcb53882 \accessed 24 January 2006\.
26. E. Kalipeni and J. Oppong, "The Refugee Crisis in Africa and Implications for Health and Disease: A Political Ecology Approach," *Social Science and Medicine* 46, no. 12 (1998): 1637–1653.
27. M.J. Toole, "Mass Population Displacement: A Global Public Health Challenge," *Infectious Disease Clinics of North America* 9, no. 2 (1995): 353–366.
28. UNHCR, *Refugee Children: Guidelines on Protection and Care*, Geneva, Switzerland: UNHCR, 1994.
29. Lila Rosenthal, Deborah P. Scott, Zeman Kelleta, Astatkie Zikarge, Matthew Momoh, Judith Lahai-Momoh, Michael W. Ross, and Andy Baker, "Assessing the HIV/AIDS Health Services Needs of African Immigrants to Houston," *AIDS Education and Prevention* 15, no. 6 (2003): 570–580.
30. Amy Hagopian, Matthew J. Thompson, Meredith Fordyce, Karin E. Johnson, and L. Gary Hart, "The Migration of Physicians from Sub-Saharan Africa to the United States of America: Measures of the African Brain Drain," *Human Resources for Health* 2, no. 1 (2004): 17–26.
31. Amy Hagopian, Anthony Ofosu, Adesugun Fatusi, Richard Biritwum, Ama Essel, L. Gary Hart, and Carolyn Watts, "The Flight of Physicians from West Africa: Views of African Physicians and Implications for Policy," *Social Science and Medicine* 61, no. 8 (2005): 1750–1760.
32. Jacqueline W. Lucas, Daheia J. Barr-Anderson, and Raynard S. Kington, "Health Status of Non-Hispanic U.S.-Born and Foreign-Born Black and White Persons: United States, 1992–95," *Vital Health Statistics* 10, no. 226 (2005): 1–20; hereafter cited as Health Status of Non-Hispanic.
33. Jacqueline W. Lucas, Daheia J. Barr-Anderson, and Raynard S. Kington, "Health Status, Health Insurance, and Health Care Utilization Patterns of Immigrant Black Men," *American Journal of Public Health* 93, no. 10 (2003): 1740–1777; hereafter cited as Health Status, Health Insurance. Jen'nan Ghazal Read, Michael O. Emerson, and Alvin Tarlov, "Implications of Black Immigrant Health for U.S. Racial Disparities in Health," *Journal of Immigrant Health* 7, no. 3 (2005): 205–212. Gopal K. Singh and Mohammad Siahpush, "Ethnic-Immigrant Differentials in Health Behaviors, Morbidity, and Cause-Specific Mortality in the United States: An Analysis of Two National Data Bases," *Human Biology* 74, no. 1 (2002): 83–109.
34. Ghazal Jen'nan Read and Michael O. Emerson, "Racial Context, Black Immigration and the U.S. Black/White Health Disparity," *Social Forces* 84, no. 1 (2005): 181–199; hereafter cited as Racial Context.
35. Douglas J. Lanska, "Geographic Distribution of Stroke Mortality Among Immigrants to the United States," *Stroke* 28, no. 1 (1997): 53–57.

36. Gopal K. Singh and Mohammad Siahpush, "All-Cause and Cause-Specific Mortality of Immigrants and Native Born in the United States," *American Journal of Public Health* 91, no. 3 (2001): 392–399.
37. K.D. Rosenberg, R.A. Desai, and J. Kan, "Why Do Foreign-Born Blacks Have Lower Infant Mortality Than Native-Born Blacks?: New Directions in African-American Infant Mortality Research," *Journal of the National Medical Association* 94, no. 9 (2002): 770–778.
38. Karen A. Bonuck, Kathy Freeman, and Michelle Trombley, "Country of Origin and Race/Ethnicity: Impact on Breastfeeding Intentions," *Journal of Human Lactation* 21, no. 3 (2005): 320–326.
39. Susan Cote, Paul Geltman, Martha Nunn, Kathy Lituri, Michelle Henshaw, and Raul I. Garcia, "Dental Caries of Refugee Children Compared with U.S. Children," *Pediatrics* 114, no. 6 (2004): e733–740.
40. Gary King, Anthony P. Polednak, Robert Bendel, and Deborah Hovey, "Cigarette Smoking Among Native and Foreign-Born African Americans," *Annals of Epidemiology* 9, no. 4 (1999): 236–244. W.S. Carlos Poston, V.N. Pavlik, D.J. Hyman, K. Ogbonnaya, C.L. Hanis, C.K. Haddock, M.L. Hyder, and J.P. Foreyt, "Genetic Bottlenecks, Perceived Racism, and Hypertension Risk Among African Americans and First-Generation African Immigrants," *Journal of Human Hypertension* 15, no. 5 (2001): 341–351.
41. Ken Sexton, John L. Adgate, Timothy R. Church, Stephen S. Hecht, Gurumurthy Ramachandran, Ian A. Greaves, Ann L. Fredrickson, Andrew D. Ryan, Steven G. Carmella, and Mindy S. Geisser, "Children's Exposure to Environmental Tobacco Smoke: Using Diverse Exposure Metrics to Document Ethnic / Racial Differences," *Environmental Health Perspectives* 112, no. 3 (2004): 392–397.
42. Sonjia Kenya, Mitchell Brodsky, William Divale, John P. Allegrante, and Robert E. Fullilove, "Effects of Immigration on Selected Health Risk Behaviors of Black College Students," *Journal of American College Health* 52, no. 3 (2003): 113–120.
43. Poston, "Genetic Bottlenecks," 341–351. D.J. Hyman, K. Ogbonnaya, N.N. Pavlik, W.S. Poston, and K. Ho, "Lower Hypertension Prevalence in First-Generation African Immigrants Compared to U.S.-born African Americans, *Ethnicity & Disease* 10, no. 3 (2000): 343–349.
44. Jing Fang, Shantha Madhavan, and Michael H. Alderman, "Nativity, Race, and Mortality: Favorable Impact of Birth Outside the United States on Mortality in New York City," *Human Biology* 69, no. 5 (1997): 689–701; hereafter cited as Nativity, Race, and Mortality.
45. E. Blair Johnson, Susan D. Reed, Jane Hitti, and Maneesh Batra, "Increased Risk of Adverse Pregnancy Outcome Among Somali Immigrants in Washington State," *American Journal of Obstetrics and Gynecology* 193, no. 2 (2005): 475–482.
46. Birgitta Essén, Bertil S. Hanson, Per-Olof Östergren, Pelle G. Lindquist, and Saemundur Gudmundsson, "Increased Perinatal Mortality Among Sub-Saharan Immigrants In a City-Population in Sweden," *Acta Obstetricia et Gynecologica Scandinavica* 79, no. 9 (2000): 737–743.

47. L.J. Melton, III, M.A. Marquez, S.J. Achenbach, A. Tefferi, M.K. O'Connor, W.M. O'Fallon, and B.L. Riggs, "Variations in Bone Density Among Persons of African Heritage," *Osteoporosis International* 13, no. 7 (2002): 551–559.
48. C. Bouchardy, P. Wanner, and D.M. Parkin, "Cancer Mortality Among Sub-Saharan African Migrants in France," *Cancer Causes & Control* 6, no. 6 (1995): 539–544.
49. A.E. Grulich, A.J. Swerdlow, J. Head, and M.G. Marmot, "Cancer Mortality in African and Caribbean Migrants to England and Wales," *British Journal of Cancer* 66, no. 5 (1992): 905–911. E.A. Haworth, V.Soni Raleigh, and R. Balarajan, "Cirrhosis and Primary Liver Cancer Amongst First Generation Migrants in England and Wales," *Ethnicity and Health* 4, no. 1–2 (1999): 93–99.
50. Hugh C. Hendrie, Adesola Ogunniyi, Kathleen S. Hall, Olesegun Baiyewu, Frederick W. Unverzagt, Oye Gureje, Sujuan Gao, Rebecca M. Evans, A.O. Ogunseyinde, A.O. Adeyinka, Beverly Musick, and Siu L. Hui., "Incidence of Dementia and Alzheimer Disease in 2 Communities: Yoruba Residing in Ibadan, Nigeria, and African Americans Residing in Indianapolis, Indiana," *JAMA* 285, no. 6 (2001): 739–747.
51. Alero Fregene and Lisa A. Newman, "Breast Cancer in Sub-Saharan Africa: How Does It Relate to Breast Cancer in African-American Women?," *Cancer* 103, no. 8 (2005): 1540–1550.
52. S.M. Gueye, C.M. Zeigler-Johnson, T. Friebel, E. Spangler, M. Jalloh, S. MacBride, S.B. Malkowicz, and T.R. Rebbeck, "Clinical Characteristics of Prostate Cancer in African Americans, American Whites, and Senegalese Men," *Urology* 61, no. 5 (2003): 987–992.
53. Christopher J. L. Murray and Alan D. Lopez, "Mortality by Cause for Eight Regions of the World: Global Burden of Disease Study," *Lancet* 349 (1997): 1269–1276.
54. Philip W. Setel, Lance Saker, Nigel C. Unwin, Yusuf Hemed, David R. Whiting, and Henry Kitange, "Is It Time to Reassess the Categorization of Disease Burdens in Low-Income Countries?," *American Journal of Public Health* 94, no. 3 (2004): 384–388.
55. Ernest C. Madu, Kelly D. Richardson, Obinna H. Ozigbo, and Dainia S. Baugh, "Improving Cardiovascular Disease Prevention and Management in Africa: Issues to Consider for the 21st Century," *Ethnicity and Disease* 13, no. S2 (2003): 71–76.
56. Amy Luke, Richard S. Cooper, T.Elaine Prewitt, Adebowale A. Adeyemo, and Terrence E. Forrester, "Nutritional Consequences of the African Diaspora," *Annual Review of Nutrition* 21 (2001): 47–71.
57. Luke, "Nutritional Consequences," 47–71. Jean-Claude N. Mbanya, J.Kennedy Cruickshank, Terrence Forrester, Beverly Balkan, Jeanne Y. Ngogang, Lisa Riste, Anne Forhan, Norma McFarlane Anderson, Franklyn Bennett, and Rainford Wilks, "Standardized Comparison of Glucose Intolerance in West African-Origin Populations of Rural and Urban Cameroon, Jamaica, and Caribbean Migrants to Britain," *Diabetes Care* 22, no. 3 (1999): 434—440. Wilks, R., N. McFarlane-Anderson, F. Bennett, H.

Fraser, D. McGee, R. Cooper, and T. Forrester, "Obesity in Peoples of the African Diaspora," *Ciba Foundation Symposium* 201 (1996): 37–48.

58. A. Luke, X. Guo, A.A. Adeyemo, R. Wilks, T. Forrester, W. Lowe, Jr., A.G. Comuzzie, L.J. Martin, X. Zhu, C.N. Rotimi, and R.S. Cooper, "Heritability of Obesity-Related Traits Among Nigerians, Jamaicans, and US Black People," *International Journal of Obesity and Related Metabolic Disorders* 25, no. 7 (2001): 1034–1041.
59. Richard S. Cooper, Charles N. Rotimi, Jay S. Kaufman, Eme E. Owoaje, Henry Fraser, Terrence Forrester, Rainford Wilks, Lisa K. Riste, and J. Kennedy Cruickshank, "Prevalence of NIDDM Among Populations of the African Diaspora," *Diabetes Care* 20, no. 3 (1997): 343–348.
60. Richard Cooper, Charles Rotimi, Susan Ataman, Daniel McGee, Babatunde Osotimehin, Solomon Kadiri, Walinjom Muna, Samuel Kingue, Henry Fraser, Terrence Forrester, Franklyn Bennett, and Rainford Wilks, "The Prevalence of Hypertension in Seven Populations of West African Origin," *American Journal of Public Health* 87, no. 2 (1997): 160–168.
61. Data from: World Health Organization, *The World Health Report 2004: Changing History* (Geneva: World Health Organization, 2004).

Chapter Three

Discourses on Health Risks and Anti-Racial Diversity in the Media Coverage of the Non-Ebola Panic

Charles T. Adeyanju

The global spread of infectious diseases with the potential risk for severe consequences has been a major focus of the media and a concern of the general public in recent years. Ulrich Beck[1] and Anthony Giddens[2] have characterized the present period as risky and existentially perilous. Proliferation of risk is partly a consequence of the processes of what Giddens calls the "sequestration of time from space" and the attendant "lifting out" of social relations from their local moorings (Giddens, 1990). The mass media play a major role in the separation of time from space. From a "risk society" thesis, the preponderance of risks in post-industrial societies precipitates anxieties (Beck, 1992).

This chapter uses the case of Canadian media coverage of a female visitor from the Congo suspected of carrying the deadly Ebola virus[3] to show how race has been constructed and sustained in Canadian society. Li's[4] insights into the current state of anxiety among Canadians over racial diversity are instructive. Li argues that, as an immigrant country, Canada has always been linguistically, ethnically, and culturally heterogeneous, but it was not until the de-racialized immigration policy of the 1960s that the presence of racial minorities has been visibly felt (Li, 2003). Li maintains that the growing presence of people of non-European descent, distinguished by their discernible physical features, has become a source of anxiety for the public that has often perceived Canada as 'White' (Li, 2003). I use the "non-Ebola panic"[5] case to argue that this isolated event tapped into the uncertainties that Ungar[6] and Beck conceptualize as sites of social anxiety in a risk society (Beck, 1992). There is a general grassroots public concern about environmental, nuclear and health risks. The media construction of the non-Ebola case around immigration and racial diversity, through a "signification spiral,"[7] merely taps into the existing sense of insecurity that is confronting ordinary Canadians. How anxieties over this concern are articulated through discourse of harm and risk in the media matters for Canadians, who may make sense of social change in relation to international migration and societal complexity through the medium of "race."

BACKGROUND

The possibility that an Ebola positive patient on a visitor's visa from the Democratic Republic of Congo was admitted to a Hamilton hospital first appeared in the print media on February 6, 2001. Newspapers indicated that while the woman was visiting an acquaintance in Hamilton on February 4, she fell ill: she was feeling unwell, could not eat, and had a rising fever. According to her host, as reported in the newspaper stories, that Sunday night an ambulance was requested to transport her to the Henderson Hospital in Hamilton. Under medical examination, Ebola was considered as a probable cause of her illness by the medical practitioners who attended to her.

The *Globe and Mail* of February 7, 2001, quoting a source familiar with the case, reported that on Monday, February 5, the woman's illness had become so severe that she was "bleeding from several sites on the body." The popular local newspaper, the *Hamilton Spectator*, published stories on how a panic-stricken community was reacting to the news of Ebola in their neighborhood. According to news media's reports, the situation had become serious enough that those who came in contact with the woman, including five ambulance workers, were immediately identified for isolation; the ambulances in which she was transported were de-commissioned; and some hospital staff who came in contact with the patient voluntarily quarantined themselves to protect their family members from contracting the virus.

As the media coverage placed emphasis on Ebola as the possible cause of the patient's illness, public reaction in the Hamilton area grew. The Heritage Front, a self-acclaimed white supremacist organization, picketed the hospital and distributed anti-immigration pamphlets in the vicinity of the hospital; hospital workers panicked and threatened legal action against the hospital for exposing them to danger; Black children in some elementary schools in Hamilton were shunned by their fellow White students; and an acquaintance of the patient in the Congolese community is reported to have lost her job and moved out of her residence.

Subsequent newspaper articles reported that after a series of medical tests, Ebola and other suspected hemorrhagic fevers were ruled out. As soon as Ebola and these other hemorrhagic fevers were ruled out by the medical experts, the news quickly dropped off the media radar. But then news reports brought to public attention that the woman's medical care had been costly; and also that she was being investigated by the authorities for diamond smuggling.

The analysis of media coverage of this case is taken up in the final portion of this chapter. In the following sections, data sources and methods for collecting data for the study are presented, followed by the study's theoretical backdrop.

METHODS

This chapter is part of a larger study on the media coverage of an Ebola panic. Data for the study are derived from content analysis of four major Canadian newspapers: the *Hamilton Spectator*, the *Toronto Star*, the *National Post*, and the *Globe and Mail.*

The four newspapers for the study were selected on the basis of their ideological positions and circulation. The *Toronto Star* is a daily newspaper, published in Toronto. Its audience is largely in southern Ontario. The *Toronto Star* caters to an economically and socially diverse group. In one study, it was argued that the *Toronto Star* is "a socially liberal paper."[8] The *Globe and Mail* is also a daily newspaper that serves the interest of the economic and political elites. It is a national newspaper, but is published in Toronto. Ideologically, the *Globe and Mail* is sympathetic to neo-liberal philosophy. The *National Post* is a daily national newspaper that caters to the nation's intellectual and corporate elites. The *National Post* is generally considered a conservative press. The *Hamilton Spectator* is the local Hamilton newspaper. It serves the Hamilton local community and neighboring towns.

Data analysis is informed by critical discourse analysis.[9] Van Dijk lays out a number of principles guiding critical discourse analysis. Most important of these principles are: one, a discourse cannot be divested from its broader social, political, economic, and ideological contexts. The analyst must pay attention to the insidious role of discourse in the reproduction of inequality and domination; and two, critical discourse analysis is not decoupled from the analyst's sociopolitical stance, and so textual analysis must be seen from the viewpoint of marginal members of society.[10]

RACE, RACIALIZATION, RACISM, AND NEW RACISM

Most social scientists now agree that the biological connotations of race are a product of the Enlightenment and modernity.[11] The human mind has a propensity to classify people or things. It is this quality of the human mind to classify that Barrett[12] refers to as a "pan-human phenomenon" that cannot be confined to time and space.

Prior to the 19th century, people were classified along religious, cultural and regional identities, and somatic features, but physical and cultural differences were not considered permanent and immutable. A scientific explanation of human variations did not emerge until the late 18th century (Miles and Brown, 2003). In the late 18th century, according to Miles and Brown, the concept of race "increasingly came to refer to a biological type of human being, and science purported to demonstrate the number and characteristics of each "race," and a hierarchical relationship between them" (Miles and Brown, 39). On this basis, the belief that the human population can be classified and organized hierarchically on the basis of genetics gained popularity in Europe from the late 18th century.

At the turn of the 20th century, the scientific conception of race was attacked and debunked by both natural and social scientists because compelling evidence emerged that classifying people into different hierarchies of "races" on the basis of the distribution of discernible physical features, such as skin color, nose shape, hair texture, and the like, in the human population is arbitrary, given that biological heredity such as skin color does not necessarily overlap with the invisible genetic attributes such as genotype.

Racism is grounded in a belief of a natural sub-division of the human population into discreet "races" that can be ranked hierarchically. Social and natural scientists of the 20th century argued that the human species was biologically and psychically related. The triumph of race as a social construction over race as a science made Banton proclaim in 1970 that, "as a biological doctrine, racism is dead" (Banton, 28). Given the fact that human relations in modern societies continue to be defined in terms of "race," Banton seemed to be overly optimistic at the time. While the scientific conception of race declined at the turn of the 20th century, the scientific explanation of race has not disappeared from either the scientific lexicon or everyday language in the West, (Miles and Brown, 45). The use of the concept of race to define social relations continues to dominate everyday discourse in contemporary society. In confirming this permeability of racial thinking in American society, Omi and Winant write: "our society is so thoroughly racialized that to be without racial identity is to be in danger of having no identity."[13] Martin Barker's notion of "new racism" has gained popularity, and his argument has shown that race still matters in the definition of social relations in the West. Barker[14] uses the term "new racism" to describe a strain of racism in Britain in the 1970s. Barker claims that anti-immigrant discourse adopted by British politicians in the 1970s was a form of racism, which he refers to as the "new racism." Barker argues that the new form of racism does not talk about race as a differentiation of human beings into hierarchical order on the basis of skin color. Rather, hierarchies of groups are expressed in terms of cultural differences. He identifies the concept of the new racism as a: " . . . theory of human nature. Human nature is such that it is natural to form a bounded community, a nation, aware of its differences from other nations. They are not better or worse. But feelings of antagonism will be aroused if outsiders are admitted. And there grows up a special form of connection between a nation and the place it lives," (Barker, 15). The new racism, as espoused by Barker, does not allude to ranking people biologically, but indirectly holds that ethno-racial diversity can lead to social problems. Drawing on a 1991 national survey, Satzewich holds that the beliefs of the new racism are widespread in Canada.[15]

Studies have also shown that an overt expression of racism has declined in contemporary Western society as a result of political correctness. With the exception of right wing white supremacist organizations,[16] public expression of scientific racism has become largely unfashionable, and is rarely expressed. Nevertheless, racism is still reproduced in different forms. In the Canadian case, Kirkham[17] claims that New Right politicians in Canada have an anti-immigrant agenda that targets non-Whites. Kirkham asserts that New Right politicians in Canada express their anti-immigration rhetoric by re-articulating race in a non-race way (243–267). In regard to the Canadian immigration policy of the 1990s, Li[18] makes related points in his analysis of racist sub-texts regarding Canadian immigration policy.

In a study of three European countries (Netherlands, Britain, and Germany), using public discourses and information from the media, Husbands[19] argues that "new moral panics" are fuelled in these countries by one or two interrelated factors that are considered as threats to "national identity." First, the rising numbers of new immigrants and refugees of perceived distinctive culture and physiognomy in the 1980s and 1990s were considered to be a cause of economic and social problems. Second, the large numbers of refugees and immigrants were perceived as diluting the "national culture," and were therefore a threat to the national identity of the various indigenous European White populations. Wodak and Matouschek[20] also claim that anxieties around the changing ethnic composition of Austria were interpreted as a threat to Austrian cultural identity by the presence of non-Austrians—Poles, Turks, Jews, etc.—in the 1990s. Their findings were based on the expression of "prejudiced discourse" by politicians, ordinary people in the street, and the Austrian media.

MASS MEDIA AND CROSS-ARTICULATION OF DISEASES AND IMMIGRATION/ RACE

Tomes'[21] comparative analysis of past and present "germ panics" in the US explicates how the articulation of immigration/racio-ethnic differences and social problems can become forged. She notes: " . . . Both germ panics coincided with periods of heavy immigration to the United States of groups perceived as "alien" and difficult to assimilate. At the turn of the 20th century, it was the "new" immigration from eastern and southern Europe. In the 20th century, it is the "new" wave of recent immigration from Asia, Africa, and Latin America. The association of immigration and infectious disease has intensified scrutiny of national border crossings. . . ." (Tomes, 195).

The mass media has also played a role in cross-articulating race/immigration with infectious disease. Power[22] claims that the news media coverage of the bubonic plague in San Francisco in the 1900s attributed its etiology to the "Chinese Other," fuelling anti-Asian sentiments. Chirimuuta and Chirimuuta[23] have also argued that race was a factor in the media construction of the Acquired Immune Deficiency Syndrome (AIDS) in the 1980s and 1990s. Dubois[24] points out that deep rooted racism in the US was the initiating factor for blaming Haitians for the emergence of AIDS: "Many, including well-intentioned doctors and journalists, have participated in racist descriptions of the Haitian people and therefore in policies which have discriminated against them. In the early 1980s, the American media, following the lead of certain scientists, blamed Haitians as the source of a then new epidemic: AIDS. In doing so, they played into prevalent stereotypes about Haiti, deepening those stereotypes and magnifying the stigmatization they cause," (Dubois, 8). The recent outbreak of the Severe Acute Respiratory Syndrome (SARS) was cross-articulated with the Chinese by the media and members of the Western public.[25] Its representation in the media took the form of visually linking SARS with images of Chinese citizens in masks even when the virus was infecting non-Asians in Canada.

Most social scientists have concluded that race involves inclusion/ exclusion paradigms. Fleras and Elliot insist that, "there is no such thing as race relations in the sense of a "race" of people who stand in a relationship to another "race." What exist instead are relations that have been defined by reference to race."[26] Miles argues that social relations become defined in racial terms through the "signification process," defined as: "the representational process by which meanings are attributed to particular objects, features and processes, in such a way that the latter are given special significance, and carry or are embodied with a set of additional, second-order features," (Miles and Brown, 70). For Miles, the signification process entails racialization, which involves situations where social relationships between people have been organized based on the signification of human physical characteristics "in such a way as to define and construct differentiated collectivities" (Miles and Brown, 75). Racialization is also a dialectical process: ascribing real or alleged biological characteristics with meaning to define the "Other" necessarily entails "Self" by the same criteria (Miles and Brown, 75). The studies of Power, (Power, 1995, 89–110), Chirimuuta and Chirimuuta (1989), Tomes (2000) and Washer (2004) presented above demonstrate instances where representations of diseases go through the process of racialization.

GLOBALIZATION AND INSECURITY

Growing anxieties over indeterminacy and fear of the unknown distinguish the "risk society" from "industrial society," (Giddens, *The Consequences of Modernity*). Beck distinguishes the two societies in the following way: "The driving force in the class society can be summarized in the phrase: *I am Hungry*! The movement set in motion by the risk society, on the other hand, is expressed in the statement: *I am afraid*! The *commonality of anxiety* takes the place of the *commonality of need*. The type of the risk society marks in this sense a social epoch in which solidarity from anxiety arises and becomes a political force" (emphasis original) (Beck, 49). According to Giddens, "time-space distanciation," (Giddens, *The Consequences of Modernity*, 14) radicalizes modernity, and connects us "with events, with actions, and with the visible appearance of physical settings thousands of miles away from where we happen to live," (Giddens, *The Consequences of Modernity*, 141). Separation of time from space, therefore, necessitates "intrusion of distant events into everyday consciousness," (Giddens, *The Consequences of Modernity*, 141). Through the process of separating time from space, health risks and other risks become unbounded, de-localized and globally intrusive.

Globalization of risk makes risks ubiquitous and contributes to modern anxiety. However, Giddens notes that the routines of life allow humans to cope with everyday risks. Humans, right from infancy, Giddens states, have always developed fortitude to cope with risks and their attendant ontological insecurity through the security system they develop, (Giddens, *Modernity and Self-Identity*). To illustrate how individuals deal with existential perils of modern life, Giddens explains the development of "self" from infancy. At an early stage, Giddens notes, the infant forges relationships with the caretaker through habit and routine. The relationships are based on basic trust. Basic trust links the self to the object-world, and others, even in their absence. According to Giddens, "basic trust is connected in an essential way to the interpersonal organization of time and space," (Giddens, 38). The basic trust invested in the caretaker makes the infant believe that the caretaker will always return after any absence. If it were not for the basic trust, everyone would be prone to anxieties about risks all the time: "The sustaining of, in a bodily sense as well as in the sense of psychological health, is inherently subject to risk. The fact that the behavior of human beings is so strongly influenced by mediated experience, together with the cumulative capacities which human agents possess, means that every human individual could (in principle) be overwhelmed by anxieties about risks which are implied by the very business of living. That sense of 'invulnerability' which blocks off negative possibilities in favor of a generalized attitude of hope derives from basic trust," (Giddens, 40). Further, in his analysis of risk and insecurity in the contemporary world, Giddens indicates that the "protective cocoon" that allows people to carry on with their daily activities in the presence of risks is a sense of "unreality" rather than "a firm conviction of reality," as the "protective barrier it offers may be pierced, temporarily or more permanently, by happenings which demonstrate as real the negative contingencies built into all risk," (Giddens, 40).

MEDIA AND MORAL PANICS: IMPLICATIONS FOR HEALTH PANICS

From the literature on moral panic, we can gain insights into the relationship between the mass media and collective behavior. Hall et al. claim that in times of social change, a discourse of moral panic, disseminated through the mass media, provides a rallying point for the power elites who seek political dominance, (Hall et al., 1978). In the course of fomenting a moral panic, they argue, less advantaged members of society become delineated as the "folk devil." Drawing on the Gramscian strain of Marxism, Hall and his colleagues argue that the media helped the British ruling class amplify a crisis in order to cement its hegemony at a time of fragile consensus in Britain (Hall et al., 1978). The media, as an indirect representative of the ruling class and its interests, constructed a crisis that paved the way for "authoritarian populism"[27] and the legitimization of a law and order state. Through what Hall and his colleagues refer to as a "signification spiral," they claim that the "folk devil" was created in the urban Black youth, who were criminalized in their entirety. The disproportional reaction to the objective harm of criminality associated with the urban youth, Hall et al.

claim, was motivated by the "signification spiral"—"a way of signifying events which also intrinsically escalates their threat," (Hall et al., 223). One of the escalating mechanisms of the "signification spiral" is "convergence," which entails cross-articulation of two or more events "so as to implicitly or explicitly draw parallels between them" (Hall, et al., 223).

In their insights on moral panics, Goode and Ben-Yehuda[28] refer to Hall et al.'s perspectives on moral panics as "an elite-engineered model": "a conscious undertaking by the elite group to generate and sustain concern, fear, and panic on the part of the public over an issue that they recognize not to be terribly harmful to the society as a whole," (Goode and Ben-Yehuda, 135). In lieu of this perspective (the elite-engineered model), Goode and Ben-Yehuda favor an articulation of what they refer to as "grassroots model" and "interest group theory." They argue that moral panic is not an ideological imposition from the top, given that the situation leading to a moral panic must be organic to a society. Thus, a grassroots model of moral panic posits that "panics originate with the general public; the concern about a particular threat is a widespread, genuinely felt-if perhaps mistaken-concern," (Goode and Ben-Yehuda, 127). However, public concerns do not lead into a panic unless they are articulated. Therefore, Goode and Ben-Yehuda state that moral panics stem from the middle rungs of society. Interest groups, they claim, such as "professional associations, police departments, the media, religious groups, educational organizations" shape "the content or timing of panics" (139).

Goode and Ben-Yehuda maintain that a moral panic founders in the absence of a grassroots endorsement, but pre-existing fears and concerns must be brought to public attention by those in the middle rungs of society: "While widespread stress or latent public fears almost necessarily pre-exist moral panics, they do not explain how and why they *find expression* at a particular time. These fears must be articulated; they must be focused, brought to public attention, given a specific outlet. And this almost always entails some form of organization and leadership," (Goode and Ben-Yehuda 141). The media play a major role in establishing a relationship between health risks and moral panics.[29] According to Seale, the media are capable of generating a "culture of fear" by inaccurately constructing diseases as dangerous, for the purpose of influencing people's opinion of the risks of modern life, (Seale, 2002). Goode and Ben-Yehuda's view of public reaction to a panic influences this study. Although the media often cross-articulates diseases with immigration / race, the elite discourse can only be effective when it resonates with people's material condition. In other words, the mass media cannot fully be held responsible for collective reaction to panics.

FINDINGS

Panic

Panic is a key theme in the media coverage of the non-Ebola case (see Table 3.1). Panics are conveyed in the choice of words in headlines (see Table 3–2). The following are some examples of the newspaper headlines with the word "Ebola": "Mystery Virus Fells Woman: Ebola not ruled out, Woman arrived from the Congo,"[30] "Doctors Fear Woman May Have Ebola,"[31] and "Ebola Fever Case Feared: Woman from Congo in Hamilton."[32] According to van Dijk, headlines have both cognitive and textual functions.[33] Most readers do not read the remainder of an article, taking with them the summarized version of the news in the headline. However, headline messages, like other media texts, do not have direct effects on people, but they are capable of influencing public opinion. While there is no indication in the early coverage that the hospital had diagnosed Ebola, the word was already embedded in some of the news headlines. Other possible infections could have been meningitis and malaria, and a broad category of hemorrhagic fevers, including Marburg, and Crimean-Congo, which were not included in the headlines.

Apart from the use of words like Ebola, another notable word inspiring panic is "mystery." Giddens distinguishes between "anxiety" and "fear": "fear is a response to a specific threat and therefore has a definite object," (Giddens, *Modernity and Self-Identity*, 43) whereas "anxiety is diffuse, it is free floating: lacking a specific object," (Giddens, *Modernity and Self-Identity* 44). While "Ebola" signifies a detectable fear, "mystery" relates to "anxiety"-an unknown enemy, no cure and something that strikes without warning. Therefore, anxiety may evoke feelings of uncertainty and insecurity. The following are some examples: "Mystery Illness Strikes Woman,"[34] "Disease Mystery Unsolved: Doctors are still bewildered by Congolese woman's illness,"[35] and "Woman with Mystery Illness on Life-Support: condition worsens."[36] Other key words in the headlines are "risk," "deadly," and "virus" (see Table 3–2).

Panics are also expressed in the body of news articles. The choice of words and statements attributed to medical authorities and individuals in the medical profession have a tendency to promote fear. The following are some examples of such expressions, comments and remarks: "Doctors say they have not been able to specifically determine what is wrong with the seriously ill woman and are assuming the worst."[37] "She is also showing at least some of the symptoms listed under the plan [Health Canada's contingency plan] such as fever, headache, sore throat, shock or bleeding.

TABLE 3.1 Frequency of Key Words in the Media Coverage

		National Post		Hamilton Spectator		Globe and Mail		Toronto Star	
Themes	Key Words	N1 %	N2 (%	N1 %	N2 %	N1 %	N2 %	N1 %	N2 %
Diseases	Ebola	20(39.2)	16 (16.5)	55 (28.1)	76 (15.4)	25 (26.6)	11 (10.4)	37(21.9)	35(26.7)
	Malaria	0(0.0)	1(1.0)	6(3.1)	13 (2.6)	1(1.1)	3(2.8)	7(4.1)	3(2.3)
	Hemorrhagic fevers	3(5.9)	2(2.1)	23(11.7)	46 (9.3)	10(10.6)	6(5.7)	20(11.8)	9(6.9)
	Meningitis	3(5.9)	1(1.0)	8(4.1)	5 (1.0)	1(1.1)	0(0.0)	2(1.2)	0(0.0)
	Lassa	2(3.9)	0(0.0)	7(3.6)	7 (1.4)	1(1.1)	0(0.0)	8(4.7)	2(1.5)
	Marburg	2(3.9)	0(0.0)	4(2.0)	5 (1.0)	2(2.1)	2(1.9)	3(1.8)	5(3.8)
	Crimean-Congo	1(2.0)	1(1.0)	5(2.6)	9 (1.8)	4(4.3)	0(0.0)	6(3.6)	3(2.3)
Panic	Deadly	5(9.8)	5(5.2)	16(8.2)	19 (3.9)	3(3.2)	5(4.7)	11(6.5)	1(0.8)
	Death	0(0.0)	0(0.0)	8(4.1)	5 (1.0)	4(4.3)	0(0.0)	8(4.7)	2(1.5)
	Bleeding	2(3.9)	0(0.0)	19(9.7)	7 (1.4)	9(9.6)	5(4.7)	10(5.9)	1(0.8)
	Mysterious illness	1(2.0)	5(5.2)	6(3.1)	12 (2.4)	1(1.1)	7(6.6)	2(1.2)	2(1.5)
	Mystery	0(0.0)	3(3.1)	0(0.0)	17 (3.4)	0(0.0)	1(0.9)	0(0.0)	6(4.6)
	Virulent	0(0.0)	2(2.1)	2(1.0)	6 (1.2)	1(1.1)	1(0.9)	0(0.0)	4(3.1)
Identity	Congolese Woman	0(0.)	8(8.2)	8(4.1)	23 (4.7)	3(3.2)	11(10.4)	7(4.1)	8(6.1)
	Congo	7(13.7)	5(5.2)	10(5.1)	35 (7.1)	10(10.6)	6(5.7)	9(5.3)	8(6.1)
	Congolese	0(0.0)	1(1.0)	0(0.0)	10 (2.0)	2(2.1)	0(0.0)	0(0.0)	2(1.5)
	Africa	3(5.9)	2(2.1)	14(7.1)	19 (3.9)	6(6.4)	3(2.8)	11(6.5)	4(3.1)

Continued

TABLE 3.1 *Continued*

		National Post		Hamilton Spectator		Globe and Mail		Toronto Star	
Themes	Key Words	N1 %	N2 (%	N1 %	N2 %	N1 %	N2 %	N1 %	N2 %
	Naming	0(0.0)	10(10.3)	0(0.0)	107 (21.7)	8(8.5)	33(31.1)	0(0.0)	20(15.3)
Suspicion/ Crime	Investigation/ Smug-gling	0(0.0)	13(13.4)	0(0.0)	24 (4.9)	1(1.1)	5(4.7)	0(0.0)	3(2.3)
Immigration	Visitor's Status	1(2.0)	11(11.3)	3(1.5)	34 (6.9)	0(0.0)	5(4.7)	10(5.9)	10(7.6)
	Screening	1(2.0)	1(1.0)	0(0.0)	1 (0.2)	0(0.0)	0(0.0)	7(4.1)	0(0.0)
	Immigration	0(0.0)	10(10.3)	2(1.0)	13 (2.6)	2(2.1)	2(1.9)	11(6.5)	3(2.3)
Total		**51(100)**	**97(100)**	**196(100)**	**493(100)**	**94(100)**	**106(100)**	**169 (100)**	**131(100)**

N1 denotes the frequencies of words in the newspaper articles in 'the Ebola period coverage': from February 6, 2001 to February 8, 2001.

N2 denotes the frequencies of key words in the newspaper articles in the 'the post-Ebola period coverage': from February 9, 2001 to March 7, 2001.

TABLE 3.2 Key Words in the Newspapers' Headlines

	National Post		Hamilton Spectator		Globe and Mail		Toronto Star	
Key Words	N1 (%)	N2 (%)	N1 (%)	N2 (%)	N1 (%)	N2 (%)	N1 (%)	N2 (%)
Ebola	4(40)	6(31.6)	3(16.7)	11(39.3)	5(55.6)	2(18.2)	5(33.3)	3(33.3)
Deadly	1(10)	1(5.3)	3(16.7)	1(3.6)	1(11.1)	2(18.2)	1(6.7)	0(0)
Risk	1(10)	1(5.3)	1(5.6)	2(7.1)	1(11.1)	0(0)	0(0)	0(0)
Congo	0(0)	1(5.3)	1(5.6)	3(10.7)	1(11.1)	0(0)	0(0)	0(0)
Congolese Woman	0(0)	1(5.3)	0(0)	6(21.4)	0(0)	3(27.3)	1(6.7)	2(22.2)
Mystery	1(10)	5(26.3)	1(5.6)	3(10.7)	0(0)	2(18.2)	1(6.7)	2(22.2)
Virus	3(30)	1(5.3)	3(16.7)	1(3.6)	1(11.1)	2(18.2)	5(33.3)	1(11.1)
***OTHER	0(0)	3(15.8)	6(33.3)	1(3.6)	0(0)	0(0)	2(13.3)	1(11.1)
TOTAL	**10(100)**	**19(100)**	**18(100)**	**28(100)**	**9(100)**	**11(100)**	**15(100)**	**9(100)**

N1 denotes the frequencies of words in the newspaper headlines in 'the Ebola period coverage': from February 6, 2001 to February 8, 2001.

N2 denotes the frequencies of key words in the newspaper headlines in the 'the post-Ebola period coverage': from February 9, 2001 to March 7, 2001.

***Other: This category is determined by empty cells that are more than four. They are smuggling/investigation, mysterious, dangerous, bleeding, and crisis.

Doctors say she is not bleeding from her ears or mouth, which are final stage signs of Ebola or other hemorrhagic fevers. However, that doesn't means (sic) she does not have one of the viruses."[38] Concerning the fear of infection by some members of hospital staff, the president of CUPE Local 794 is quoted: "They are scared to death. They're scared not just for themselves, but for their children."[39] On a related note, the *Hamilton Spectator* comments: "A Hamilton X-ray technician exposed to a Congolese woman with a mystery virus has cancelled her wedding in the Caribbean because she can't leave the country," (Frketich, A6). In a similar vein, the *National Post* writes: "Five people are considered to be at the highest risk for contracting the unknown infection, including two friends or family members who had contact with her when she arrived, one ambulance attendant and two Henderson staff members who were splashed with the woman's blood, urine, mucus or vomit. They remain on the job," (Vallis, Woman with Mystery Illness). The fact that those "who were splashed" with the bodily fluids of the patient remain on the job is "scary" as it implies a possible spread of an "unknown" infection.

ARTICULATION OF IMMIGRATION AND HEALTH RISKS

Beck has indicated that risk consciousness in a risk society is rampant and that conflicts over risk get displaced. The displacement model of risk leads Beck to suggest that the risk society is a "scapegoat society" (Beck, 75).

Unlike the other newspapers, the *Toronto Star* brings up the issue of immigration and health early in its coverage of the case. In the other newspapers, the issue of immigration and health does not get coverage until later. One of the early *Toronto Star* news articles, published on February 6, 2001, begins by stating that the patient arrived from Africa. The second paragraph adds: "The woman, whose identity and nationality is not known, arrived at Toronto's Pearson International Airport on Saturday from the Congo via New York, where she stayed Friday night."[40] The article concludes by bringing up the topic of her immigration status in a way that connotes disfavor: "Immigration officials noted that Canada does not do medical screening for legitimate visitors to the country, unless they appear ill on arrival." The news article closes by quoting an immigration official as saying: "There is no way you can insulate Canada from the rest of the world" (Talaga, A04).

In another news report of February 7, 2001, the *Toronto Star* reports that the "news that the female patient is a visitor to Canada prompted calls by Ontario Health Minister Elizabeth Witmer to review the federal immigration screening program, which appears to be allowing people with serious illness into the country."[41] One of the *Toronto Star*'s headlines reads: "*Can't 'Shrink Wrap' Borders, Caplan Says: Witmer stresses importance of 'safety of the public'*"[42] This news article "moderates" a debate between the Ontario Minister of Health and the Citizenship and Immigration Minister, Elinor Caplan. The latter is quoted as saying: "Medical screening of all visitors to Canada wouldn't be realistic." The news report adds: "'It is impossible to shrink wrap our borders,' Caplan told reporters who asked about her department's handling of visitors who might be sick." Further the federal minister is quoted as saying: "We live in a global world, Canadians are on the move and traveling internationally. Hundreds of thousands of people visit Canada each year for short periods of time," (Thompson, A06).

The news article presents the position of the Ontario Minister of Health as follows: "At Queen's Park, Ontario, Minster Elizabeth Witmer said there needs to be an immediate review of the federal immigration screening program." She is quoted as saying, "We need to carefully review the current procedures that are in place and take a look at what additional measures may be required to ensure the safety of the public. . . . It is important that we protect the public."

News reports on medical coverage and immigration come later in other newspapers. The suspected case is also used to criticize the health care system and inadequate funding for the hospitals. The *Globe and Mail* uses the case to recall that residents also do not pay their bills. Its headline of March 14, 2001 reads: "Ontarians Leave Trail of Hospital Debts Too: Suspected Ebola victim's tab unpaid, but official says residents also fail to pay up." The article makes the following comments: "But the unpaid bills for the uninsured visitor to Canada—who was given experimental drugs and treated for 27 days in an intensive-care unit—have become news despite the fact that many hospitals deal with bad debts from Canadian residents every day."[43] The spokesman for the Hamilton Sciences Corporation is quoted as saying: "At the end of the day, we have more bad debts from Ontario residents than from visitors . . . visitors are part of the problem, but not the whole problem," (Foss, A16). This case has provided a space for expressing the public's dissatisfaction with the reigning political economy of neo-liberalism. This indicates that the media are not simply a "mouth piece" for the powerful.

The case also leads to a call for immigration reforms. This concern is expressed through the President of the Ontario Medical Association in the *National Post*: "the expensive case has the president of the Ontario Medical Association calling on the federal government to take responsibility for visitors it allows into the country and to cover the costs."[44] The president of the Ontario Medical Association is further quoted as saying: "We don't have any policy in this country to make sure visitors from abroad carry medical insurance of any sort." It continues, "When our government decides to receive people here in the country, they need to make sure they've made provisions for care," (Canadian Press, A08). The news article further comments that: "The federal and provincial governments never pay for the health care of foreign visitors, who are expected to pay for themselves. However, nothing is done before they enter the country to ensure they have health coverage or the money to pay for medical emergencies. The issue is significant because hospitals do not have extra cash to cover the outstanding bills. They have to pay for it out of their tight annual budgets," (Canadian Press, A08). The spokesman for the Hamilton Health Sciences Corporation is quoted as saying: "our budgets are so razor-thin that we're committed to funding $15-million in [cost] savings," said Jay Robb, spokesman for the Hamilton Health Sciences Corporation. "There isn't a whole lot of money to go around." The newspaper makes additional comments: "it is unknown exactly how much this case will cost the corporation but the bill is currently $60,000 and growing," (Canadian Press, A08). The frustration over inadequate health care funding is deflected to the immigration/visitor status of the patient. The patient thus becomes a symbolic expression of public concern and anxiety over the declining social welfare under the regime of neo-liberalism.

ANTI-RACIAL DIVERSITY SUB-TEXTS

There is no single reference to "race" or "Black" in the media coverage. The terms of reference are "Congo" and "Africa," and they occur in connection to the etiology of Ebola and other "deadly" diseases (see Table 3.1). It is not unusual for the media to couch views of anti-racial diversity in non-racial terms. Li has addressed this in his analysis of anti-immigration rhetoric in public consultations organized by Canadian Immigration and Citizenship. In his analysis of opinion polls, government documents and the media, Li argues that intolerance for the immigration of people of non-European descent is expressed in race neutral ways: "To study racial discourses involves accepting racism as an everyday phenomenon that is manifested in a benign version, often without the label of racism. This version is communicated in coded language so that on appearance it is not race or racism at stake, but in essence it carries a message about unbridgeable differences of people premised upon values, traditions, and ways of life subsumed under skin color or other superficial features," (Li, The Racial Subtext, 81.) A word like "diversity" and a phrase like "visible minorities" serve as a sobriquet for racially different groups. Li states that: "Racism can be articulated in an elusive and covert manner in a democratic society precisely because the construction of race is not scientifically grounded, and the absence of a scientific standard provides flexibility in racial signification" (Li, The Racial Subtext, 79). However, van Dijk has noted that texts with racist undertones can be detected by a technique he refers to as "implications": "meanings (propositions) that are not explicitly expressed in the text but may be inferred from words or sentences in the text, as well as from the mental models constructed during understanding. Indeed, it is sometimes more important to specify what is *not* said by the text than what is actually expressed. In many respects, media texts are ideological icebergs, of which only the tip is visible to the reader."[45]

In this case, direct allusions are not made to Blacks or racial minorities as a problem. However, the racist connotations of the coverage can be detected by the "implications" of some expressions and ideas. For example, the *Toronto Star* of February 6, 2001 comments: "It was a turn-around for a department that kept quiet when a man from the Dominican Republic with multi-drug resistant tuberculosis exposed more than 1,200 people in Hamilton to the deadly disease." By implication, the subtext from the above newspaper text is that non-Whites pose risks to the lives of Canadians. To be specific, it is more probable that a national from the Dominican Republic would be of African or Hispanic descent. The readership would rarely think of the "man" as White.

Like Li, (The Racial Subtext) Miles[46] shows in his study of Britain's post war immigration policy that racism can be coded by politicians and the public in non-racist terms. With a specific reference to Enoch Powel, who launched a campaign against 'colored immigration' in the late 1960s, Miles maintains in his analysis that racism was tactfully articulated in the public sphere by the politician with minimal reference to "race." Miles claims that: "As an element of commonsense, the idea of 'race' needs not necessarily be explicitly articulated for it to have real effects on the political process. By definition, commonsense is all those "taken for granted" ideas and "facts" which shape the manner in which problems are defined and solutions are sought. This can be done without the idea of 'race' ever being articulated. And even when the idea of 'race' is explicitly articulated, its commonsense status ensures that such usage does not require legitimation or explanation," (Miles, "Beyond the 'race' Concept," 13). The following newspaper quote is an archetypal example of "race neutral" expressions of racism, in the coverage of the non-Ebola panic: "A source said one of the community members who might be at risk attends a downtown Hamilton school. A staff member at École Notre Dame, a French elementary school, said they have two students who recently arrived from Congo—but neither had been contacted by public-health officials. In Hamilton there are as many as 300 residents originally from the Democratic Republic of Congo, according to a representative for the Settlement and Integration Services Organization."[47] Although there is no direct reference to race or "Black" in the above quote, it has some racial connotations. The reference to "two students," who just arrived from the Congo who are in the community implies that the public should look out for every "Black-looking kid," as the audience would imagine the Congolese to be Black rather than White or Asian. However, since it is very difficult to identify the Congolese from other Blacks, for the purpose of isolation, it then implies that every Black person in Hamilton is a potential carrier of the deadly virus.

Van Dijk notes, "much of the information in discourse, and hence also in news reports, is implicit, and supplied by the recipients on the basis of their knowledge of the context of the world."[48] Derogatory or denigrating statements about racial minorities in the media are not explicitly stated, "because of social norms, and for reasons of impression management. For instance, many negative things about minorities may not be stated explicitly, and thus are conveyed 'between the lines,'" (van Dijk, New(s) Racism, 40). The newspapers examined do not categorically claim that the Congolese are carriers of the deadly disease. However, it is implicit in some of the media texts. The following is an example. In regard to whether her illness is caused by malaria or some more serious virus, the *Hamilton Spectator* writes: "she was diagnosed with malaria, but tropical disease specialists concluded she had to be suffering from something else as well." The newspaper quotes a doctor as saying: "It's unlikely that everything she has would be caused by that degree of malaria. Apparently in that part of the world (Africa), it's not unusual for people to be entirely healthy walking around like you or I with that level of a parasite load."[49] In medical parlance, people get exposed to the malaria plasmodium/parasite if they live in an environment where malaria-carrying mosquitoes are rife. However, this quote seems to imply that the risk that the patient poses is greater because visible signs of the problem may remain latent longer among some populations rather than others. The statement "that part of the world" implies the "othering" of the disease in a way that Canadians are believed to be at greater risk than people from "that part of the world." Moreover, the comparison makes it look like Africans are natural hosts of deadly viruses, as compared to you or I, the Canadians, as the statement implies. Whatever scientific validity that this statement may have, it may unwittingly reinforce in the public the perception of racial differences and attribute contagious diseases to phenotype variations.

AGENDA SETTING: EDITORIALS AND LETTERS TO THE EDITOR

Two letters to the editor are published by the *Hamilton Spectator*: one by the *Toronto Star;* two by the *National Post;* and none by the *Globe and Mail.*

On the 9th of February 2001, the *Hamilton Spectator* published two "letters to the editor"; one from Niagara Falls, Ontario and the other one from Calgary, Alberta. They take somewhat different standpoints. The first letter sets to oppose Immigration Minister Elinor Caplan's comments on the case, opening as follows: "With respect to concerns over the latest disease carrier entering Canada, Immigration Minister Elinor Caplan has said: 'it's impossible to set up a policy of testing everyone. We have over 200 million people crossing our borders annually. It is impossible to shrink-wrap our borders.'" It continues: "Agreed. But the immigration minister can take effective action far short of that." The writer then identifies two groups with "the highest probability of being carriers of new and deadly diseases to Canada." They are: "refugee claimants released into the general population as soon as their initial paperwork is done"; and "those arriving from high-risk locations." The letter concludes: "both groups are identifiable" and states that it is imperative to protect Canada from the danger posed by these groups. "Refugees/refugee claimants," singled out by this writer, can be read as substitution for racial minority immigrants. Just as Li (Li, *Destination Canada*) asserts that in the folk version of an immigration problem "there is a considerable overlap between the concepts 'immigrants' and 'non-whites' or 'visible minorities,'" (Li, *Destination Canada,* 46) this writer may be using "refugee claimant" as a code phrase for racial minorities. "High-risk locations" refer to non-Western countries of Asia and Africa where it is presumed that deadly diseases are preponderant. The subtexts of the letter writer's proposition are that "immigration" of non-Whites to Canada is a threat to Canadians. This writer seems to advocate racial profiling as an effective measure for guaranteeing Canadians' safety.

The second letter acknowledges the reality of crossing borders in the global age, and the possible presence of contagious diseases in Canada. In a letter titled "Let's start from overseas," the writer states: "For our protection in Canada, we must treat victims overseas as well as here." The writer believes infectious diseases, such as Ebola, TB, malaria and HIV/AIDS are related to poverty and underdevelopment. The letter supports increased government spending on foreign aid for the eradication of "poverty: basic education, primary health care and nutrition."

The letter to the editor published by the *Toronto Star* on February 9, 2001, points out "the difficulty of 'shrink wrapping' the Canadian border," as expressed by Witmer. In the view of the writer, "shrink wrapping" the border is not commercially viable. However, the writer states, "I do, however, believe that it would be possible to target high-risk areas, which to me, seem to include The Democratic Republic of Congo." The letter then identifies those who need not be screened by the Canadian government: "You cannot expect to screen everyone who comes across the border from the U.S., or flies in from Europe and other such locations," it then adds, "It is not economically feasible and would definitely not help tourism." The letter is concluded with the following comments: "Canada is as multicultural as countries come, and with borders becoming more open, such as those within the European Union, the fact remains that diseases are an ever-present threat, where the only means of protection is to target the high-risk areas." This discourse is consistent with Miles' notion of "race/immigration dualism," (Miles, Beyond the 'race' Concept). In this case, threat of a disease is equated to the immigration of people from certain parts of the world. The subtext is that immigrants and visitors from "high-risk areas," like the Democratic Republic of Congo, are anathema to the health of Canadians and are *ipso facto* an "immigration problem." The panacea to this immigration problem is their de-legitimization through border control.

Letters to the editor are normally a reaction to op-ed, including the editorial, and "hard news" that are previously published by the newspaper. The day prior to the publication of the above letters to the editor, February 8, 2001, the *Hamilton Spectator* ran an editorial. Although an editorial lacks the journalistic ideals of "objectivity" and "balance," it exerts considerable influence over how readers "make meaning" of the events around them. Van Dijk claims that editors in Western countries use the editorials to speak to the White audience, (*Elite Discourse and Racism*, 266). If so, this editorial may be aiming to set an anti-immigration agenda in the way it constructs a discourse of health insecurity around immigration. It opens with the following: "Fear and anxiety for ourselves, our children, and neighbors. Growing unease about our government's ability to keep us safe from new and frightening diseases. Immeasurable stress on our already stretched health system. Intolerance and mistrust of people from other parts of the world . . . and at the centre, a critically ill woman who came to Canada on business, perhaps carrying a deadly passenger." The editorial continues: "surely, this isn't what Marshall McLuhan had in mind when he talked about the global village." Further, it states: "News that a seriously ill Congolese woman being treated at Henderson General Hospital is probably not suffering from the Ebola virus is welcome, but doesn't lessen the gravity of this situation . . . the clinical specifics of this case are less important than the lessons we can take from it."

The editorial spells out two lessons that need to be learned. One is that while globalization has made the world smaller and more interdependent, diseases like Ebola are still a threat because they are closer to "home" (Canada). The editorial compares the possible devastation of diseases like Ebola to the one wrought on the Aboriginals of North America by the Europeans centuries earlier: "like North American Aboriginal people exposed to small pox and influenza by European visitors hundreds of years ago, we are players on the global health stage, whether we like it or not." The subtext of this message is that just as the European visitors' incursion to North America was deadly to the population, contemporary immigration and visitors signal a related danger to the Canadian population. The second lesson that can be gleaned from this case is that the "crisis" must be used as a learning experience "to improve public policy and raise awareness." It also suggests that "stereotypes, fear, or intolerance" should not prevent people from discussing the issue. The editorial concludes with a note of warning: "There will be a next time. This may be a North American first, but it won't be the last time a community struggles with a situation like this. Let's set a good example." This conclusion sounds "apocalyptic" in the way it predicts a future tragedy. Moreover, the term "community," as it is used by the editorial, is ambiguous and seldom clear.[50] Its usage in this editorial allows readers to take the term in different ways. Some may see it in terms more exclusionary than others.

Unlike "hard" news texts, opinion discourses have a potential to recruit newsreaders because they "possess a unique idiomatic character that 'speaks' directly to the readership in a way that is familiar, habitual, and reliable."[51] The use of pronouns such as "we" and "our" in the *Hamilton Spectator's* editorial is a direct appeal to members of society. These pronouns are meant to tap into their collective conscience of external threat. Thus, the *Hamilton Spectator*'s editorial appeals to average members of society—parents, neighbors and citizens.

According to Beck, risks pertain to anxiety about the future. He indicates that "risks have something to do with anticipation, with destruction that has not yet happened but is threatening, and of course in that sense risks are already real today," (Beck, 33). The statement "there will be a next time" echoes Beck's notion of risks regarding the possibility of future danger, judging from the present. Unlike the editorial of the *Hamilton Spectator,* the editorial of the *National Post* of February 9, 2001, aims to allay the fear of the public, but like the former it also sounds its own note of warning about future risks. Its opening statement is: "Breathe easy. Lab results released this week indicate that a Congolese woman receiving treatment in a Hamilton, Ont. hospital does not, as first feared, suffer from the dreaded Ebola virus." Following these sentences, like the editorial of the *Hamilton Spectator*, it warns of impending health risks through international migration: "But it is probably only a matter of time before a visitor to Canada does. And when that happens, it is important we avoid hysteria." Two points are worthy of note here. First, the statement "only a matter of time before a visitor to Canada does" bring a deadly disease excludes the possibility that the potential carrier could be a Canadian. Second, the editorial's allusion to a possible future presence of viruses like Ebola in Canada, like that of the *Hamilton Spectator*, is a call for state intervention in the form of immigration control and screening of certain immigrants.

Knight notes that alternative points may compete with dominant values in the media, but both work towards an attainment of hegemony: "Hegemony entails the need to appear objective, so the media sometimes allows dissenting voices to offer alternative or oppositional definitions of an event or issue that break with the dominant definition by primary sources."[52] Knight's point is relevant to the analysis of the two letters to the editor carried by the *Hamilton Spectator*. As discussed above, the two letters do differ in perspective. Contrary to the position of the first letter, the second one introduces discourses of "development" and "hygienization" to dilute the dominant discourse of immigration and health. It proposes increased foreign aid and eradication of poverty as a solution to global health risks and insecurity.[53] Nevertheless, the letter is consistent with the dominant terms of reference; that is, a perception of deadly disease from the "outside." This letter coupled with the "anti-racial diversity" letter may give an impression of journalistic neutrality or impartiality to the *Hamilton Spectator*: publication of two letters with opposing views. However, the letters do not divest the newspaper of its ideological project. Apart from converging on the point that Canada is a possible target of foreign deadly diseases, differing positions in the newspaper may exonerate it of partiality. This is essentially ideological or hegemonic, according to Knight, (The Mass Media).

CONCLUSION

On the surface, it appears that the four newspapers examined have varied ideological orientations and differentiated audiences and market niches. For example, the *National Post* is popularly considered to be more critical of immigration and racial diversity than other newspapers, (Henry and Tator, 2002). But beneath the surface there do not appear to be appreciable differences in coverage among the newspapers. While some words and themes appear more or less frequently in the newspapers, they all single out the "Other"—an alien/immigrant as the problem, and celebrate the persecution of the categorized "racial Other" in the image of the woman in question. Their seemingly different accounts of events, nevertheless, converge to reproduce the dominant stereotypes of the "Other." In regard to this convergence, Hall et al.'s view that the media do not necessarily represent "the vast pluralistic range of voices," but "a range within certain distinct ideological limits" is relevant to this case, (*Policing the Crisis*, 61).

Some have argued that racism comes from the top and trickles down to the bottom. The concept of "elite racism" implies that ordinary people succumb to the dominant ideology of race, (van Dijk, *Elite Discourse and Racism*). One may be tempted to believe that media representation of events has a direct relationship on how people behave. From this line of reasoning, the representation of the specific non-Ebola event has a direct effect on the Canadian public. Though the media may have a powerful influence on public opinion, they do not impose their views on the readership. Rather, people relate to media content based on their fragmented subjective positions or identities. Joffe's illustration of how research participants interpret the origins of HIV/AIDS in relation to their racial and sexual subject positions is instructive. Her illustration shows that people interpret events and phenomena based on their social identity and broader life experience.[54]

An elaborate explanation of how the ideology of race manifests in ordinary people's practices has been provided by Miles and Brown, albeit from a neo-Marxist perspective. Miles and Brown have argued that working class racism in the specific historical formation of Britain was not an ideology that was imposed from the top; rather, racism was used by the working class to make sense of their social world and experiences in times of "capitalist production and the decay of the urban infrastructure."[55] Concerning the racist reaction of the British working class to Caribbean and Asian migrants, Miles and Brown assert that: "The idea of 'race' is used to define the Caribbean and/or Asian migrants as an illegitimate, competing Other whose presence has either caused or intensified the struggle for housing, social services and employment, from which it is concluded, apparently logically, that the problems could be resolved by excluding the Other. For this reason, this specific instance of working-class racism does not have to be explained by proposing a capitalist conspiracy or by identifying small groups of people who gather to celebrate Hitler's birthday and can only see Jewish and 'black' people as biologically degenerate" (Miles and Brown, 106). Racism is not imposed from the top by institutional authorities, such as the political, judiciary, educational or media branches, as van Dijk claims,

(*Elite Discourse and Racism*). It is a means for people with a racial capacity to make sense of the world and selves in times of societal complexities.

Using the Gramscian notion of "traces," Hall[56] illustrates how old stereotypes about Africa and Blacks have been modified to suit contemporary actualities. These traces have their source in slavery, colonial discourse, and observable material imbalances between Europeans and Africans. The media's constant reference to a "Congolese woman" with "Ebola" can reinforce in the public an image that may already exist; thus further reinforcing existing stereotypes. While content analysis cannot make a linkage between these "traces" and a contemporary event like the Ebola coverage, the structure of the coverage privileges a particular way of viewing the issues of immigration, race and diseases, and as such, provides the audience with information that is already ideologically inflected. Ideology functions at the moment when it finds resonance with the experiential consciousness of the people. Gramsci refers to the moment where ideology finds this resonance "feeling passion," (Knight, Hegemony). Ideology becomes effective at recruiting its audience when it can relate to people's feelings and emotions. The media does not impose dominant ideology; Canadians have what Barrett refers to as a "pan-human psychological propensity" that makes them think racially, (Paradise, 1994).

NOTES

1. Ulrick Beck, *Risk Society: Towards a New Modernity*, (New York: Sage, 1992).
2. Anthony Giddens, *Modernity and Self-Identity: Self and Society in the Late Modern Age*, (Stanford: Stanford University Press, 1991); hereafter cited in text as Modernity and Self-Identity. Anthony Giddens, *The Consequences of Modernity*, (Cambridge: Polity Press, 1990); hereafter cited in text as The Consequences of Modernity.
3. Ebola is a virus named after a river in the Democratic Republic of Congo, formerly Zaire, where it was first recognized in 1976. The Ebola virus and the Marburg are two members of a family of viruses called "Filoviridae," and they can cause severe hemorrhagic fever in humans and nonhuman primates. The Ebola virus can be deadly; its mortality rate ranges from 50 to 90 percent. Its etiology is unknown.
4. Peter Li, *Destination Canada: Immigration Debates and Issues*, (Oxford: Oxford University Press, 2003); hereafter cited in text as Destination Canada.
5. "Non-Ebola" denotes non-incidence, from a bio-medical viewpoint, which nevertheless had serious consequences on the community.
6. Sheldon Ungar, "Moral Panic versus the Risk Society: the Implications of the Sites of Social Anxiety," *British Journal of Sociology*, vol. 52, no 2, (2001): 271–291.

7. Stuart Hall, Chas Critcher, Tony Jefferson, John Clarke and Brian Roberts, *Policing the Crisis: Mugging, the state, and law-and-order,* (London: Macmillan, 1978).
8. Graham Knight, "Prospective News: Press Pre-Framing of the 1966 Ontario Public Service Strike," *Journalism Studies*, vol. 2, no 1, (2001): 73–91.
9. Teun van Dijk, "Principles of Critical Discourse Analysis," *Discourse & Analysis*, vol. 4, no 2, (1993): 249–283; Frances Henry and Carol Tator, *Discourses of Domination: Racial Bias in the Canadian English-Language Press*, Toronto: University of Toronto Press, 2002.
10. As an immigrant from Nigeria, West Africa, in Canada, I concur with van Dijk's assertion that "theory formation, description, and explanation, also in discourse analysis, are sociopolitically 'situated,' whether we like it or not" (van Dijk, 2001: 353). However, in spite of my proclivity to take particular points of view because of my subject position, I adhere strongly to Becker's (1967) recommendation, "to make sure that, whatever point of view we take, our research meets the standards of good scientific work, that our unavoidable sympathies do not render our results invalid" (Howard Becker, "Whose Side are We On?" Social Problems, Vol 14, no. 3, 1967,pg. 249.).
11. Robert Miles and Malcolm Brown (ed.), *Racism*, (London: Routledge, 2003); Joseph Mensah, *Black Canadians: History, Experiences, Social Conditions*, (Halifax: Fernwood Publishing, 2002); Audrey Smedley, "'Race' and the Construction of Human Identity," *American Anthropologist*, vol. 100, no 3, (1999): 690–702; Vic Satzewich, "Race, Racism and Racialization: Contested Concepts," in Vic Satzewich (ed.), in *Racism and Social Inequality in Canada*, (Toronto: Thompson Educational Publishing, Inc., 1998), 25–45; Michael Banton, "The Concept of Racism," in S. Zubaida (ed.), *Race and Racialism,* (London: Tavistock, 1970).
12. Stanley Barrett, *Paradise: Class, Commuters, and Ethnicity in Rural Ontario*, (Toronto: University of Toronto, 1994); hereafter cited in text as Paradise.
13. Michael Omi and Howard Winant, "*On the Theoretical Concept of Race,*" in Cameron McCarthy and Warren Crichlow (eds.), Race, Identity and Representation in Education (New York: Routledge, 1993), 5.
14. Martin Barker, *The New Racism*, (London: Junction Books, 1981).
15. Vic Satzewich, "Race and Ethnic Relations," In Robert Brym (ed.), *New Society: Sociology for the 21st Century*, (Toronto: Thompson Educational Press, 1998, 219).
16. Peter Li, "Racial Supremacism Under Social Democracy," *Canadian Ethnic Studies*, vol. 27, no 1, (1995): 1–17; Stanley Barrett, *Is God a Racist? The Right Wing in Canada*, (Toronto: University of Toronto Press, 1987); Stanley Barrett, "White Supremacists and Neo-Fascists: Laboratories for the Analysis of Racism in Wider Society," *Canadian Ethnic Studies*, vol. 16, no 1, (1984): 1–15.
17. Della Kirkham, "The Reform Party of Canada: A Discourse of Race, Ethnicity and Equality," In Vic Satzewich (ed.), *Racism and Social Inequality in Canada*, (Toronto: Thompson Educational Publishing, Inc., 1998), 243–267.

18. Peter Li, "The Racial Subtext in Canada's Immigration Discourse," *Journal of International Migration and Integration*, vol. 2, no 1, (2001): 77–97; hereafter cited in text as The Racial Subtext.
19. Christopher Husbands, "Crises of National Identity as the 'New Moral Panics': Political Agenda-Setting about Definitions of Nationhood," *New Community*, vol. 20, no 2, (1994): 191–206.
20. Ruth Wodak and Bernd Matouscheck, "'We are dealing with people whose origins one can clearly tell just by looking': Critical Discourse Analysis and the Study of Neo-Racism in Contemporary Austria," *Discourse & Society*, vol. 4, no 2, (1993): 225–248.
21. Nancy Tomes, "Public Health Then and Now: The making of a Germ Panic, Then and Now," *American Journal of Public Health*, vol. 90, no 2, (2000): 191–198.
22. Gerard J. Power, "Media Dependency, Bubonic Plague, and the Social Construction of the Chinese Other," *Journal of Communication Inquiry*, vol. 19, no 1 (spring), (1995): 89–110.
23. Richard Chirimuuta and Rosalid Chirimuuta, *AIDS, Africa and Racism*, (London: Free Association Books, 1989).
24. Laurent Dubois, "A Spoonful of Blood: Haitians, Racism and AIDS," *Science as Culture*, vol. 6, no 1, (1996): 7–43.
25. Peter Washer, "Representations of SARS in the British newspapers," *Social Science & Medicine*, vol. 59, (2004): 2561–2571.
26. Augie Fleras and Leonard Elliot, *Unequal Relations: An Introduction to Race and Ethnic Dynamics in Canada,* 4th Edition, (Toronto: Prentice Hall, 2003), 34.
27. See Graham Knight, "Hegemony, The Media, and the New Right Politics: Ontario in the Late 1990s," *Critical Sociology*, vol. 24, no1/2, (1998): 105–129; hereafter cited in text as Hegemony.
28. Erich Goode and Nachman Ben-Yehuda, *Moral Panics: The Social Construction of Deviance*, (Oxford: Blackwell, 1994).
29. Kevin Dew, "Epidemics, Panic and Power: Representations of Measles and Measles Vaccines," *Health*, vol., 3, no 4, (1999): 379–398; Clive Seale, *Media and Health*, (London: Sage Publications, 2002).
30. Joanna Frketich, "Mystery Virus Fells Woman: Ebola not ruled out, Woman arrived from the Congo," *Hamilton Spectator*, February 6, 2001, 1.
31. Tanya Talaga, "Doctors Fear Woman May Have Ebola," *Toronto Star*, February 6, 2001, A04.
32. Ken Kilpatrick and Krista Foss, "Ebola Fever Case Feared Woman from Congo in Hamilton," *Globe and Mail*, February 6, 2001, A1.
33. Teun van Dijk, *Racism and the Press,* (London: Routledge, 1991), 50.
34. "Mystery Illness Strikes Woman," *Toronto Star*, February 6, 2001, A04.
35. Joanna Frketich, "Disease Mystery Unsolved: Doctors are still bewildered by Congolese woman's illness," *Hamilton Spectator*, February 10, 2001, A1.
36. Mary Vallis, "Woman with Mystery Illness on Life-Support: condition worsens," *National Post*, February 9, 2001, A15; hereafter cited in text as Woman with Mystery Illness.
37. Suzanne Morrison, *Hamilton Spectator*, February 6, 2001, A1.

38. Joanna Frketich, *Hamilton Spectator*, February 7, 2001, A1.
39. Joanna Frketich *Hamilton Spectator*, February 9, 2001, A6.
40. Tanya Talaga, *Toronto Star*, February 6, 2001, A04.
41. Tanya Talaga, *Toronto Star*, February 7, 2001, A1.
42. Allan Thompson, *Toronto Star*, February 7, 2001, A06.
43. Krista Foss, *Globe and Mail*, March 14, 2001, A16.
44. Canadian Press, *National Post*, March 13, 2001, A08.
45. Teun van Dijk, *Elite Discourse and Racism*, (Newbury Park: Sage Publications, 1993), 256; italics original; hereafter cited in text as Elite Discourse and Racism.
46. Robert Miles, "Beyond the 'race' Concept: The Reproduction of racism in England," in Marie de Lepervanche and Gillian Bottomley (eds.), *The Cultural Construction of Race*, (Sydney: University of Sydney Press, 1988), 7–31; hereafter cited in text as Beyond the 'race' Concept.
47. *Globe and Mail*, February 8, 2001.
48. Teun van Dijk, "New(s) Racism: A Discourse Analytical Approach," in Simon Cottle (ed.), *Ethnic Minorities and the Media,* (Buckingham: Open University Press, 2000), 40; hereafter cited in text as New(s) Racism.
49. Joanna Frketich, *Hamilton Spectator*, February 9, 2001, A06.
50. Luin Goldring, "Blurring Borders: Constructing Transnational Community in the Process of Mexico-US Migration," *Research in Community Sociology*, vol. 6, (1996): 69–104.
51. Joshua Greenberg, Opinion Discourse and the Canadian Newspapers: the Case of the Chinese "Boat People," *Canadian Journal of Communication*, vol. 24, no 4, (2000): 8.
52. Graham Knight, "The Mass Media," in Robert J. Brym (ed.), *New Society: Sociology for the 21st Century* (2nd edition), (Toronto: Harcourt Brace Canada, 1998), 116; hereafter cited in text as The Mass Media.
53. Laurie Garrett, *Betrayal of Trust: The Collapse of Global Public Health*, (New York: Hyperion, 2000).
54. Helene Joffe, "The Shock of the New: A Psycho-dynamic Extension of Social Representational Theory," *Journal for the Theory of Social Behavior*, vol. 26, no 2, (1996): 202–203.
55. Robert Miles and Malcolm Brown, *Racism* (2nd edition), (London: Routledge, 2003).
56. Stuart Hall, "The Whites of their Eyes: Racist Ideologies and the Media," in George Bridges and Rosalid Brunt (eds.), *Silver Linings: Some Strategies for the Eighties*, (London: Lawrence and Wishart, 1981), 7–23.

Chapter Four

"Predatory Globalization?": The World Trade Organization, General Agreement on Trade in Services, and Migration of African Health Professionals to the West

Obijiofor Aginam

> Several characteristics of the global political economy shape the tactics and aspirations of progressive social forces: extreme hierarchy and unevenness of circumstances, acute deprivation and mass misery among the poor; erosion of autonomy at the level of the state as a consequence of the play of non-territorial capital forces
>
> —Richard Falk.[1]

I: THE CRUX OF THE ARGUMENT

In 1979, the World Health Organization (WHO), a specialized agency of the United Nations with a membership of 192 countries, published a detailed 40-country study on the trans-border migration of health professionals. In the study, the Organization found that close to 90% of all the migrating physicians were moving to just five industrialized countries: Australia, Canada, Germany, United Kingdom, and the United States.[2] In recent years, the migration of highly skilled health professionals, especially from Africa to the industrialized countries of the West, has emerged as an extremely controversial, complex and complicated phenomenon in the process of economic globalization. In ways not yet fully explored and understood either in scholarly literature or policy dialogues, the neo-liberal World Trade Organization (WTO), supported by the US and other leading western industrialized countries, has since 1995 adopted the General Agreement on Trade in Services (GATS), part of which might further undermine the already precarious health sector in most African countries as a result of the migration of trained physicians and nurses from Africa to the West.

This chapter assesses aspects of the exceedingly complex GATS agreement that would likely have serious implications for migration of health professionals out of Africa. I argue that GATS would most likely further undermine the precarious health sector in most of Africa by facilitating the migration of African physicians and nurses to the West, and would open up the health services sector in Africa for foreign investment by corporate health care providers. In recent years, an intense debate has raged between the proponents and critics of GATS on the likely impact of the agreement on poor countries. Within this debate, there is now a distillation of powerful arguments that international trade in services, as articulated and codified in the GATS agreement, will be exceedingly complex and problematic for developing countries.[3] As a majority of the African countries are already member states of the WTO which has the mandate to enforce GATS and other international trade agreements on a global scale, how would these African countries address any foreseeable predatory impact that GATS might have on outward migration of health professionals? Regardless of one's point of view in the debate on liberalization of trade in services that is now firmly anchored on the GATS agreement, the fundamental questions, as articulated by one Afro-centric epidemiologist and demographer, remain: should skilled migration, and by extension migration of health professionals, be left entirely to the forces of the global market? Should some form of intervention be negotiated? If so, what possible options could effectively and equitably work to the advantage of developing countries, especially in Africa?[4] In exploring these questions, it is important to situate the GATS discourse squarely on the legitimacy deficits of the emergent global political economy, the South-North asymmetry and inequalities, and the privileged prominence of the WTO as an indispensable component of the engine of economic globalization. Using the metaphor of "global apartheid," Falk observed:

> . . . several characteristics of the global political economy shape the tactics and aspirations of progressive social forces: extreme hierarchy and unevenness of circumstances, acute deprivation and mass misery among the poor; erosion of autonomy at the level of the state as a consequence of the play of non-territorial capital forces. . . . If these critical differences are appreciated, the global apartheid metaphor seems useful. It confronts the moral and political complacency of the North. . . . The metaphor of global apartheid, then, represents a warning as well as a provocative line of critique, suggesting the urgency of taking far more serious steps to overcome the North-South cleavage. (Falk, 13, 17)

To situate the debate on migration impact assessment of GATS in Africa, I proceed to highlight the evolution of the GATS agreement within the WTO architecture, based on the neo-liberal dogma of free trade and liberalization, the links between GATS and the health sector in developing countries, and how African countries would likely be helpless if indeed the GATS agreement, as predicted by some, facilitates outward migration of health professionals from the continent. Africa's helplessness in the evolving framework of global economic relations is inexorably linked to the contemporary South-North asymmetry in the predatory global order.

II: THE EVOLUTION OF GATS IN GLOBAL TRADE ARCHITECTURE: AN OVERVIEW

> The General Agreement on Trade in Services is a multilateral framework agreement that restricts government actions affecting services through legally enforceable constraints backed up by trade sanctions. The GATS is one of the numerous agreements that were adopted in 1994 as part of the newly established World Trade Organization system that apply to all WTO members. The GATS is an extraordinarily ambitious and quite complex agreement. (Sinclair, GATS, 3)

The General Agreement on Trade in Services (GATS) is one of the trade agreements that emerged from the end of the Uruguay Round of multilateral trade negotiations that ended with the creation of the World Trade Organization (WTO) in 1995. Although most scholars are right to observe that global services trade has expanded considerably in recent years, there are divergent views on whether trade in services should be regulated the same way as international trade in goods.[5] Before 1995, the governance architecture of international trade, dating back to the post World War II period, focused exclusively on the cross-border movement of goods based on the "loose" rules codified in the General Agreement on Tariffs and Trade (GATT) 1947. These rules operated largely on the principle of reciprocity between countries and trading partners. This meant that countries—rich or poor—could, based on the principle of comparative advantage, pick and choose areas where they could negotiate better tariffs on goods with their trading partners based on reciprocity.[6] An important feature of the Uruguay Round of trade negotiations was the radical transformation of the GATT-driven trading system into a rules-based global trading system anchored on the governance architecture of the new World Trade Organization (WTO). In just ten years after the emergence of the WTO, immutable trade norms have crystallized through its powerful adjudicatory dispute settlement system, with an unprecedented speed unparalleled in the post World War II practice of Westphalian international organizations. The establishment of the WTO witnessed a radical expansion of global trade from "goods" to complex areas such as services, intellectual property, sanitary and phytosanitary measures, and technical regulations on labeling and packaging. As observed by Malhotra et al,

> The transformation of the General Agreement on Tariffs and Trade (GATT) into the WTO in 1995 marked a paradigm shift, resulting in significant differences between the two regimes. The GATT system was primarily about negotiating market access for traded goods. But the WTO's extension into new substantive areas, intrusiveness into domestic policy-making, 'single undertaking' mandate, explicit linkage of trade with the protection of investment and intellectual property rights, and strict enforcement of disputes and cross-retaliation have extended its authority into areas of domestic regulation, legislation, governance and policy-making central to the development process. Recent agreements under the trade regime commit members not just to liberalizing trade in goods but also to making specific policy choices on services, investment and intellectual property. These choices can affect human development through their effects on employment, education, public health, movements of capital and labor and ownership of and access to technology.[7]

As one of the agreements that emerged with the paradigm shift from GATT to the WTO framework, GATS seeks progressively to liberalize global trade in services through four modes of supply: (i) cross-border supply of services, that is, from the territory of one WTO member into the territory of another member; (ii) consumption of services abroad, i.e. movement of consumers to the home country of the service supplier; (iii) supply of service by a WTO member, through the commercial presence in the territory of another member, i.e. foreign investment and movement of capital; and (iv) supply of service through the movement of natural persons across the territories of WTO members, i.e. cross-border migration of skilled labor. Although these four modes of supply services under GATS, based on existing literature on services trade, involve aspects of migration, it is Mode Four—"movement of natural persons" that bears the most significant impact on outward migration of skilled health professionals (doctors and nurses) from Africa. This paper therefore focuses on GATS Mode Four and its implications for health care delivery, and flight of human capital out of Africa.

III: THE FLIGHT OF HUMAN CAPITAL FROM AFRICA: OUTWARD MIGRATION OF DOCTORS AND NURSES

The problem is grievously compounded by the practice of "poaching," and the resulting brain-drain from Africa to the outside world. Some of the drain goes to other countries in the region—South Africa or Botswana, for example—but they, too, lose professionals in the predominant flow to the United Kingdom, the United States, Australia and Canada. It's rancid behavior on the part of the West—Stephen Lewis.[8]

Migration, especially in the case of health professionals, is a complex phenomenon to study and analyze with intellectual rigor. First, we need to concede that people, especially skilled professionals, have the right to decide freely to leave their countries of birth to make a living elsewhere. Second, migration patterns have shown that there is also South-South migration; from one developing country to another as in the case of Nigerian doctors who migrate to Southern Africa (Botswana and South Africa), the Caribbean (Jamaica, and Trinidad and Tobago), or the oil-rich Persian Gulf countries (Saudi Arabia, Kuwait, Quatar, and United Arab Emirates). In all of this, as Lewis rightly observed, "people have the human right to move to better jobs, with better pay, better benefits, better working conditions," (Lewis, 47). However, in the past two decades at least, outward migration of doctors and nurses from Africa has never been wholly a voluntary decision taken by these professionals in the absence of "inducement" from the West. Highly skilled African nurses and doctors are actively "poached" by Western countries that are eager to address the occupational shortages and deficits in their national health sectors. It is estimated that there are more Malawian doctors in the city of Manchester than in Malawi, more Zambian doctors in the city of Birmingham than in Zambia, (Lewis, 48). Data from international organizations and other scholarly studies on migration of health professionals from developing to developed countries is alarming. Rupa Chanda, an Indian scholar, and one of the leading policy analysts on GATS and health services, reported that as a result of the various visa schemes implemented by the United States government aimed at recruiting skilled health migrants from abroad, there were 150,000 foreign-trained doctors in the U.S in 1993, and 110,000 foreign-trained nurses living and working in the U.S. in 1996.[9] The World Bank, in 1993, estimated that developing countries accounted for 56% of all outward migration of physicians.[10] Using secondary data and collaborating with the World Bank, a joint study published by the United Nations Conference on Trade and Development (UNCTAD) and the World Health Organization (WHO) in 1998 stated that 56% of all migrating physicians come from developing countries, and that the figure for nurses is likely to be higher.[11] In Ethiopia, it is reported that between 1984 and 1994, 55.6% of the pathology graduates from the Addis Ababa Medical School left the country.[12] In Ghana, of the 65 doctors that graduated from the University of Ghana's Medical School in 1985, only 22 remained in the country by 1997.[13] In South Africa, about 10,000 health professionals emigrated from the country between 1989 and 1997.[14] It is estimated that more than 10,000 Egyptian medical and biotechnology experts have emigrated from the country.[15] In 1997, it was estimated that there are over 21,000 Nigerian doctors practicing in the United States.[16]

As developed countries actively recruit skilled health professionals from the major labor exporting African countries, South Africa, Nigeria, and Ghana, for instance, these countries would always strive to replace lost human capital in their health sectors by recruiting from the poorer countries. As Woodward observed, "Developed countries actively recruit health professionals, primarily from developing countries, and some facilitate immigration, to compensate for shortages arising from inadequate training programs. This provides the momentum for a chain of migration of medical professionals, as developed countries recruit from lower-income countries (e.g. South Africa and Nigeria), who in turn recruit from still poorer countries to off-set the resulting shortages."[17] The ultimate victims of this negative chain of events are the poorest African countries with very weak capacity to train enough doctors and nurses in their national educational institutions. Outward migration from the more intensive labor exporting African countries like Nigeria, Ghana, and South Africa to the West, and internal migration within Africa to replace lost human capital in these countries, taken together, seriously complicates health care delivery in all of Africa. In 2002, the World Health Organization estimated that in comparison with Eastern and Central European and some upper-middle-income countries with 200–400 medical doctors per 100,000 population, most Sub-Saharan[18] African countries have fewer than 10 doctors per 100,000 population.[19] In the midst of the precarious end result of outward migration by skilled health professionals, how then does the GATS agreement stand to complicate or ameliorate an already bad situation?

IV: CO-OPTING THE SOUTH-NORTH MIGRATION PATTERNS OF HEALTH PROFESSIONALS BY GATS AND THE WTO

Corporate pressure is nothing new in WTO negotiations. Such pressure, largely exerted by U.S.-based firms, is widely acknowledged to have been a driving force in the negotiations resulting in the original GATS within the broader package of WTO agreements, (Sinclair, GATS, 22).

Evidence from existing literature and data has invariably shown that migration patterns of skilled health professionals are predominantly from the developing to the western industrialized countries. Focusing on Mode Four of services trade under GATS—movement of natural persons—how would the ongoing GATS negotiations at the WTO protect Africa by ensuring that GATS commitments do not co-opt and "legalize" the present realities of South-North migration patterns to the advantage of developed countries? Conversely, as outward migration has proved to be a serious problem in the health sectors of most African countries, would GATS commitments further aggravate this problem by effectively legalizing these migration patterns and bring them within the architecture of international trade law enforced by the powerful WTO? Like other WTO agreements, GATS requires WTO member states to liberalize international trade in services by making commitments on market access, national treatment, and most favored nation principles for specific service sectors within their countries. Under Article XVI of GATS, market access requires that each WTO Member shall not discriminate between services and service suppliers of other member states. GATS provision on market access is sweeping and complex because once a commitment is made by a WTO Member, that member is precluded from setting limits on the number of service providers, service operations, transactions, employees, value of transactions and assets, restrictions on the types of legal entity through which services may be traded, or participation of foreign capital in their ownership. National treatment under Article XVII requires a WTO member to treat service providers from other WTO member countries no less favorably than its own domestic/national service providers. This precludes national policies that modify conditions of competition in favor of domestic providers. Commitments on market access and national treatment principles may be full, unbound, or partial.

GATS allows each WTO member the discretion to decide in which sectors to make commitments on, including the terms and conditions of such commitments. Commitments in each sector may be made in any or all the four modes of supply of service. The health services sector under GATS is divided into four sub-sectors: medical and dental services, nursing and midwifery, hospital services, other health services. WTO member states are allowed to make the so-called horizontal commitment that could apply to all service sectors instead of picking and choosing which sectors to open up to foreign competition.[20] Once a WTO member makes a commitment on a sector, such a commitment may, under very stringent and onerous conditions, be modified or withdrawn at any time after three years have elapsed from the date the commitment entered into force.[21]

On the surface, it appears as if GATS is a remarkably flexible agreement that allows a WTO member, especially developing countries, the discretion to choose which sectors of their economies to open up to foreign competition. This argument has been strongly canvassed by leading GATS proponents, especially the WTO secretariat.[22] However, like other WTO agreements like TRIPS, developing countries lack the capacity and economic clout to negotiate equitable and favorable trade rules with industrialized countries. Most GATS critics have argued that the scope of GATS is broad. Given the stark inequalities between WTO members as well as corporate pressure behind the position of most industrialized countries in international trade negotiations and global economic diplomacy, GATS poses a serious risk to the protection of public goods in most developing countries. Commenting on GATS 2000 negotiations, Scott Sinclair, a well-known Canadian GATS critic, puts the point succinctly,

> Global business interests are seeking binding, global and irreversible rules on services. It should come as no surprise that multinational corporations, as they expand and extend their global reach, increasingly have a strong interest in reducing the cost of complying with the regulations they face in different countries. . . . On behalf of predominantly northern-based multinationals, the U.S., Japan, the European Union and Canada, the so-called Quadrilateral governments, will be pressing developing countries for guaranteed, irreversible access to southern markets. They will also seek from each other more privatization and commercialization of public services such as education and health care, and further deregulation of publicly regulated sectors such as media, publishing, telecommunications, energy, transport, financial, postal and other services. (GATS, 3.8)

Commenting further on the link between GATS, corporate interests and the WTO, Sinclair observed that, "Powerful international interests have shaped the GATS agenda. . . . The potential for conflict between local government regulation in the public interest and the multinational corporate interest may arise in many and varied areas. Protecting the public interest by preventing further commercial encroachment in hospital food services, for example, may conversely be viewed as an unwarranted infringement on corporations' market access in the health care or food services field," (Sinclair, GATS, 26).
As African countries continue to navigate the *Scylla* of opening up their sectors (including the health services sector) to GATS and the *Charybdis* of

stemming the outward migration of nurses and doctors to the West, a sustained and robust building of capacity is needed to guide them, in carefully evaluating how to proceed with commitments on GATS Mode Four—movement of natural persons as it pertains to the health services sector. Mistakes in WTO's GATS negotiations could be costly and will most certainly co-opt and legalize the present patterns of South-North migration of African doctors and nurses to the West. If a mistake is made, modifying or withdrawing any such GATS commitment could prove stringent and onerous, and could also trigger the "dreaded" WTO dispute settlement mechanism.

V: POSTSCRIPT: BEYOND GATS—AN ARGUMENT FOR HUMANE ECONOMIC GLOBALIZATION

The monumental influence of the WTO in global economic relations between countries is now both enthusiastically supported and scathingly critiqued by scholars on both sides of the debate. In the GATS and public health context, this debate exemplifies what some scholars have aptly called a "tale of two treaties;" it is the best of treaties and the worst of treaties.[23] Specifically, on GATS and migration of doctors and nurses, it has been observed that, "the implications of trade via movement of health service providers are similarly mixed in nature. From the sending country's perspective, increased mobility of health care providers can help promote the exchange of clinical knowledge among professionals, help upgrade their skills, and raise the standard of health care in the home country, provided these service providers return to the home country. There are also gains to the sending country from remittances and transfers."[24] The World Bank and the WTO have, in different ways, argued in support of aspects of this observation. A World Bank sponsored study stated that in 2001, the value of remittances from emigration of skilled workers stood at $72.3 billion.[25] Assessing health services under GATS, the predominant view at the WTO has recognized that the interest of low-income countries hinge on attracting foreign investment inflows (Mode 3), and sending health professionals abroad in order to gain from remittances (Mode 4). Taken together, foreign investment in health services represents a positive transfer of resources with positive effects on other sectors.[26] However, the argument in favor of remittances and the potential for GATS to facilitate cross-fertilization and exchange of clinical and scientific knowledge between countries seems to be flawed. There is no reliable data and detailed empirical studies have not comprehensively examined the co-relation between remittances, the cost of training these skilled health professionals, the positive and negative impact of their emigration, and the effects of such migration on the health sectors of most developing countries. Until such empirical studies are undertaken, which will prove extremely difficult, we do not have a complete and holistic picture of how remittances from the migration of African doctors and nurses advances the health sector or contributes to the economic development of African countries.[27] As several developing countries seek Mode 4 commitments from developed countries, it has been rightly observed that the benefits to the exporting countries in form of remittances and acquired technical competencies and expertise may not off-set losses, and "temporary" providers of health services admitted to importing countries may eventually become permanent residents, (Schrecker and Labonte, 412). The relevant question, therefore, is not whether economic globalization and international commerce anchored on global free-trade agreements like GATS would contribute to the economic development of developing countries. There is no doubt that, in an ideal world, fairly-constructed trade norms and policies would serve as engines of economic growth. The real question is whether the present orthodoxy of free trade, driven by the interests of the leading industrialized democracies, could maximize the potential for humane globalization, given the glaring asymmetry between Africa and the developed world. It is now perceived that economic globalization (which the WTO is a part of) constrains the capacity of the state to finance social safety nets for the protection and provision of public goods.[28] This is the basis of Howse's construct of the "democratic deficit" at the World Trade Organization.[29] For GATS and outward migration of skilled doctors and nurses from Africa, committing to the GATS is just not enough. GATS must be situated in a broader global social policy context, and globalization needs to be humane. Managed migration ought to bring benefits to source countries without crippling their health and other sectors. Some of the proposals made on ethical recruitment of doctors and nurses from developing countries will most likely be trumped by the intrusive provisions of GATS and the WTO trade regime.[30] If the experience from other WTO agreements, especially TRIPS, proves anything in international economic relations, it is that global multinational corporate giants, hiding under the veil of their home governments, drive the agenda of economic globalization. It is therefore doubtful, and indeed only time will tell, if the GATS agenda will be any different. Africa is seriously marginalized in the international economic system, and will likely be powerless to influence the outcome of GATS negotiations.

NOTES

1. Richard Falk, *Predatory Globalization: A Critique* (Cambridge: Polity Press, 1999), 13.

2. A. Mejia, H. Piyurki, and E. Royston, *Physician and Nurse Migration: Analysis and Policy Implications* (Geneva: WHO, 1979).
3. See for instance, John Hilary, *The Wrong Model: GATS, Trade Liberalisation and Children's Right to Health* (London: Save the Children, 2001); Scott Sinclair, *GATS: How the World Trade Organization's "New Services" Negotiations Threaten Democracy* (Ottawa: Canadian Centre for Policy Alternatives, 2000); hereafter cited in text as GATS. Scott Sinclair and Jim Grieshaber-Otto, *Facing the Facts: A Guide to the GATS Debate* (Ottawa: Canadian Centre for Policy Alternatives, 2002).
4. Omar B. Ahmad, "Brain Drain: The Flight of Human Capital" (October 2004) Vol 82 (10) Bulletin of the WHO 797.
5. See generally, D. Woodward, "The GATS and Trade in Health Services: Implications for Health in Developing Countries" (2005) Vol.12 No.3 *Review of International Political Economy* 511–534; S. Zarrilli & C. Kinnon, *International Trade in Health Services: A Development Perspective* (Geneva: United Nations/World Health Organization, 1998); N. Drager & C. Vieira, *Trade in Health Services: Global, Regional, and Country Perspectives* (Washington, DC: PAHO, 2002); Rupa Chanda, "Trade in Health Services" (June 2001), Working Paper for the Commission on Macroeconomics and Health (Geneva: WHO).
6. For a comprehensive history of international trade law, See J. Jackson, *The World Trading System: Law and Policy of International Economic Relations* (Cambridge, MA: MIT Press, 1997); M.J. Trebilcock & R. Howse, *The Regulation of International Trade* (London: Routledge, 1999).
7. Kamal Malhotra, et al, *Making Global Trade Work for People,* (London: Earthscan, 2003), 3.
8. Stephen Lewis, *Race Against Time* (Toronto: House of Anansi Press, 2005), 47.
9. Rupa Chanda, "Trade in Health Services," Paper No. WG4:5, Commission on Macroeconomics and Health (Geneva: WHO, June 2001), 64.
10. World Bank (1993) *World Development Report, 1993: Investing in Health*, Washington, DC: World Bank.
11. O. Adams & C. Kinnon, "A Public Health Perspective," in S. Zarrilli & C. Kinnon, eds., *International Trade in Health Services: A Development Perspective* (Geneva: United Nations/WHO, 1998), 37.
12. S. Ababulgu, "Problem of Physician Migration in Ethiopia" (Unpublished Document) cited in O. Adams & C. Kinnon, 37.
13. Volta Regional Research Team, "The Doctors Are Out—Where are They?" Accra, Ministry of Health, 1997 cited in O. Adams & C. Kinnon, 37.
14. D. Kaplan, J. Meyer, and M. Brown, "Brain Drain: New Data, New Options" (unpublished paper), citied in Rupa Chanda "Trade in Health Services," 22.
15. A. Khalil, "Unchecked Exodus" (Unpublished Paper, April 1999), cited in Rupa Chanda, "Trade in Heath Services," 22.

16. A. Oyowe, "Brain Drain: Colossal Loss of Investment for Developing Countries" (Unpublished Paper), cited in Rupa Chanda, "Trade in Health Services," 22.
17. D. Woodward, "The GATS and Trade in Health Services," *Review of International Political Economy*, Vol.12 No.3 (2005): 511–518
18. I use the term "sub-saharan Africa" only in direct reference to a seminal work where the term is used. The term, now firmly embedded in most global development discourses, balkanizes the African continent by cutting off its Northern part and projects most of Black Africa as poor, undeveloped, and a reservoir of diseases, wars and conflicts. I agree with Molefi Asante that, there is neither an Africa north of the Sahara nor an Africa south of the Sahara . . . the Sahara is in Africa and human populations have inhabited the Sahara for thousands of years. It is as useless to speak of Africa separated by deserts, as it is to speak of separations by rain forests. See Molefi K. Asante, *Kemet, Afrocentricity and Knowledge* (Trenton, J.J: Africa World Press, 1990), 33.
19. WHO (2002) *WHO Estimates of Health Personnel: Physicians, Nurses, Mid-wives, Dentists and Pharmacists (around 1998)* (Geneva: WHO).
20. See generally, World Trade Organization, (1998) *An Introduction to the GATS* (Geneva: WTO Secretariat).
21. Article XXI GATS Agreement.
22. WTO (2001), *GATS: Facts and Fiction* (Geneva: WTO Secretariat).
23. D. Fidler, N. Drager, C. Correa, & O. Aginam, "Making Commitments in Health Services Under the GATS: Legal Dimensions," in C. Blouin, et al, eds., *International Trade in Services and the GATS: Current Issues and Debates* (Washington, DC: World Bank, 2006), 141–143.
24. Rupa Chanda, "Trade in Health Services," 20. See also Rupa Chanda, "Trade in Health Services," in N. Drager & C. Viera, eds., (2002) *Trade in Health Services: Global, Regional and Country Perspectives* (Washington, DC: PAHO, 2002), 35–44.
25. D. Ratha, "Workers' Remittances: An Important and External Source of External Development Finance," in *Global Development Finance 2003: Striving for Development in Global Development Finance* (Washington, DC: World Bank, 2003), 157–175.
26. R. Adlung & A. Carzaniga, "Health Services under the General Agreement on Trade Services," In N. Drager & C. Viera, eds., (2002) *Trade in Health Services: Global, Regional and Country Perspectives* (Washington, DC: PAHO, 2002), 12–31.
27. See generally, T. Schrecker & R. Labonte, "Taming the Brain Drain: A Challenge for Public Health Systems in Southern Africa" (2004) Vol.10 No. 4 International Journal of Occupational and Environmental Health 409 at 410; S. Bach, "International Migration of Health Workers: Labour and Social issues," Working Paper, International Labour Office, Geneva, July 2003, 13.
28. See generally, D. Rodrik, "How Far Will International Economic Integration Go?" (Winter 2000) 14 *Journal of Economic Perspectives*, 177–186;

D. Rodrik "Governance of Economic Globalization," in J.S Nye & J.D. Donahue, eds., *Governance in a Globalizing World* (Washington, D.C: Brookings Institution, 2000), 347; John Hilary, *The Wrong Model: GATS, Trade Liberalisation and Children's Right to Health* (London: Save the Children, 2001); Robert Howse & Makau Mutua, *Protecting Human Rights in a Global Economy: Challenges for the World Trade Organization* (Montreal: Rights and Democracy, 2000).

29. Robert Howse, "How to Begin to Think About the 'Democratic Deficit' at the WTO," available online at: http://faculty.law.umich.edu/howse (accessed 27 September, 2005).
30. For some of the proposals on ethical migration for both exporting and importing countries, See O. Ahmad, op cit; T. Shrecker & R. Labonte, op cit.; S. Bach, op cit.; Commonwealth Secretariat, *Companion Document to the Commonwealth Code of Practice for International Recruitment of Health Workers* (London: Commonwealth Secretariat, 2003).

Chapter Five

Searching the World: Following Three Graduating Classes of a Nigerian Medical School

Ike Anya[1], Chikwe Ihekweazu and Enyi Anosike

Much research has been published about the career pathways of medical graduates in the industrialized world,[2] but very little is known about medical graduates from developing countries.[3] In an increasingly globalized world, there has been much debate about the ethics of recruiting doctors from developing countries to work in wealthier industrialized countries.[4] Various estimates have been made of the number of medical professionals who migrate each year, generally, yet very little empirical data exists to quantify the rate of migration or destination of medical graduates from developing countries.[5] As members of three separate graduating classes from the College of Medicine of the University of Nigeria, currently working in the United Kingdom (UK), we decided to examine the career pathways of our former classmates.

In this chapter, we examine three consecutive graduating classes of the College of Medicine of the University of Nigeria (UNN). There are fifteen accredited medical schools in Nigeria, of which UNN is the third oldest (World Directory of Medical Schools). This chapter begins with setting the personal context. It explores how and why we became interested in this topic and discusses methodological and practical challenges faced in carrying out this study, from conceptualization to publication of the preliminary results. In the final section, we examine and discuss our findings, their implications and our plans for further research.

PERSONAL CONTEXT

To examine our interest in this topic, it is necessary to understand the backgrounds of the authors. We are members of three successive graduating classes of the University of Nigeria, the third oldest of Nigeria's medical schools. All three of us are currently at various stages of public health specialist training and have arrived in the United Kingdom via several routes. While the first author arrived in the UK, having worked in Nigeria for more than five years, the second and third authors have each spent less than three years of their working lives in Nigeria. The seeds for what would become this research were sown at a social gathering not long after the last of us had arrived in the U.K. In one conversation at the gathering, a Nigerian colleague marveled at the number of people from our medical school who were present and said he was sure that three quarters of his graduating class were now living outside Nigeria. This led to a conversation in which we noted that with the exception of ourselves (two of the three authors then specializing in public health), most of those present were training as specialists in psychiatry. A chance comment from one of us predicting a potential glut of Nigerian psychiatrists in the future when all these people returned home led to some vigorous discussion about the needs of the Nigerian health system and the role that we would play in it. One thread of the discussion questioned the assumption that all these doctors planned to return to Nigeria on completion of their specialist training in the United Kingdom; another examined the possible reasons for the popularity of psychiatry as a specialty for Nigerian doctors in the United Kingdom. From these conversations, there were anecdotal suggestions that psychiatry was chosen because of the relative ease with which training posts in that specialty could be obtained, but there was little empirical evidence to support or refute this claim. Following that meeting we tried to identify the available evidence on the career choices and pathways of medical doctors from Africa and from developing countries more broadly, working in the Western world. While we found a fair amount of literature describing the factors driving medical migration from the developing world[6] and some evidence suggesting that doctors in the UK who had trained abroad were more likely to become consultants in specialties that had been traditionally hard to fill,[7] we found very little quantitative evidence to support these studies. Finding ourselves in a fairly unique position as three members of successive graduating classes from one of Africa's major medical schools working within the same specialty in the same area, we resolved to carry out a study to answer some of our questions.

DESIGNING THE STUDY

In defining our study questions, we were conscious of several potential limitations. We wanted to know:

- What proportion of our graduating classes had emigrated?

- Why had they made the decision to emigrate (or not to emigrate)?
- What had been their career paths in their host country?
- What factors had influenced their career choices?
- What were their immediate, short-term and long-term career plans?

We determined that our study should utilize both quantitative and qualitative methods. Our choice of a quantitative aspect was rooted in our discovery during our literature review that various studies had estimated the numbers of medical doctors migrating to the West but that many of these studies were outdated and had severe limitations. As to the qualitative aspect of the study, we found that while there had been several qualitative studies of graduates of Western medical schools, very few similar studies had been published looking at African medical schools. In effect, our adoption of a dual methodology approach was intended to seek answers to the questions posed at our initial discussion months earlier. While the quantitative approach would support or refute the assertion of one of our colleague who contended that three quarters of our classmates were now living and working abroad, the qualitative approach would help us understand the decisions around choice of specialty and the long term career plans of our study subjects.

Having decided that we wanted to adopt both qualitative and quantitative approaches we were faced with practical questions. We agreed that a questionnaire survey, while not comprehensive, would begin to outline the broad picture, which we could then follow up with focus groups to begin to fill in the fine details. Our choice of a questionnaire survey was pragmatic as all three authors at the time were fully employed in non-research positions, so work on this project would need to fit into our spare time.

Having agreed on a questionnaire survey and our study questions, we set ourselves three tasks:

- Obtain valid graduating class lists for each of our three graduating sets to enable us to identify what our denominator population was.
- Design a questionnaire that would capture the information we required in as unambiguous a manner as possible.
- Identify how we could contact members of our graduating classes and begin to build a database of addresses.

OBTAINING VALID GRADUATING CLASS LISTS

Our initial thoughts had been to use the graduating class yearbooks for the years 1995, 1996 and 1997 to provide us with comprehensive class lists. We also owned copies of our respective class yearbooks as this would have been a fairly easy option. We soon realized, however, that this would be inaccurate as subscriptions to the yearbook were optional and so would not necessarily capture all the members of a given graduating class.

Having discarded the idea of using the yearbooks, we next considered using the official class lists of the graduates for each set obtained from our medical school. We were apprehensive of following this path for a number of reasons. First, communication with the school was notoriously poor—letters often went unanswered and email, telephone and fax facilities, while available, were extremely unpredictable. The only sure way of getting what we wanted (as we had learned when we required any documentation from the school) was to go there in person. As we were all nearly three thousand kilometers from the school, going there physically was not feasible. We were however able to enlist the services of one of our classmates, now a staff member at the medical school, who after several attempts managed to obtain permission from the administrative staff at the medical school. Finally, after nearly a year we were able to get graduating class lists for the relevant years.

Having obtained the class lists, we were faced with a new dilemma. At our medical school, it was not uncommon to find a number of students who had almost met the requirements for graduating barring one or two papers. This often meant that the final graduating class list bore no resemblance to the original entering class, as it was a mixture of students from the original class combined with a scattering of students from previous years with one or two papers outstanding. Faced with the inability to define a distinct graduating class, we made the decision to use the official class lists strictly, regardless of any inconsistencies they contained. We felt that this was the most practical approach that addressed the problem of defining the three graduating classes.

DESIGNING A QUESTIONNAIRE

When we started our study, two of the three authors had completed (or were in the process of completing) Master's degree programs in public health in which study design was a major component. We were thus able to apply these skills to the design of our study questionnaire. Again, we faced the competing tensions of collecting strictly quantitative information and therefore strictly applying closed questions with little scope for personal opinions. We realized however that while we had tried for instance to list as many factors as possible that had influenced subjects' decisions to emigrate, there was still the potential that our listed options would not capture the full range of factors. We therefore decided to give participants the option of filling in any other factors that we may have missed.

We also faced the challenge of deciding how to distribute the questionnaires, as this would determine the design of the questionnaire to aid the ease of completion. Our initial instincts were to avoid using a classic postal questionnaire given what we expected to be the diversity of locations with varying levels of efficiency of postal services. There were also anecdotal indications that many of our subjects were geographically mobile and therefore using fixed postal addresses would undermine response rates. We therefore chose to utilize e-mail as our primary means of dissemination of questionnaires. The reasons for this decision and the consequences will be discussed in the next section as it is closely related to the challenges of building a database of subjects with their contact details.

BUILDING UP A DATABASE OF ADDRESSES

Having obtained our original class lists and having agreed on the criteria for inclusion, our next task was to locate the various members of the graduating classes and obtain their contact details. We decided to build a database of class members with their contact details including country of location with each investigator taking responsibility for his class. We hoped to utilize our class e-mail groups, which had been set up to provide a means for classmates to keep in touch. However, we found that the most recent graduating classes tended to have a more complete mailing list than the earlier graduating classes. We also found that there was a bias in the memberships of the various e-groups, with these being dominated by members of the graduating classes who were currently based outside Nigeria.

Having obtained the contact details of class members via the e-mail groups, we were faced with the challenge of obtaining contact details for class members who were not on the e-group mailing list. To achieve this, we adopted a variety of methods including a snowballing process in which we contacted class members and asked them if they had contact details for other class members, the use of Internet search engines with follow-up e-mails and telephone calls and occasionally by pure serendipity. Over a period of months we were able to obtain contact details for between 40 and 60 per cent of the three graduating classes.

Since obtaining contact details was proving to be a slow and unsatisfactory process, we began to re-examine our methodology and study objectives. In the process of trying to obtain the contact individuals of old classmates we were often told “I don’t have her details, but she’s somewhere in California,” or Kano or Johannesburg. We soon found that while we could not always obtain the contact details for each individual, we could often pinpoint which country they were based in at the time. As a result of this discovery, we resolved to set the more achievable goal of populating our database with the location of each of our study subjects. This proved a useful decision, as we were subsequently able to locate 90 per cent of the cohort producing preliminary results, which were published in *The Lancet*[8] and are discussed in the next section.

OUR PRELIMINARY FINDINGS

We located 90% of the graduates of the three sets dispersed in 16 countries. Graduates from the three graduating classes could be found in a variety of countries including Nigeria, the United States of America, the United Kingdom, the Republic of Ireland, South Africa, and Trinidad and Tobago. The graph below shows the percentage and numbers of graduates by current country of residency and based on all three graduating classes combined.

From the class lists provided by the College of Medicine, there were a total of 152 graduates in the 1995 graduating class, 171 graduates in the 1996 class and 145 graduates in the 1997 class, making a cohort of 468 graduates in total. The locations of 46 graduates (9.8%) were unknown and 6 graduates were deceased. Of the six deceased graduates, the causes of death included road traffic accidents in Nigeria, complications of sickle cell anaemia and asthma, and a soft tissue malignancy.

We found that across all three classes, about 40% of all medical graduates were living abroad, and when we looked specifically at female graduates, we found that 50% of female graduates were living abroad at the time of the study. The foreign countries with the highest number of graduates were the USA followed by the UK and Ireland. These three countries received 33—38% of graduates across all three sets. The proportions of graduates in these three destination countries, plus Nigeria, were consistent across the three years. We concluded that this trend appeared representative of the University of Nigeria medical school as well as others in the country.

TABLE 5.1 Percentage and Numbers of Three Graduating Sets of the University of Nigeria's College of Medicine by Present Country of Residence

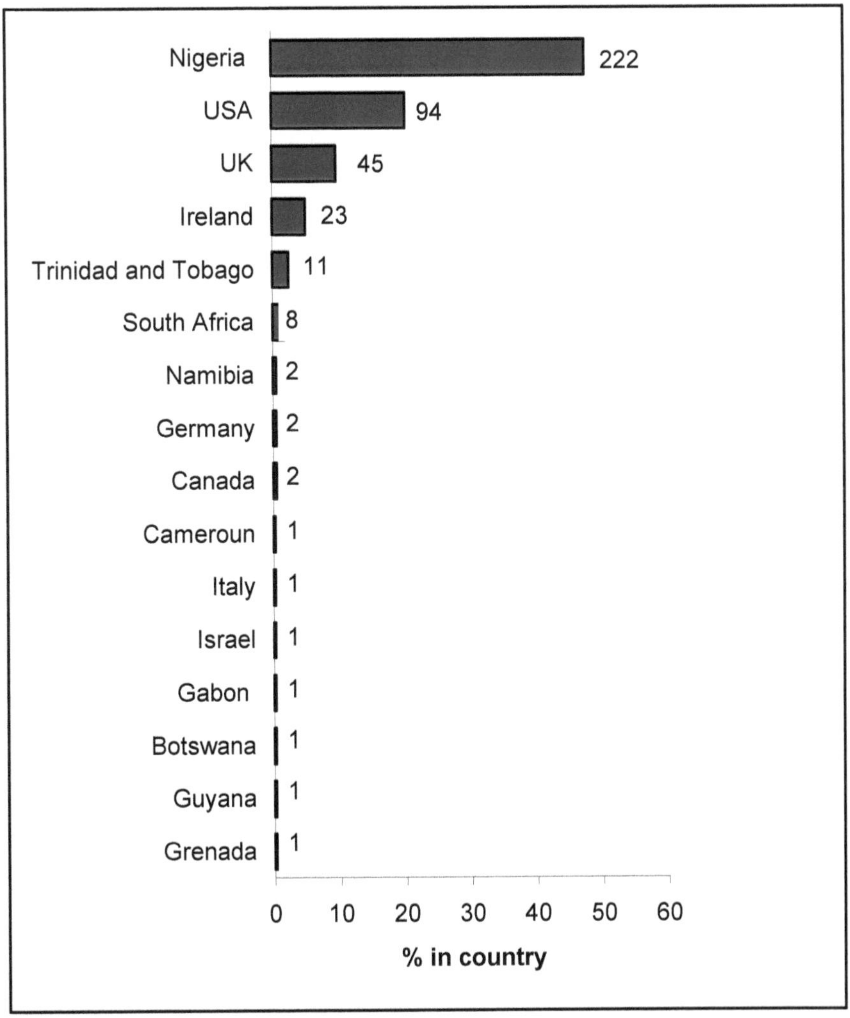

DISCUSSION

Our study as far as we know was one of the first attempts in recent history to attempt to credibly quantify the proportion of medical graduates who migrate from a developing country's medical school.[9] Our finding that 40 per cent of the graduates from a Nigerian medical school had migrated ten years after graduation is a significant finding, particularly in light of anecdotal information suggesting that the trends are higher for more recent graduates.

Medical education in Nigeria is subsidized by the state, which underlines the importance of these findings as they indicate a significant investment loss that could have severe implications for health services in the source country.

Reimbursement of donor developing countries by recipient countries has been suggested as one way of redressing this imbalance produced by the loss of medical staff, (Stilwell et al, 2004). Our findings indicated the scale of resources that would be required to put such a mechanism into practice. The finding that the bulk of migration, at least from Nigeria, is to only a few countries, suggests that discussions on how to address this issue can be focused on a handful of primary recipient countries.

CONCLUSION AND NEXT STEPS

When we embarked on this study we did not realize the extent to which our classmates were dispersed across the world. The challenges posed by this diversity were also largely met through the same instruments that had created them. The technological advances that have made it easier for skilled professionals to move in search of career fulfillment have also made it easier to track these movements. Using Internet search engines such as Google, we were able literally to search the world and locate old classmates within a very short time, far more easily than we would have been able to in a different age. Our class e-mail group lists were invaluable in our being able to embark on this study. And yet it would be misleading to imagine that the world of Google and the Internet that we searched is comprehensive and analogous to the real world. It is still circumscribed and limited as illustrated by the difficulties we faced in tracing and contacting colleagues and classmates based in Nigeria.

The next phase of our study will be an e-mail questionnaire based study that will focus on those members of the graduating classes based outside Nigeria. The questionnaire will seek to examine their motivations for migration, their career pathways and their plans for the future. As we progress in this study, we will continue to search the real and virtual worlds in seeking answers to these questions.

NOTES

1. Bristol North Primary Care Trust, King Square House, Bristol, UK
2. P. J. Moss, T. W. Lambert, M. J. Goldacre, and P. Lee, "Reasons for Considering Leaving UK Medicine: Questionnaire Study of Junior Doctors' Comments," *BMJ* 329 (2004): 1263 and E. Ryten, A.D. Thurber, and L. Buske, "The Class of 1989 and Post-MD Training," *CMAJ* 158 no.6 (1998): 731–7.

3. Y. M. Dambisya, "The Fate and Career Destinations of Doctors who Qualified at Uganda's Makerere Medical School in 1984: Retrospective Cohort Study," *BMJ* 329 (2004): 600–601.
4. V. Patel, "Recruiting Doctors from Poor Countries: The Great Brain Robbery?" *BMJ* 327 (2003): 926–928, and M. L. Scott, A. Whelan, J. Dewdney, and A.B. Zwi, "'Brain Drain' or Ethical Recruitment?" *Med J Aust.* 180 no. 4 (2004): 174–6.
5. B. Stilwell, K. Diallo, P. Zurn, M. Vujicic, O. Adams, and M. Dal Poz, "Migration of Health-Care Workers from Developing Countries: Strategic Approaches to Its Management." *Bull World Health Organ.* 82 no. 8 (2004): 595–600.
6. A. Mejía, "Migration of Physicians and Nurses: A Worldwide Picture." *International Journal of Epidemiology* 7 (1978): 207–15, A. Mejía, H. Pizurki, and E. Royston, "Physician and Nurse Migration: Analysis and Policy Implications," Geneva: World Health Organization, 1979, and Stilwell et al 2004.
7. M. J.Goldacre, J. M. Davidson, and T. W. Lambert, "Country of Training and Ethnic Origin of UK Doctors: Database and Survey Studies," *BMJ* 329 (2004): 597.
8. C. Ihekweazu, I.Anya, and E. Anosike, "Nigerian Medical Graduates: Where Are They Now?" *Lancet* 365 (2005):1847–8.
9. *Lancet* Editorial, "Migration of Health Workers: An Unmanaged Crisis," *Lancet* 365 (2005): 1825.

REFERENCES

Dambisya, Y. M. "The Fate and Career Destinations of Doctors who Qualified at Uganda's Makerere Medical School in 1984: Retrospective Cohort Study." *BMJ* 329 (2004): 600–601.

Goldacre, M. J., Davidson J. M, and Lambert T. W. "Country of Training and Ethnic Origin of UK Doctors: Database and Survey Studies." *BMJ* 329 (2004): 597

Ihekweazu, C., Anya I., and Anosike E. "Nigerian Medical Graduates: Where Are They Now?" *Lancet* 365 (2005):1847–8.

Lancet Editorial. "Migration of Health Workers: An Unmanaged Crisis." *Lancet* 365 (2005): 1825.

Mejía, A. "Migration of Physicians and Nurses: A Worldwide Picture." *International Journal of Epidemiology* 7 (1978): 207–15.

Mejía A, Pizurki H, and Royston E. *Physician and Nurse Migration: Analysis and Policy Implications*. Geneva: World Health Organization, 1979.

Moss P. J., Lambert T. W, Goldacre M. J., and Lee P. "Reasons for Considering Leaving UK Medicine: Questionnaire Study of Junior Doctors' Comments." *BMJ* 329 (2004): 1263.

Patel, V. "Recruiting Doctors from Poor Countries: The Great Brain Robbery?" *BMJ* 327 (2003): 926–928.

Ryten E, Thurber AD, and Buske L. "The Class of 1989 and Post-MD Training." *CMAJ* 158 no.6 (1998): 731–7.

Scott M.L, Whelan A, Dewdney J, and Zwi AB. "Brain Drain" or Ethical Recruitment? *Med J Aust.* 180 no. 4 (2004): 174–6.

Stilwell B, Diallo K, Zurn P, Vujicic M, Adams O, and Dal Poz M. "Migration of Health-Care Workers from Developing Countries: Strategic Approaches to Its Management. *Bull World Health Organ.* 82 no. 8 (2004): 595–600.

World Directory of Medical Schools, http://www.who.int/hrh/ (accessed January 15 2006).

Chapter Six

A Group of Twenty Nurses and the Pan African Struggle for Liberation

Sifiso Mxolisi Ndlovu

> *It was right* ukuhamba ngiye e Tanzania *because now I am very happy that I contributed in uplifting health services* zakwamanye amazwe e Africa. *I am very happy that I managed* ukuba ngifunde ibehaviour zabantu kwamanye amazwe. *It was also a contribution to our struggle for liberation. Again,* nokubuyisa *our organisation's (ANC) morale even though* abantu bakithi be *oppressed* bayabona ukuthi banalo usizo kwabanye abantu akusho ukuthi *they are useless. . . .* [1]

INTRODUCTION

Early in December 1961 before the official proclamation concerning the armed struggle and the existence of Umkhonto we Sizwe, the military wing of the African National Congress, a group of 21[20?] African nurses left South Africa into exile. This was before the first large contingent of MK cadres went into exile in 1962. These nurses were recruited by the ANC from the Cape, Natal and Transvaal provinces. The names of these nurses are as follow:

1. Edith Ncwana
2. Finess Luke
3. Sinah Jali
4. Edith Thunyiswa
5. Kholeka Thunyiswa
6. Edna Mgabaza
7. Mary Mwandla
8. Celia Khuzwayo
9. Nicolene
10. Georginah Masusu

11. Gertrude Nzimande
12. Mavis Motha
13. Mary Jane Socenywa
14. Natalie Msimang
15. Hilda Bonqo
16. Victoria Magodla
17. Moni de Swardze (Dutch/Scandinavian husband surname)
18. Nosipho Mshumpela
19. Neo Raditladi
20. Edna Miya

Unsung heroines as the twenty nurses were, and still are, they were members of a colonized indigenous society whose silent workers nobly raised, nursed, cared for and mothered the gamut of the white population in South Africa. Popular history finds it easier to record the story of the main actor and dominant race in racist societies such as South Africa, and sadly ignores the compelling story of the ordinary people and the subjugated, whose stories are equally valuable in human experience and history. In 20th century history and literature, there was a move towards social history as represented by the downtrodden; these writings consciously aimed at focusing on plebeians and the oppressed, instead of kings, thanes, chiefs, dukes and earls. I am continuing with this tradition by focusing and foregrounding my paper on freedom fighters-in this instance represented by ordinary African women who were part of the Pan African struggle for liberation. But one can also argue that these heroines were not necessarily ordinary because their role in the Pan African struggles for liberation was extra-ordinary.

The First Conference of Independent African States held in Accra on 15–22 April 1958, passed the following resolution:

> We, the African States assembled here in Accra, in this our first Conference, conscious of our responsibilities to humanity and especially to the peoples of Africa, and desiring to assert our African personality on the side of peace, hereby proclaim and solemnly reaffirm our unswerving loyalty to the Charter of the United nations, the Universal Declaration of Human rights and the Declaration of the Asian-African Conference held at Bandung. We further assert and proclaim the unity among ourselves and our solidarity with the dependent peoples of Africa as well

> as our friendship with all nations. We resolve to preserve the unity of purpose and action in international affairs which we have forged among ourselves in this historic Conference; to safeguard hard won independence, sovereignty and territorial integrity. . . . Desirous of mobilising the human resources of our respective countries in furtherance of social and cultural aspirations, we will endeavour to promote and facilitate the exchange of teachers, professors, students, (and other professionals including nurses and doctors). . . . [2]

Therefore, by sending the twenty nurses to Tanzania, the ANC was pro-actively responding to the declarations and resolutions of the First Conference of Independent African States held in 1958. This was because the ANC, together with the nurses, was conscious of its responsibilities to humanity and especially to the peoples of Africa. It was also an effort to preserve unity, and to establish and cement friendship with African nations and countries.

This chapter is based mainly on the life histories and experiences of extra-ordinary people, Edna Miya, Mary Jane Socenywa, Kholeka and Edith Thunyiswa—four of the twenty nurses. The choice of these four nurses rests on the fact that they are the only ones we could trace and who were available for oral history interviews.[3] Some of the nurses have passed away in exile. They include Georginah Masusu, Finess Luke and Edna Mgabaza. Their families in South Africa did not have the opportunity to bury them. Others such as Moni de Swardze have settled and married abroad; they visit South Africa, occasionally. While in exile and based in West Germany, Khuzwayo married a fellow South African whom she had met in Botswana when the nurses were en-route to Tanzania. They later met in Germany and decided to marry and Khuzwayo helped her husband to complete his university studies. He changed totally after completing his studies and he ill-treated his wife and mother of his two children. Later they were divorced. Moving on with her life, Khuzwayo settled in England and chose to visit South Africa regularly during holidays. Similarly, others like Natalie Msimang and Mary Mwandla settled abroad (in England) and only visit family members in South Africa during holidays. Kholeka Thunyiswa is married to a Tanzanian; she and her family have settled in Dar es Salaam. None of the nurses knows what happened to Mavis Motha—they last heard about her after she married an African- American in Tanzania and they went to settle in the United States. Neo Raditladi has retired and returned from abroad and settled in Botswana—her home country. Edith Thunyiswa has also returned to South Africa and works for the ANC. She is now based at Luthuli House. Victoria Magodla and Nosipho Mashumpela left

Tanzania and later went to work and settle in Kenya. The last time Kholeka Thunyiswa went to visit the two in Kenya, Magodla, who was married to a Ugandan, was very sick, Thunyiswa doubts whether she is still alive.

THE EARLY HISTORY OF NURSING AND THE TRAINING OF AFRICAN NURSES

A cursory glance at the timeline of a course about the History of Nursing in South Africa, under the title 'The Growth of Non-White Nursing in South Africa,' suggests that the profession began in 1810. These lecture notes, authored by Jane McLarty, the matron at Baragwanath Hospital, formed part of the three year nursing course. A book authored by Charlotte Searle claimed that the profession began in 1652. Both authors note that when Jan van Riebeck landed at the Cape, he had some knowledge of medical matters, and tried to organize some care of the sick in the colony.[4] However, McLarty and Searle fail to mention the fact that there were qualified experts dealing with the sick prior to the arrival of the white settlers. They had been caregivers for centuries and had amassed valuable expertise and an impressive nomenclature of medicinal plants and herbs. Glancing through Searle's book and McLarty's lecture notes and teaching material reminds one of deliberate racist omissions, biases and silences in the teaching of South African history, particularly the History of Medicine, Primary and Public Health, wherein the enormous contribution of the indigenous peoples, indigenous lore and indigenous knowledge systems are ignored and ridiculed. It is as if there were no indigenous knowledge systems focusing on health systems and medicines prior to the arrival of white settlers.[5]

Various missionaries, mainly the American, British and Swiss, conducted the training of the first professional African nurses in the beginning of the 20th century. Shula Marks argues that, like colonial authorities, the missionaries saw western medicine as part of an onslaught against black 'savagery' and 'ignorance'; in the first decade of the 20th century; whatever the denomination or nationality, the message was the same. In the eyes of Dr. James McCord of the Congregationalist American Board of Mission, who was the first to train African nurses in Natal, the '"witch-doctors" have a profound influence [of] evil on the social and religious life of Africa.' Similarly, for Neil Macvicar, the Free Church of Scotland mission doctor who pioneered western training for African nurses in the Eastern Cape's Lovedale Institute, 'the hospital stood for science against superstition, for fresh air, cleanliness and temperance, as against over-crowding, dirt . . . infestation[,] and for Christian helpfulness and simple trust in God as opposed to the fear, the selfishness, the malevolence of heathenism.'[6]

Situated at Lovedale, the Victoria Hospital was the first medical mission hospital in South Africa which was opened in 1898, but was closed during the Boer War. It was reopened during 1902–1903 and Dr. Macvicar was the first doctor and Mary Balmer the hospital's first matron. The hospital was small with only 16 beds, and although the training of the white nurses was still in its infancy, a course was developed for the training of Africans. To begin with, only two ex-school teachers named Mina Colani and Cecilia Makiwane enrolled for the course, which lasted for three years. Both women received the Hospital Proficiency Certificate at the end of the three years. Makiwane further enrolled for a year and passed the professional nursing examination of the Cape Colony Medical Council. She was then registered as a professional nurse and became the first African woman to be registered by the state as a qualified professional in her field. Dr. McCord followed suit in 1906 and implemented a 3-year hospital certificate for Africans at McCord Zulu Hospital in Durban. In 1924 the state funded the training of African nurses at this hospital, and training for midwives began. Beatrice Msimanga became the first African woman to hold certificates in General Nursing and Mid-wifery. From 1925 there was rapid progress in the training of African nurses. In 1925 Dr. Macvicar was called to Pretoria and discussions were held about the training of African nurses at the government Hospital. Also in 1933, the Frere Hospital in East London began the training of African nurses. In 1939, three more hospitals began training African nurses: the Pretoria General Hospital, Somerset Hospital in the Cape, and the non-European[7] Hospital in Johannesburg. In 1948, the training school at Baragwanath Hospital in Soweto opened with 180 students. In 1933 six African nurses passed the final nursing examination and were placed in the state register. In 1959, there were 458 nurses who had passed the examination and were registered and over the following years the growth only accelerated.[8]

In the ideological battle between superstition and enlightenment, fear and fresh air, that permeated the syllabus and content, the African nurse was supposed to be 'the ally against magic and superstition.' This was not to be the case, as during the late 1950s, Edna Miya, one of the nurses who later went into exile and settled in Tanzania and Zambia, saw beyond the ideological battle. She was trained at McCord Hospital and subsequently worked at a TB hospital before she went into exile. She recalls the following about the politics of fresh air, cleanliness, racism and discrimination in terms of salaries whilst employed at King George V Hospital in Durban:

kodwa ubumnyama bami angiboni mahluko phakathi kwami nalowayana (white nurse) ngoba senza *the same job* uyabona *in fact even more* ngoba uMatron uma efikelwe ama*visitor from the* United States of America ubewaletha e wardini ethi thina maAfrica ngobu clean (siyancomeka) asho wona (white) amavistors athi niyazi ukuthi yini eyenza ukuthi ama (hospital) *ward* abe clean, kube khona i*fresh air, cool* and fresh, its *cleanliness* kodwa ke manje uma sekufika kuma *salaries* hayikhona, uma kunemihlangano *niks* asibizwa abelungu bodwa, yikho konke lokhu okwangikhathaza, angiboni i*difference* phakathi kwami nalona ngoba sonke senza *the same job, the skin, its only pigmentation* eyenza sihlukane, kodwa nje, nje ngengqondo siyafana.[9]

DISTURBANCES AT HOSPITALS: THE SOUTH AFRICAN NURSING ACT(S) OF 1944 AND 1957

During the 1940s there were a number of strikes by African nurses. For example, in 1941 African nurses went on strike at the Sir Henry Elliot Hospital at Umthatha in the Transkei. Marks noted that the main cause of these strikes appears to have been the authoritarian way in which the hospital authorities dealt with the nurses' complaints of food shortages, around which wider and deeper political and social discontents condensed. In 1947, all the nurses who went on strike for twelve days at the Alexandra clinic were dismissed by the Management Board, and then reappointed. On the 15th of July 1949, a confrontation occurred between senior staff and 'non-European staff nurses' at Baragwanath Hospital. The most serious of these disturbances took place at Lovedale Hospital in 1949, when a nurses' strike was followed by nearly three months of defiance. The proximity of Victoria Hospital to the school at Lovedale and to the University of Fort Hare was of great relevance to the upheavals of 1949, (Marks, 1994). These strikes coincided with the ANC Youth League's 1949 program of action. There were a lot of hands that were involved in producing what eventually became the program of action in 1949, and the main message of that program was mass action, civil disobedience and strikes. These were all mentioned as veritable methods that could be used in the struggle for the liberation of the oppressed. Henry Makgothi, a prominent member of the Youth League, recalled the nurses' strike and some of his colleagues who supported a united front between the nurses and the ANC's Youth League and those who did not:

There was one year, I forget when that was probably 1948/49, the nurses at Lovedale hospital had a strike and the ANC Youth League

> mobilised . . . support for that strike and we took out the nurses on strike. It was something unheard of and we got them to go out on strike and they spent (two) weeks outside (after being expelled from their rooms). They couldn't go home, but we encouraged them and we brought our own blankets from the College so that they could sleep out in the open for weeks, they slept in the open (on the hospital lawn), so that they could get some concessions from the administration of the hospital. This was the time when the Youth League Manifesto, the Manifesto of the Youth League was being debated in the Youth League circles and it was . . . we were eager that it should be part of the ANC policy and strategies and so on. And we were . . . you know, we were engaged in such debates. I was at one stage secretary of the ANC Youth League at Fort Hare and the Youth League was very popular at Fort Hare, we virtually ruled Fort Hare and we opened our doors to not only students from South Africa but students from what we today call Zimbabwe were members of the African National Congress. I wish I could say the same about Mr Robert Mugabe, but he was there at that time too, but he was more of a withdrawing person and a deep thinker yes, but he did not actually join like most of his other colleagues, the Nkomos (Joshua Nkomo) and so on (who supported the nurses strike), who became members of the African National Congress Youth League. But I think he (Mugabe) had reservations about it and he never really joined.[10]

The nurses convened their meetings at the nearby the Tyumie River. One of the ANC Youth League members who formed part of the vigil with the striking nurses was the young Robert Sobukwe. At first Sobukwe, who was President of the Fort Hare's SRC, had reservations and was reluctant to join the strike, and said he was too busy with his studies. But his fellow students persuaded him to join the strike—convincing him that the nurses were his sisters and he had a duty to help them. Eventually he did become involved and together with the nurses and representatives assumed a leadership role. He fell in love with one of the striking nurses, Zodwa Veronica Mathe, who later became his wife.[11]

Before 1944, the South African Medical and Dental and Pharmacy Act No 13 of 1928 exercised control of the nursing and midwifery profession in South Africa. Certain provisions of the 1928 Act affecting nurses and midwives were however incorporated in the Nursing Act No. 45 of 1944, the first Nursing Act of South Africa. This Act led to formation of the South African Nursing Association (SANA), which consisted of all registered nurses and midwives, and mandated compulsory membership. SANA was governed by a Board to which, theoretically, any nurse, regardless of racial background, could be elected. Simultaneously, the South African Nursing Council (SANC) was established. Its major role was to protect the public by regulating examinations, issuing standardized nursing certificates and acting as a disciplinary body and a watchdog among other things. As the 1944 Act read, all registered nurses and midwives, irrespective of race, had the right to stand for nomination as members of the SANC and of SANA and to take part in elections. Thus the Act implied that that all nurses and midwives, irrespective of race, were compelled to become members of SANA, and the control of the association was vested in the executive consisting of ten nurses and midwives elected by the members of the association. While the association usually met only every second year, meetings of the executive were held every year. In terms of the powers granted to it by the Act, the executive divided the association into 36 regional branches, and the resolutions adopted at branch meetings were referred to the executive for consideration.[12]

As far back as 1943, many white nurses and midwives objected to the fact that no provisions were made to maintain the Color Bar. These protests were, however, to a certain extent allayed by a statement from the authorities that in view of the fact that the number of qualified African nurses was insignificant, there need be no fear that the Color Bar would not be maintained. The basis for the white nurses' fear was confirmed by the fact that as a result of trade union action, seven blacks were elected as members of the committee of the Witwatersrand branch of the Nursing Association, which consisted of 12 members. Effectively, the black nurses were in control of the Witwatersrand branch, (Assembly Debates, 1957). Shula Marks observed that even before the amended Nurses' Act of 1957 was passed to impose segregation by statute, twenty-five of the thirty-three regional branches of SANA precluded black membership. Half of the remaining eight had formed separate 'non European discussion groups,' and two, the Western Cape and the Witwatersrand held mixed meetings which were in any case made more difficult by the state's ban on mixed meetings under the Group Areas Act. The integration of black nurses in the Witwatersrand branch of SANA led to the formation of a separate Witwatersrand Private Duty Nurses' Discussion group by white nurses. This group agitated vociferously for the use of Afrikaans and for the full implementation of apartheid policies in the profession, and particularly for the change of the 1944 nursing legislation, (Marks, 1994, 149–150).

During the late 1940s, the Nursing Amendment Bill was referred to a Select Committee for inquiry that was empowered to take evidence, to call for papers and to submit an amended Bill. Theoretically, this meant that representations could be made for as long as the committee, chaired by Dr. Carel De Wet, was prepared to receive further evidence. Professional nurses and other members of the public including experts (whites in particular) could use their personal rights as citizens in making their views known to their members of parliament before the matter was debated in the House of Assembly. The amendment clauses dealing with the principle of racial discrimination sharply divided the nurses. Many of the amending clauses were of an administrative nature and were non-controversial. Sections dealing with the proposed enrolment and control of auxiliary nurses and midwives were generally accepted as necessary in the interest of the public. As far back as 1948, certain draft amendments to the 1944 Nursing Act were proposed by both SANA and SANC. As this was the year that marked the ascendancy of the apartheid government, the Minister of Health added further amending clauses, limiting membership of the boards of both SANA and SANC to white South African citizens.[13]

The apathy with which many nurses regarded this vital question was demonstrated in February 1950, when the Board of SANA referred it to its white dominated branches for an expression of opinion. Eight thousand, seven hundred and sixty five members were entitled to vote, but only two thousand, four hundred and ninety five votes were recorded, of which 1,390 were in favour of excluding blacks from the SANA board and the Council, and 1,104 against. Thus, by a small majority of two hundred and eighty six, forming part of only 28% of SANA members who voted, gave their approval to a proposal that was introduced without consulting them and one which proposed a fundamental change in the 1944 Nursing Act. The Board of SANA, confronted with a proposal that would exclude black members, and having had this proposal endorsed by the majority of those who voted, they proceeded to consider ways and means of replacing the lost privilege by some type of representation. From these deliberations and consultations that included black nurses came proposals that the Board of SANA would include one member elected by registered black nurses and midwives. This member, according to the government apartheid policies, was expected to be white. A suggestion was also made for the establishment of a 'non-European Standing Committee' to advise the Board of SANA, (Amendment to the Nursing Act).

These proposals were widely discussed by black members of SANA. Judging by some of the evidence given to the Select Committee, the majority of black members completely rejected these discriminatory proposals, including the racism and racial policies they propagated. They refused to nominate candidates, and in fact they proposed to dissociate themselves from a Nursing Association in which they no longer had full membership rights in common with other registered nurses and midwives.

When the apartheid government realized that the number of registered black nurses in 1944 was merely 842, while by 1957 it had increased to 3,099, they saw that it was time to act. The increase also factored in the increase of African nurses, which was the result of the extension of the training facilities for Africans so as to support the government policy of apartheid and separate development. These policies were implemented in order to encourage Africans to serve 'their own' communities and societies as health professionals. It therefore meant that in terms of demographics, African nurses would in the foreseeable future outnumber white nurses. The danger inherent in the failure of the Nursing Act, No. 45 of 1944, to provide for the maintenance of the Color Bar in the nursing profession, could readily be understood by those in power.[14]

Apart from the serious effect which the election of blacks as members of the body responsible for the control of nursing had, the mingling of the racial groups at SANA's meetings and social gatherings connected with such meetings, particularly in the Witwatersrand and the Western Cape, also led to serious friction within the nursing profession. Charlotte Searle, the Directress of Nursing Services for the Transvaal Province, was forthright about the fact that if she had known government policy was just the opposite, she would not have agreed to the introduction of the Bill (without racial discrimination) as it was introduced in 1944. In 1955 she elaborated as follows to the Select Committee that was drafting the Nursing Act Amendment Bill: "We would have fought it to the last ditch. We certainly would not have liked something that would ultimately have wrecked the European nursing services in South Africa. At any event, because there were no problems at the time, it was decided that there would be no colour bar."[15] Regarding the possibility of non-Europeans swamping Europeans, and the ominous possibility of white nurses serving under Africans, Searle gave evidence to the committee that: "I found that to be the position in one of my hospitals in 1947, again in 1948, and again in 1949 when I found that it was being tried out in a hospital. It only lasted for half an hour after I arrived on the scene," (Marks, 1994). It was therefore not surprising that the chairperson of the Select Committee, Dr. Carel De Wet, together with his colleagues, would submit provisions in the Bill to limit membership of the Nursing Council and of the executive of SANA to white South African citizens permanently residing in the Union or in South West Africa. In addition, the Nursing Act Amendment Bill also provided for the limitation of the franchise in regard to the election of members to of SANA and SANC to whites. Although black nurses were expected to have no say in the election of members, provision was made for the establishment of Advisory Committees exclusively reserved for Coloreds and Natives. This was a variation that was not different from the earlier proposed establishment of a non-European Standing Committee. The members of these Advisory Committees were also expected to be exclusively Coloreds and Natives, respectively, who would be elected by Colored and Native nurses and midwives. The function of these Advisory Committees would be to advise the white Nursing Council in regard to matters affecting nurses and midwives belonging to their respective race groups. As a form of control, the Bill also provided for the presence at the Advisory Committee meetings of the white president or vice-president or any member of the SANC. This issue was vividly captured by De Wet in 1957 during a parliamentary debate about the proposed Nursing Act Amendment Bill:

> In regard to the white nurses, I want to say that the absolute assurance is now being given—and it has been necessary for a long time—that in the Nursing Council and in the Nursing Association the control will be in the hands of the White nurses. That being the case, we are now giving certainty where in the past there was uncertainty, which was to the detriment of the profession. Secondly, it will remove difficulty that non-Whites will be put in charge of White nurses. This is also a very important matter. Where there a[?] Nursing Council which has to apply disciplinary measures and take steps against nurses who have committed a contravention of the rules, this Act will prevent a non-White sitting in judgement over a White nurse. (Assembly Debates, 1957)

De Wet further argued that the legislation as expressed in the proposed Bill would prevent social integration and equality in the profession. Black nurses were not passive, however, and relentlessly protested against the Amendment Act. As an example, on the 9th of December 1954, the 'non-European group' of the Witwatersrand branch of SANA held a meeting at the non-European Hospital in Johannesburg and voiced their objection against the proposed Bill. The meeting resolved to submit a memorandum to the board of SANA. This memorandum listed the black nurses' opposition to the Nursing Act Amendment Bill. They rejected the proposals because of the following reasons:

a) It is unethical to debar non-European nurses from becoming members of the South African Nursing Council and of the Board of South African Nursing Association.

b) It is contrary to the International Code of Nursing Ethics adopted by the International Council of Nurses, which states: "Need for nursing service is universal. Professional nursing is therefore unrestricted by considerations of nationality, race, creed, colour, politics or social status."

c) It will cause suffering to humanity, through damaging good professional relationships, where European and non-European medical and nursing staff work together. Where professional relationships are bad, patients suffer.

2. Infiltration of politics into the Nursing Profession is strongly opposed by the non-European nurses-disease knows no colour.

3. We therefore move that all clauses in the Nursing Amendment Act debarring non-Europeans from becoming members of the South African Nursing Council and of the Board of the South African Nursing Association be deleted, and that non-European nurses by virtue of their professional qualifications, service and experience be eligible for election to the Council and the board, and not debarred because of their colour.[16]

On 8 May 1957, both the Federation of South African Women (FEDSAW) and the ANC's Women's League entered the fray and noted with deep concern the discriminatory and virulent racism embodied in the proposed Nursing Act Amendment Bill. In a letter addressed to the authorities, both organizations protested and condemned the callous indifference of a government 'which deliberately sacrifices the health of the nation to achieve the perpetuation of white supremacy.' These organizations commended the constructive role played by African women in maintaining the high standards of nursing despite poverty and their struggle for education. These women, as nurses, responded magnificently to 'the call of womanhood to come forth and nurse the sick, to restore to health the people of South Africa.' Therefore, there was no evidence to support the claims of the white dominated SANC that black nurses, principally Africans, could not absorb the training common to all nurses. On the contrary, black nurses had proven to be a valuable and indispensable asset to the nursing profession. Against this, the SANC was prepared not only to sacrifice its own profession, but to violate its own integrity by proposing lower standards of training for non-white nurses, with the inevitable results of lowering nursing standards in the hospital and at home.[17]

These spirited protests fell on deaf ears as the apartheid government finally enacted the South African Nursing Act, No 69, of 1957, on the 24th of June. Race was to be the main determining factor in appointing members of the SANC. Part 1 of the Act, referring to the South African Nursing Council in paragraph (c) of sub-section (1) of section (4) proclaimed, 'no person shall be appointed or elected as a member of the council-who is not a South African citizen and a white person permanently resident in the Union or the territory.' In addition, certain paragraphs of sub-section (2) of section (3) noted the following about the election of Council members:

> (h) one female registered nurse . . . elected by female registered nurses who are white persons resident in the area concerned;
>
> (i) one registered midwife . . . elected by registered midwives who are white persons resident in the area concerned;
>
> (j) one male nurse registered nurse elected by male registered nurses who are white persons; one person registered both as a nurse and as a midwife, elected by student nurses and midwives registered under section fourteen, who are white persons;
>
> (k) one person who is registered both as a nurse and as a midwife, elected by the advisory board for coloured persons; one person who is registered both as a nurse and as a midwife, elected by the advisory board for natives.18

Part 2, Section 16, of the Act with reference to Advisory Boards for Coloured Person and Natives confirmed: "As from the date to be fixed by the Minister by notice in the *Gazette*, there shall be established an advisory board for coloured persons and an advisory board for natives, to advise the council on such matters relating to nurses or midwives who are coloured persons or natives, as may be referred to such board by the council, or upon which any such board may wish to report to the council." Furthermore, Section 20, subsection (2) of the Act recorded that: "The president and the vice-president of the council and any other member thereof designated by council, and the registrar or any officer of the council designated by him may attend any meeting of an advisory board as an observer and adviser but shall have no vote," (Nursing Act, 1957).

It really did not matter that the SANC's white representative had no vote as a member of the Advisory Committee because whites dominated as the final arbiter, the Nursing Council itself. In 1957, a notice suddenly appeared in every hospital warning nurses that since they were 'public servants,' those who took part in political activities were liable to dismissal. Certain hospitals directly threatened their staff that if they took part in such marches they might be expelled. This arose because of a proposed national conference of nurses to discuss 'the changed conditions brought about by the promulgation of the Nursing Act, 1957.' The conference organizers also proposed 'to co-ordinate efforts to maintain the status of the Nursing Profession in South Africa.' The secretary of the organizing committee for the conference of nurses was G. Khala. She was a nursing professional based at the Orlando Municipal Clinic in Soweto. The proposed date of the conference was the 2nd and 3rd of November 1957, and the venue was at Johannesburg. In addition to discussing the 1957 Act, Advisory Board and Committee, syllabus, uniforms and salaries, item seven of the agenda proposed the discussion of a 'possibility of forming a non-discriminatory nurses' organization, with direct affiliation with the International Nursing Council.'[19]

The seriousness of the situation became obvious in November 1957, when 200 nurses held the conference in which they voiced their protest against the Act. The conference was largely successful and the venue was decorated with banners declaring, "No apartheid in Nursing' and 'Disease Knows No Color Bar." The conference attendants were mainly black nurses and one of the resolutions adopted by the conference was a unanimous vote of no confidence in SANA. Another result of the conference was the formation of a new non-racial body, the Federation of South African Nurses and Midwives, (Jarrett-Kerr, 1960). The white authorities feared that South Africa would be expelled from the international body if this federation sought direct affiliation with the International Nursing Council. SANA officials frantically worked behind the scenes to avoid this damaging situation—to a large extent it was successful.

Acts of discrimination and racism became the order of the day at various hospitals after the passage of the 1957 Nursing Act. For example, the Boksburg-Benoni was caught up in such a storm in 1957. This hospital provided training for both black and white nurses, though separately. During mid-1957, white nurses protested against the poor quality of food provided to its student nurses and boycotted the dining hall. The authorities did not punish these students and the Matron, a Miss D.E. Weldon, attended to their grievances. But the latter was later forced to resign apparently because of complaints from Afrikaans speaking nurses who accused her of being 'partial to the English language.' When in November 1957 African nurses complained about the quality of their food to the hospital's Assistant Matron, the hospital authorities dealt with their complaint unsympathetically. No improvement took place and on 12 December the African nurses decided to stage a food boycott. The new Matron, a Miss Rainus, in order to 'maintain discipline and to set an example,' chose twelve senior student nurses for dismissal and gave a twenty-four hour notice to leave. All these senior students were due to write their final examinations in a few months' time. The Superintendent of the Boksburg-Benoni Hospital confirmed their dismissal, extending the notice to leave to one month, expiring on 16 January 1958.[20]

Both white and black nurses unsuccessfully appealed to the Matron to be less severe in her punishment of the twelve nurses. She refused to accept a joint apology from the twelve African nurses, insisting on individual apologies and letters. Her divide and rule strategy succeeded as seven nurses complied and apologized for not attending breakfast. Six of them were allowed to complete their training at the hospital and the remaining one was advised to apply elsewhere. Four other nurses refused to comply with this demand, considering it undignified and unnecessary. The twelfth nurse was traumatized by the Matron's treatment and subsequently hospitalized. She was jailed and released in the custody of her mother and her case was heard in court on 10 January 1958. On 13 December 1957 the nurses requested SANA to intervene, but their representative refused as she considered this issue to be 'a domestic matter' concerning only the Boksburg-Benoni Hospital. As a result, the Rand Nurses' Professional Club and the Federation of South African Nurses and Midwives, however, decided to help the expelled nurses, (as FEDSAW papers, 1137/Cc6).

Late in 1957, in a government Gazette published a few days before New Year, the apartheid government announced the introduction of separate racial Registers for South African Nurses from the 1st of January 1958. Hence, as a result of this move, both the ANC's Women's League and FEDSAW decided that their major campaign in 1958 would be in support of the opposition of nurses' passes. The organizations also proposed to organize mass demonstrations involving non-nursing women of all races to march to hospitals to protest against matrons who compelled nurses to produce identity numbers. The Women's League and FEDSAW argued that it was the intention of the Nationalist government not only to compel African nurses to carry passes, but to introduce passes for African women into the cities and larger towns, where Verwoerd, the Minister responsible for Native Affairs, had not yet dared to send the pass units. It was clear that this the apartheid government's strategy was that if African nurses were compelled to produce identity numbers which could only be obtained from pass books, the example of nurses would easily be followed by other African women, who held their educated sister in high esteem. The acceptance of passes by the African nurses would be a defeat for the African women's resistance to apartheid policies. These struggles were defined by the 1956 women's march to Pretoria, and the subsequent women's anti-pass struggles in Zeerust, Winburg, Nelspruit, Lichtenburg, Pietersburg, Rustenburg, Barberton, Venterspost, Standerton, Boons, Heidelburg, Balfour, Driefontein, Potgietersrust, Sekhukhuniland and Dewildt.[21]

On 14 March 1958, the *Rand Daily Mail* reported that African nurses at Baragwanath Hospital—nearly 750 of them—were living in fear of losing their jobs as a result of being forced to carry passes by the apartheid government. In February the SANC sent forms to nurses, entitled "Keeping of Separate Registers for White Persons, Coloured Persons, and Natives, The Nursing Act, 1957." African nurses were required to state on the separate register their names, their race classifications and their identity numbers. They flatly refused to provide the authorities with this information and, subsequently, meetings were held between the two groups. Also, the Native Commissioner was called by the hospital authorities, to address the nurses about the importance of the issues at stake. Again, the nurses refused to sign the forms as they vehemently objected to separate classification defined in the register. The state officials threatened these nurses with dismissals and informed them that if they did not sign the forms, two hundred and forty trained nurses would not be registered as qualified professionals at the end of 1958. They would thus be barred from practicing as nurses. In essence, unless they signed the forms, a total of five hundred student nurses would have wasted three and half years training. Moreover, twenty nurses were already in that dilemma, as they had just completed their professional training. To complicate issues further, twenty-five nurses who were about to commence their professional training would not be allowed to do so. These nurses had already signed the forms on 11 March 1958, but because of the pending strike, demanded them back on the 12th of March. An irate official from the hospital declared, "if they do not sign by April, they will be barred from training." As expected, this official, an apologist of the apartheid government, assumed the nurses were receiving threats of physical violence and burning of their homes if they carried passes. He criticized the nurses and referred to them as ignorant for they thought that signing the separate register would mean that they would have to carry passes. He commented, "if they would only realize that the signing of these forms has nothing to do with the issuing of passes."

Nevertheless, African nurses and their supporters disagreed with this self- serving viewpoint and argued that the signing of the SANC forms had everything to do with subjugation of the oppressed African women. It was therefore not surprising that women belonging to both the ANC's Women's League and FEDSAW staged their anti-pass protest outside Baragwanath

Hospital on the 22nd of March 1958. The protestors included women who were not necessarily classified as Africans and professional nurses. There were a number of Special Branch officers on duty and a number of African policemen were armed. From the air, police riot cars could be seen patrolling Orlando East and nearby townships in strength. All police leave in the Johannesburg precinct was cancelled on the day of the protest march until 'further orders' from their superiors. This was in case of trouble arising from women of all races demonstrating against the signing of race classification registers at Baragwanath Hospital. Such was the fear of women by the state because two years previously they had stormed the Union Buildings protesting against the passes. To some of us, the Pretoria march symbolizes and was akin to the storming of the Bastille—without the help and presence of men. Shortly after 10 A.M. small groups of African women wearing the ANC uniform of green blouse and black skirts with gold decorations began to assemble opposite the hospital. Among them were a number of European women dressed in the same manner. They were later joined by lorry loads of women and other groups who marched down the road to the hospital. A deputation of nine women represented by Africans, Indians, Coloured and white women met the matron, Miss A. Simpson and Dr. I. Frack, the Superintendent of the Baragwanath Hospital and voiced their protest.[22]

This deputation presented a memorandum to the hospital authorities. In this memorandum they highlighted that passes meant that families of African nurses would be broken up when they were arrested and jailed under the pass laws. It meant that children would be left uncared for and helpless, and that mothers would be torn from their babies for failure to produce a pass. This suffering would also be felt at the hospitals, where patients would suffer the consequences of pass laws being extended to African nurses. Women and young girls would also be exposed to harassment and degradation at the hands of male police searching their passes. Also, African nurses, as women, would lose freedom of movement in their own country. The women also protested against the introduction of different standards of training, as enacted in the Nursing Act of 1957. Like Bantu Education, the standards set for the training of African nurses would be determined by their race. According to the protestors, death and disease knew no color bar: "We fear the effect of the differential standards of training that may be imposed upon nurses, and those of us who are non-European women claim the right to make this protest, for it is **our** children, **our** families, who would be nursed by those who would receive an inferior training. We say for you and the world to know, that a life is a life, and a child is a child, no matter what the colour of the skin. Death and disease know no colour bar."[23]

As is always the case in such situations some African nurses dissented. They supported the racist policies of the apartheid government as defined by the 1957 Nursing Act. The Port Elizabeth branch of FEDSAW labeled the actions of these dissenters as treacherous. Among the nurses named as "sell-outs doing the dirty work for the Nationalist Party" were Mrs. Gcule and Miss Jayiya. They were dubbed the "Pretoria Gang" and accused of representing nobody but themselves as they assembled in Pretoria during October 1958 "to act as midwives while the Nationalist Apartheid Monster was labouring to give birth to its deformed and diseased baby." Gcule and Jayiya supported and attended an apartheid conference organized by the state authorities in order to implement the 1957 Nursing Act. A pamphlet issued by FEDSAW noted that these nurses, "rather than make breast of it," and apologize for their inexcusable act of treachery, sought to drag everybody "into the sticky mud in which they were wallowing." Before their apartheid conference took place, they invited the illustrious Dorah Nginza to come and "bless their unholy work." Unhappy that she did not attend the state sponsored conference, but determined to cover up for their shameful conduct, the 'Pretoria Gang' decided to entice Nginza by offering to present her with an illuminated address. It was therefore not SANA that sought to honor Nginza but this gang that exploited those Africans they had deceived, to degrade, and not to honor her. These pro-apartheid African nurses described as "Self seekers without pride," were behind the sinister plot,

> (to) besmirch the glorious name of one of our most deserving pioneers in this field of work. (The plotters were) shamelessly attempting to drag her (Dorah Nginza) down to their own moral level. The women behind this were from East London and Uitenhage . . . their leaders were boasting if they managed to entice the Sister their evil plans would be graced by her presence (Dorah Nginza) at a function they plan to stage on the 30th at Uitenhage. Last month we exposed the treacherous plans of this type of self seeker who has pride-neither professional nor national, nor personal pride for that matter.[24]

In Pietermaritzburg, a group of nurses calling itself "The Society of Young Africa," and who were part of the All-African Convention and the Non-European Unity Movement, issued a call to black nurses to put up a united front against a common enemy and racism. This rallying call was imperative and addressed to all the nurses in general and to the Edendale Hospital in particular. This was because of obvious racial division between African, Colored and Indian nurses employed at this hospital. It had been brought to the notice of members of the Society of Young Africa that a certain group of Indian nurses at Edendale hospital were responsible for practicing racialism. African nurses were barred at a certain party organized to celebrate the Hindu festival, as only Indian and Colored nurses were invited. Objections from nurses who were members of the Society did not arise from the fact that Africans were denied access 'to the fun and pleasure that normally accompany parties,' but rather from the fact that they, as nurses, were excluded because they were Africans.[25]

Certain Indian nurses were alleged to have confided in their "dear" white Matron that African nurses were excluded from the Hindu celebrations because they were "rowdy." The opportunistic pro-apartheid Matron, on hearing this, and noticing the hostility between the different groups, seized the opportunity and encouraged student nurses to form separate branches as stipulated by the 1957 Nursing Act. But however despicable the role of the Matron was, even worse was the role of those nurses who supported the Matron and apartheid government in forming separate branches. The Indian and Colored nurses at Edendale Hospital concurred with the matron and formed their separate branches and baptized their creation by a fancy name "Colind," short for Colored and Indian. The Society of Young Africa concluded that no amount of talk could brush aside the fact that the formation of Colind was an act of supreme betrayal to the cause of Unity, and hence to the cause of freedom of the oppressed in South Africa, (United We Stand).

Elsewhere, in Durban to be particular, Edna Miya and her colleagues' protests against racial discrimination, disparity in salaries and exploitation at her place of employment was captured in various newspaper reports. This occurred when nurses at King George V Jubilee Hospital went on strike in August 1961. A forced mealtime color bar among African, Colored and Indian nurses was one of the main grievances listed in a memorandum handed to the hospital superintendent, Dr. B.A. Dormer on 9 August 1961. African nurses were served stale bread and lower quality meat while in a separate dining room, exclusive meals of higher quality were served to the Indian and Colored nurses who received fresh meat and vegetables, newly baked bread and butter. African nurses were also expected to provide their own eating utensils. All the black nurses, however, disagreed with the way segregation, in an already segregated hospital, was being enforced. They asked authorities that all nurses should eat together. African nurses also pointed out that some of them were paying more for board and lodging than nurses who received better food. In fact, African staff nurses were paying more for cramped lodging than white, Indian and Colored nurse aids who, they claimed, received better food rations. Through the Durban Hospital Workers Union the nurses demanded a minimum wage of R3.00 a day for assistant staff nurses and clerical workers; a minimum wage of R2.00 a day for hospital laborers, nurse aids and maids; uniforms and shoes without deductions from salary; an unemployment insurance fund for Africans, similar to that for Europeans and compensation for the family of an African worker who dies after contracting TB in the hospital. African nurses, previously offered no employers' protection from TB, were also demanding some form of protection from the disease. They also demanded that the right to maternity leave be extended to unmarried pregnant women.[26]

When the hospital superintendent failed to respond to their memorandum, about 300 Indian, Colored and African nurses marched in protest and also began a food boycott campaign. At about 1:00 p.m., the nurses filed away from the main office block and returned to their hostel. On the way they collected loaves of bread and other food delivered to them by SACTU officials. Members of the Durban non-White Hospital Workers' Union also alleged that eleven African student nurses were caned by a White matron, a Mrs. Malan, on 3 August because these nurses could not answer questions during a lecture. The protesting nurses demanded the immediate dismissal of Malan. Also, during the protest gathering, three senior police officers visited the hospital. The Bantu Affairs Commissioner of Durban dismissed the nurses' strike and claimed that their complaints were politically inspired. He also argued that neither he nor the hospital superintendent could do anything about the demand for higher pay because 'that is laid down by the Government.' On 11 August 1961, Stephen Dhlamini, the chairperson of SACTU Durban branch, was arrested in the vicinity of King George V Hospital for a pass offence and held in custody for nine hours before being released on bail of R10.00. SACTU members, Dlamini, Billy Nair, Curnick Ndlovu and Memory Vakalisa assisted the nurses throughout this period.[27] Edna Miya, who was married to Vakalisa, was the link between SACTU and the striking nurses at King George V Hospital: "ngikhumbula kunestrike eKing George yimi ebengi *contacta ioffice* (SACTU) *because I was in charge of the ward* ucingo *was at my disposal* akukho umuntu ozongibuza ukuthi ngishayelaphi *so* ngishayele e ofisini (leSACTU) ngibatshele, isimo sesinje, sesinje."[28]

Apart from complaints relating to corporal punishment meted out by the white tutor, African nurse aids also complained bitterly about the conduct of their racist white supervisor, a Mrs. Van Niekerk, who habitually assaulted, insulted and used derogatory names to refer to Africans. According to Miya, matters reached such a pitch of unpleasantness that three victimized African nurse aids resorted to burning the hospital's linen-room. The three were soon arrested and spent 18 months in jail after one of them had confided in her sister, who was married to a police constable. The result was that one of the African nurse aids joined MK subsequent to her release from jail. Whatever the rights and wrongs of the episode, these incidents suggested the fragility of social relationships in the hospital; in fact, according to Edna Miya, discontent had been simmering for some time at King George V Hospital:

> kwakukhona isikhathi umlungu owayephethe *ilinen room*, uMrs Van Niekerk owayedlala ngama Nurse aids amaAfricans, ewaphethe kabi, igenge ewu 2 , uyaphila lo omunye, omunye ushone *last year* beza kimi bathi sifuna ukushisa ilinen room sicela usitholele ipetrol, ngathi kubo ngizobatholela, ngawuthola lopetroli. *I advised them* ngathi ningawutheli ngaphandle lopetrol, . . . bakwenza lokho, yasha yanqonqa ilinen room, *the aim* bekuwukuthi akesihluphe lelibhunu u Van Niekerk lizoke lihlale umsebenzi lingenawo. Yasha yanqoqa *ilinen* room, kanti bafake lo owesithathu labantwana, uyabona igroup of three ayikaze yasebenza i *odd number* ngoba *these other two* ba *close*, kanti lo uzojika ayiveze indaba ku dadewabo owayeshade nephoyisa, baboshwa ke labantwana, badonsa 18 months ejele, kanti yingalesikhathi sesizokuhamba ke (into exile), lomunye wayojoyina uMkhonto weSizwe (after her release from jail). UVan Niekerk wayebabiza *all sorts of names* (including kaffirs) kukhona nokuthanda ukushaya . . . *my sister who comes after me was a Nurse Aid there, she was also complaining.*[29]

Luckhardt and Wall note that a major achievement during the strike was the display of unity among workers inspired by the leadership of these militant young African nurses, who were undeterred by the intimidation from police and hospital authorities. Though they did not succeed in getting Malan and van Niekerk dismissed, they did gain some worthwhile improvement in the working conditions of African hospital workers, and raised the consciousness of African workers in general through their actions. Tremendous solidarity from international organizations saved the nurses from massive retrenchment, and only twenty one nurses were dismissed. Dorner was later refused entry by the Nigerian government to attend an international conference of scientists in January 1962, (Luckhardt and Wall, 1980). Three months after the strike at King George V Hospital, Edna Miya (and others) made a conscious decision to go into exile.

FAMILY, EDUCATIONAL QUALIFICATIONS, WORKING EXPERIENCES: EDNA MIYA, MARY JANE SOCENYWA, EDITH AND KHOLEKA THUNYISWA

Edith and Kholeka Thunyiswa were born in Korsten in Port Elizabeth. Edith was born in 1927 and Kholeka was born in 1936, and the family later settled with their redoubtable mother in New Brighton after their parents were separated. Both sisters were qualified teachers before they joined nursing. Edith Thunyiswa, the elder sister, only taught for a year at a primary school in New Brighton and in 1948 went to McCords Hospital to train as a nurse. She did not like the place and resigned after three months; she went back home where she managed to get a teaching post in one of the primary schools in Cradock. Because she liked nursing very much it was not long before she decided to quit her teaching post in 1951 and enrolled at the Baragwanath Hospital as a trainee nurse. She completed her nursing course in 1954 after which she worked for a year at the same hospital and resigned. She went to work at the Pretoria General Hospital for another year and again resigned and went back to Port Elizabeth to train in midwifery. Edith completed her training and returned to Johannesburg where she was employed at the Shanty Clinic in Soweto as a midwife until December 1961, prior to her journey into exile.

Similarly, Kholeka Thunyiswa taught for a short period at a primary school before enrolling for her general nursing diploma at King Edward Hospital in Durban in 1957. Kholeka described leaving home for Durban as an enjoyable learning experience that allowed her to broaden her horizons. After attaining her professional qualifications in 1959, just like her sister Edith, she returned to Port Elizabeth to train and work as midwife until December 1961, prior to her journey into exile.

Edna Miya was born in 1927 at the Mahlongwa Mission Station where she grew up. This Mission Station belonged to the American Mission Board. Miya began training as a nurse at McCords Hospital in 1942, completing her training in 1945. Miya experienced the deteriorating health and painful death of her mother and took a conscious decision to become a nurse. Her mission was to help human beings, as personified by her ailing mother, whom she believed deserved better. She recalled that her professional training was underpinned by religion because of the missionary zeal of, amongst others, Dr. Alan Taylor and Ms. Cooper at McCords. This might be the main reason why Edith Thunyiswa resigned from her nursing training course after three months. As a fully qualified nurse, Miya went to work at a private clinic in Mooi River for six months. She then got a post at Ladysmith Provincial Hospital where she worked for about two years. In 1948 she was employed at King George V Hospital in Durban. This was a specialist, TB Hospital, serving the region. She worked there as a staff-nurse and later she was one of the three African nurses to be promoted as a nursing sister. She worked at King George until December 1961, prior to her journey into exile.

Mary Jane Socenywa was born at Dikeni in Alice in 1924. Her parents later migrated to Port Elizabeth and the family relocated to New Brighton.

Like all the other nurses, her role models were professional nurses within local communities. They were respected and regarded with awe by local residents. Socenywa went to Johannesburg to commence her training at the non-European Hospital. Socenywa was part of the group transferred to Baragwanath Hospital when the nursing training institute was opened in 1948. She was among the first nurses to be trained at Baragwanath, and she worked there after completing her nursing diploma. She worked at Baragwanath until December 1961 when she was recruited to join the group from the Eastern Cape that fled into exile. This occurred while she was on leave, visiting home in New Brighton.

POLITICAL CONCRETIZATION, RECRUITMENT AND REASONS FOR LEAVING

Although Edna Miya was married to Memory Vakalisa, a SACTU trade unionist based in Durban, it was Idah Mazibuko, one of her best friends, who awakened her political consciousness. Mazibuko was married to Harry Jordan, an executive member of the Natal Indian Congress. She continually pestered Miya about joining her in attending public meetings organized by the ANC and addressed by Chief Albert Luthuli. It was not long before Miya gave in to her friend's request and decided to attend one of these Sunday meetings. She was not disappointed. Thereafter, Edna Miya and her colleagues at work consciously fought against apartheid policies and exploitation at their workplace. The African nurses at King George V Hospital organized themselves against blatant racism and disparity in terms of salaries. They sought advice from the Municipal Workers Trade Union that was affiliated to SACTU. Edna Miya met her future husband during consultations for advice on trade union matters.

When Mary Jane Socenywa was still living in New Brighton Township in Port Elizabeth, she religiously attended political meetings and rallies organized by the ANC. She was recruited and personally asked by Govan Mbeki to join the group of nurses from the Eastern Cape going into exile. This occurred while she was visiting home early in December 1961. Conscious of the negative affects of the Nursing Act of 1957, Socenywa did not hesitate. Earlier she had played an important role in the nurses' struggles against pass laws and other forms of discrimination while based at the Baragwanath Hospital.

When Edith Thunyiswa completed her teacher's course she was approached by Dr. Njongwe, a medical practitioner who was also a senior member of the ANC in Port Elizabeth, to join the ANC. Dr. Njongwe was the family practitioner; hence the Thunyiswa family was close to him and used to attend ANC meetings at his house in New Brighton. The family also organized and participated in fund raising events for the ANC. Together with her younger sister Kholeka, Edith and her family were friendly with the ANC leadership that included Govan Mbeki and Raymond Mhlaba, who were instrumental in organizing the nurses from the Eastern Cape to go into exile. Kholeka Thunyiswa recalled: "uTata Govan Mbeki *wathi* he wanted highly disciplined people who wont let him down . . . so he picked me up here from the family . . . this happened without knowledge that Edith (who was based in Soweto) had been recruited because if Mama knew, I would not have gone, we were the two sisters left at home, the elder sister was already married. . . ." Edith Thunyiswa worked with Albertinah Sisulu at the Shanty Clinic. The latter recruited the Johannesburg-based nurses. Thunyiswa remembered organizing some of her friends:

> At Shanty Clinic umaSisulu approached me to organise some nurses whom I was staying with, that is, Georginah Masusu. I also organised others. I was staying at the nurses' quarters at the Shanty Clinic. . . . I really do not know how umaSisulu knew that I was political . . . but in fact . . . Lilian Ngoyi used to come to the clinic to ask for some donation for the ANC and we used to give out some money and maybe umaSisulu saw that and maybe that is what made her approach us . . . umaSisulu did explain that Tanzania was getting independence in 1961 and all white nurses had threatened to leave by then most of them had already resigned. . . .

While this process was in place, Edith Thunyiswa was unaware that her younger sister was being recruited by Govan Mbeki and others, and was part of the group from the Eastern Cape. She was shocked when she met her sister at a safe house in Fordsburg. They had a fierce argument: "When I heard that my sister was here, I was shocked . . . we were arguing and I told her, 'we can't go, the two of us, you must remain behind,' she refused point blank. She told me if I want to stay behind I must stay behind because she was determined to go. I was thinking of the old lady (our mother) because she was the only one left behind with the eldest sister. I thought it would be too much for her to be left with the family alone . . . my younger sister refused to remain behind." Kholeka Thunyiswa recalled the following about the event:

> so when Edith came I did not know that she was in the same group . . . a friend of hers saw me . . . the group from Johannesburg came, came in first, and when Edith's friend saw me she hardly

> greeted me and she went out of the house and told her, 'hey you will meet a big surprise,' so Edith was wondering what is this surprise, she did not tell her too, and when she saw me she said 'hawu, are you in this dangerous trip? you better go back home, how would mama feel if anything happen to one of us.' So I said to Edith 'you see that I am already in Johannesburg and I do not even know that the boss (mother) already knows that I have already left, so you better remain behind because you are still in Johannesburg—hey and people in Johannesburg do not know you have been recruited so I think you better remain behind,' that is the conversation which happened between me and Edith. Apparently there was a report that people were not supposed to bring friends and boyfriends, fiancé (to the point of departure-for farewells) because of the secretive nature of the whole trip. You could only confide in a parent because they keep secrets . . . I told Edith she better remain behind because she was (working) in Johannesburg it was a different situation for me because I had travelled thus far . . . she refused to take the advise, so eventually we left together, there was no way out . . .

What the Thunyiswa sisters and the other nurses did not know was that Georginah Masusu's PAC-aligned boyfriend had followed them in his car to Fordsburg. He later leaked the news about the nurses' trip into exile to the newspapers-hence jeopardizing their lives. Mary Jane Socenywa remembered the lighter side of their trip from Port Elizabeth. They were still young and full of life and energy. They were wearing their fashionable clothes and high-heels and when Edith Thunyiswa met her in Fordsburg, she was so elated and said, "chomie you are here too!" and Socenywa replied, "yes and we took everything lightly, it was not serious although we knew that there was a possibility that we might be arrested."

INTO EXILE

In her review of psycho-social literature on migration and exile, Zonke Majodina[30] and others identify the following distinct stages:

- perception of threat
- deciding to leave
- the period of extreme danger and flight

- reaching safety
- the camp experience

The first four stages are relevant to this study but the last is not precisely because the nurses were not placed in refugee camps or ANC military camps such as Kongwa. Needless to say, the contemporary South African Diasporas are differentiated and their relations are mediated by the inscriptions of gender, generation, race, class and political ideology.

The ANC, in its efforts to promote and facilitate the exchange of professionals between itself and African countries, recruited the nurses from the Cape (Port Elizabeth), Natal (Durban) and Transvaal (Johannesburg/Soweto) provinces. The group from Durban was organized by Johnny Makhathini with the help of Radebe and Vakalisa from SACTU. It included Edna Miya, Hilda Bonqa, Mary Mwandla, Gertrude Nzimande, Finess Luke, Celia Khuzwayo and Mavis Motha. The group from Port Elizabeth included Kholeka Thunyiswa, Victoria Magodla, Nosipho Mshumpela and Mary Jane Socenywa. The bulk of the group came from Johannesburg and was recruited by Sisulu. They included, among others: Edith Thunyiswa, Neo Raditladi, Sinah Jali, Georginah Masusu and Edna Mgabaza. For security reasons and as a precaution, the majority of the nurses did not inform their family members that they were leaving the country. Edna Miya told her sister that she was leaving on the very day that she was supposed to depart.

The nurses from the Eastern Cape met for the first time as a group when they boarded the train to Johannesburg at the Port Elizabeth railway station. They were met at their destination by an ANC contact. According to Kholeka Thunyiswa, this contact did not have to introduce himself as they were briefed what to do upon reaching their destination. From the Johannesburg railway station, the Eastern Cape group proceeded to the safe house in Fordsburg. The Soweto group left from Duma Nokwe's house in Orlando West and was driven by Nokwe to the safe house in Fordsburg. This is where they met their colleagues from the Eastern Cape and also where they met for the first time the bus driver who would transport them to Bechuanaland.[31] He was disguised as a priest and could fool the guards at the border gate but he could not fool his passengers as Kholeka Thunyiswa reminisced:

> There was a white student from Wits University who was wearing a collar as a Minister. He was driving us; I do not remember his name (his name was Alan Lipman, a white student from the University of

> the Witwatersrand who was a member of the African Resistance Movement.[32]) . . . at the border gate he said to the guards, 'I am transporting a group of nurses who are going to a funeral of their colleague, these are all nurses;' so, because he was a church minister, they just opened the gates and we went through, they never asked for passports, whatever, nothing, we just went through . . . and then the priest after that he disappeared after dropping us at Fish Keitsing's place (in Lobatse) . . . we are still looking for this priest . . . the most important thing that we noticed at the border gate while he was talking to the guards was that he was not a priest . . . this was because the dog collar was tied (clumsily) with a big pin at the back . . . he could not tie his collar correctly . . . we did not ask him about his true identity because he had successfully completed his mission.

The Natal group was not part of the bus trip to Bechuanaland as they arrived late in Johannesburg. It was after their colleagues from Transvaal and the Eastern Cape had departed. They were driven from Durban to Johannesburg in a car organized by the Durban branch of the ANC. Their contact in Johannesburg was Nokwe who drove the nurses to the Johannesburg Station where they boarded a train to Bechuanaland. Nokwe, an ANC activist and a banned person, had to drop them at the station before the train's departure. Before he left, he warned the nurses to be constantly on guard and also to create 'sob stories' to be told to the ticket inspectors who would request traveling documents, which they did not possess. When the time arrived for the nurses to produce the documents they pretended that they were part of a religious choral music group whose other members who had traveled by road would be meeting them at the other side of the border with the necessary documents. To prove their point, they sang religious songs on top of their voices the moment they saw ticket examiners and conductors. Their plan was successful and they were not bothered by officials. When the train arrived at Lobatse the next day, Fish Keitsing[33] took the nurses to the government house in Gaborone, where their colleagues were accommodated.

The total number of nurses who arrived in Dar es Salaam in January 1962 was twenty. One nurse had to return to South Africa because she was pregnant. She confided in some of her colleagues and it was felt that the journey would be too hazardous for her, (Interview, Miya). The remaining twenty nurses were expected to be in Tanzania before the independence celebrations of December 1961. Unfortunately they were kept in Bechuanaland longer than anticipated, as the Tanzanian government failed to secure the plane that was supposed to transport them to their destination. Joe Modise, Fish Keitsing and Thomas Nkobi, as foreign based ANC activists, were the nurses' contacts in Bechuanaland. The three coordinated the nurses' trip to Tanzania and provided the link with the ANC office in Dar es Salaam. The twenty nurses had to stay in Bechuanaland for about a month and only left on 18 January 1962. Staying for a month in Bechuanaland brought its own problems. First, there was a security problem and there was a possibility that security agents from South Africa could kidnap them. Apparently Georginah Masusu's boyfriend had sold the story about their journey into exile to newspapers and it was widely reported in various press that the nurses had gone to join the ANC in exile. Actually the nurses read about their 'escape' into Bechuanaland in South African newspapers available in Lobatse, Gaborone and Francistown.

The nurses had to negotiate relations with their particular country of origin, and their country of trans-migration, in this instance Bechuanaland. There were difficulties relating to their accommodation in Francistown; the nurses were moved from the Gaborone government house, relocated and transferred to Francistown so as to be nearer to the airstrip. They were unhappy about their new accommodation where they crammed into a small house and had to sleep on the floor sharing small mats. In addition, the nurses were running out of money as they used their own money to fend for themselves. However, senior nurses like Miya and Mgabaza had enough cash at their disposal and therefore helped ease the situation. Others, like the Thunyiswa sisters tried to establish contact with their mother as they were now cash strapped. Regardless of the hard times, the nurses rather than stay indoors at their safe hours, enjoyed the social life that Francistown offered. Most of them jokingly pointed out, "we were still young and full of life-we could not allow ourselves to be miserable in Bechuanaland." Lastly, this breach of security was very demanding to both Modise and Nkobi who were probably happy when the airplane from Tanzania finally arrived and the twenty nurses proceeded to Dar es Salaam. Modise and Nkobi could now focus their energies on arranging the pending trip into exile of the first large batch of MK cadres.[34] Tanganyika African National Union (TANU) officials and the ANC leadership warmly welcomed the nurses when they arrived in Tanzania early in 1962.

IN TANZANIA

Tanzania formed part of what was called German East Africa until after the First World War, when it became a British Mandate area under the name of Tanganyika. In 1964 Tanganyika amalgamated with the Island of Zanzibar and became the United Republic of Tanzania. The early British supervision was initially undertaken by the League of Nations and, after the Second World War by the United Nations. In the mandate agreement the British were accorded full legislative, executive and judicial power. Tanganyika had a small immigrant population that was very dominant in the economic and political sphere. The planning for development in Eastern Africa in the 1950s was influenced by subtle conflicting policy considerations in the Colonial Office in London and in Africa that were further complicated by economic and administrative needs of the territories. Colonial budgets reflected goals of economic growth, but the juggling of priorities by those concerned with education, public health and agriculture showed the presence of political motives as well.

The focus on Western modernization for the British colonies after the Second World War implied attempts to establish a development process similar to that of Britain, by which industrialization based on capitalist agriculture and the expansion of a modern urban sector was given priority over development of the traditional rural sector. While policy statements indicated a strong emphasis on the priority of self-government, it was, in reality, economic aims that were heavily pursued. This was reflected in the adopted educational policies, as modernization competed with and, in certain areas, took prominence over adaptation in order to secure the transfer of the full range of skills and norms for the envisaged development process. While Education for Adaptation was provided solely for Africans, Education for Modernization was provided disproportionately for Europeans and Indians in competition with the select few native Africans. The importance of the actual provision for the different communities related to the fact that the modern sector was small and that fluency in English was a precondition of African participation in the central political system. The lack of African access to Education for Modernization, therefore, also limited their influence in economic and political life. This included health, training and education policies. At the time of independence in December 1961, Europeans and Asians together constituted around 87% (Africans 13%) of the highest-level graduate professionals, senior administrators and senior managers in industry and commerce. They formed in all 70% (Africans 30%) of the next level of technicians, sub-professional grades, and executive grades in the civil service, middle management in industry and commerce and teachers with secondary education but without a university degree.[35]

The level of education of the African population restricted their political opportunities and this included their continued limited access to opportunities in the expanding modern sector of the economy. Of the African population of 8.7 million in 1957, less than 500,000 were in paid employment, of whom around 199, 000 were working on agricultural areas, earning approximately 38% of all wages paid to Africans. During 1948–57, more than 60% of Asians, who numbered around 100,000, continued to monopolize wholesale and retail trade. Others established themselves as capitalist owners of plantations or were engaged in public and other services. Of the approximate 20,000 gainfully employed Europeans, about half were in the public and other services primarily as administrators and technicians. Approximately 20% were employed in agriculture, forestry and fishing, and a small number were owners or managers of agricultural estates or engaged in commerce or industry. After independence in 1961, the total number of employees at the two highest professional employment levels was 17,142, of whom Africans constituted 4,468, Europeans 4,309 and Indians 8,365. These numbers were reflected in the small attendance of Africans at the secondary and post-secondary school level. Although the overall size of the African system was immense compared with both the European and Indian systems, more Indians (9,505) than Africans (6,031) received secondary education in 1961. Respectively, 80 and 95 percent of the European and Indian age groups were enrolled in primary and secondary education in 1956, whereas African enrolment in primary and middle schools, which was virtually equal to enrolment in the whole system, represented 8.5% of the age group. The obvious social differentiation along racial lines, which resulted from the unequal provision of education, was accompanied by gender inequalities as well, (Bucheret, 1994).

During the late 1950s, TANU fought successfully for recognition as the major representative of Africans and, by 1958, had won the right to present candidates for district councils and ultimately for the Legislative Council. Their success influenced the Colonial Office in advancing the timetable for independence, and this, again, led to changes of strategy in the governor's office. Like Nyerere, TANU's leader, they favored transfer of power without violence, which would allow development plans to continue after 1961. Throughout these years of delicate maneuvering, the Medical Department (Department of Health) seemed to continue its regular work without paying too much attention to the general political atmosphere. In 1956, it drafted its five-year plan without reference to potential political changes. It assumed that medical policy must continue without interruption. In its draft outline of 1956–1961, it listed the steady flux of territorial revenue as one uncertain factor that might affect its performance. But from the medical point of view, it stressed continuity.

The 1956 Plan assigned the largest capital outlay to the new general hospital in Dar es Salaam, which replace the Sewa Haji Hospital that dated back to the German period. Other hospital construction projects included the Mwanza area which was the most densely populated outside Dar es Salaam. Improvements at district hospitals and the allocation of funds for hospital personnel, and last but not least for rural medical aids (including nursing assistants), would absorb the remainder of the funds.[36]

By the time Tanzania became independent in 1961, the program left Tanzania's health services where they had been in 1956, with the exception of two larger and improved hospitals, and an embryonic program for rural health development. In this way the, an imbalance between curative and preventive health care was built into the scheme immediately before independence. The disparity was further aggravated by its dependence on territorial revenue even though total cost was estimated at no more than 10% of the total funds. If the anticipated revenue should not materialize, however, allowance for its modification was made. In that case, it was stated, reduction of the rural services was anticipated.

The 1956–61 Tanzanian health plan did not necessarily abandon preventive medicine. Its statement on the future function of health centers pointed to new alternatives. Their role would enhance and transcend more preventive needs. They were to play a role in educating and reaching out to the surrounding communities, in order to influence people's living conditions in their own homes. Social development was part of health development. Finally, the Medical Department (Department of Health) was asked to set up a special health education section. In 1961, a committee was appointed by the Ministry of Health (Titmus Committee) to examine the existing state of the Tanzanian medical services and to suggest the maximum possible improvements within a five-year period. Though critical of the slow movement of the past programs, it acknowledged their good intentions. It found, however, that the previous programs and plans were lacking in one basic respect: namely, the avowed intention to provide a vast network of curative and preventive centers for more than eight million people in the country. Valuable ideals had gone into the planning process for the last ten years, the report conceded, but they were not based on economic and demographic realities. Titmus and his colleagues set out to devise a more realistic program and submitted their report in 1963, but the economic and political structure of the new state underwent more radical changes than the Titmus Committee could anticipate, (Beck, 1981). The services were not interrupted, but their growth depended in this stage on a new economic base.

IMPACT OF DEVELOPMENT HEALTH PLAN: TANZANIA DURING THE COLONIAL PERIOD AND AFTER 1961

(from Beck, 1981).

Government Budgets for Health Expenditure in Tanzania

1950–1956: Proposed Budget was 1, 780, 000 British Pounds
1961–1964: Budget was 954, 000 British Pounds
1964–1969: Budget was 13, 98

Development of Rural Health Centers: The Colonial Period in Tanzania

1926 8, 000 British Pounds Marks the beginning of a rural dispensary system. 'Tribal' dressers with three months of training.

1930 Training period for dressers extended to eighteen months to three years in four schools at Tabora, Misoma, Bukoba, and Tukuyu.

1945 Training concentrated in one school at Mwanza.

1949 The rural medical stations are placed under medical inspection controlled by district medical officers.

1950 Rural medical aids grouped according to training:

Grade 1- Educational standard X, three years of training.
Grade 2- Educational standard VIII, not less than two years of training.
Grade 3- Less than the minimum education from grades 1 and 2, little or no medical training.

Rural Dispensaries in 1950 (from Beck 1981)

Number of Stations 416
Rural Medical Aides 445
Total Patient Att. 3, 665, 248

Functions of Rural Centers

To serve a population of approximately 50,000 persons.
To provide supervision of dispensaries in its area, to organise preventive campaigns, environmental sanitation, and nutrition among other things.

Functions of Dispensaries

To provide service for communities of approximately 10,000 people
The minimum standards, not considered satisfactory by 1964, subject to continued revision and improvement.

TABLE 6.1 Rural Medical Facilities, Medical Assistants and Rural Medical Aides in Tanzania: 1961-1969

Type	1961	1969
Dispensaries	736	1, 362
Rural Health Centres	22	50
Medical Assistants	200	250
Rural Medical Aides	200	450

When the twenty South African nurses arrived in Tanzania in 1962 they found a health system whose problems were defined by financial restrictions, by a lack of qualified and well trained indigenous personnel, by investment of capital in hospitals instead of rural centers, by emergency situations during epidemics, and by infectious and parasitic diseases. The system also depended largely on foreign, expatriate personnel for expertise and planning. All these factors absorbed the resources of the state's medical budget and the subsidies of the development funds. These were some of the challenges facing the health system in their adopted country. Planning for a comprehensive health scheme in the 1960s focused on the extension of medical facilities throughout all rural areas and was bound to link with health policy closely with the state corporative and *Ujamaa* movement.

At first, the South African nurses were placed at the central hospital at Dar es Salaam during the first two weeks after their arrival in Tanzania. They worked at the general hospital so as to familiarize themselves and were then relocated to different stations around the country. Kholeka Thunyiswa and Hilda Bonqo were posted to the rural area, Iringa, where eight white expatriate nurses were stationed. These nurses stayed for not more than three months after the arrival of the South Africans. They left a job that was being done by eight people to only three, namely, a Tanzanian administrator, Thunyiswa and Bonqo. Kholeka Thunyiswa observed that most of the foreign white nurses were not doing their jobs conscientiously. They would arrive at work and hardly do anything, 'come eight o'clock in the morning, they are already taking breaks, smoking and drinking coffee'—life was easy. When one went to visit the wards, 'you will find the place smelling, patients sleeping in beds smelling of urine.' There were no professionally qualified African nurses but there were nurse assistants employed in most of the rural hospitals.

According to Kholeka Thunyiswa and Bonqo, the Tanzanian nurse assistants also did not carry out some of their duties properly. As an example, they did not wash the patients in order to maintain good hygienic conditions at the hospitals and rural health centers. Thunyiswa and Bonqo challenged the Tanzanian nurse assistants about their responsibilities and insisted that the maintenance of high standards of cleanliness was an essential part of their mission as health workers. As a group, they then decided to organize themselves in order to tackle the various challenges facing them at Iringa. It was also part of their emancipation from mental slavery. When the white matron took rounds after a month she commented about the improving standards in terms of hygiene. She insinuated that the Tanzanian nurse assistants were now productive because of the presence of newly arrived African nursing sisters from South Africa. But, Thunyiswa and Bonqo disputed such patronizing sentiments and explained to the Matron that the Tanzanian nurse assistants were diligent and prepared to carry out their job properly if they could be provided proper supervision by their superiors. It did not matter to them whether the superiors were white or black. The South African nurses had to assume a leadership role as professionals because, as Kholeka Thunyiswa claimed, 'when lives of patients were at stake, like good nurses, what else can you do, we would rather overwork.' These nurses were conscious of their responsibilities to humanity and especially to the peoples of Africa. The infrastructure at Iringa was very poor like that at most rural hospitals. There was a severe lack of materials such as cotton and medicines. There would be no bandages if you wanted to do dressing; therefore as a nurse, you had to improvise. The white expatriate nurses could not be bothered and did not care, (Interviews, Thunyiswa).

Besides the lack of medicines and other crucial items, the nurses from South Africa observed that there were various health related problems where they worked. The most urgent problems facing East African countries were nutrition and environmental sanitation. Diseases caused by malnutrition were prevalent and so were those influenced by environmental sanitation. Other challenges included malaria, tuberculosis, yellow fever, rabies, yaw, bilharzias, onchocerciasis, trypanosomiasis and leprosy. The question of water was probably the most serious. Communities did not have adequate supply of safe drinking water and therefore the attempts to prevent tropical diseases such as bilharzias and amoebic dysentery remained largely ineffective. In planning control measures against any of these diseases, another problem of fundamental importance arose—lack of sufficient medical and auxiliary personnel.[37]

Edith Thunyiswa was stationed at Mbeya together with a colleague, Mavis Motha, who left after a short period. Motha got married to an African-American whom she met at Mbeya and subsequently returned with him to the United States. Edna Thunyiswa, meanwhile, was diligent with her work inside the hospital ward but faced different challenges because of matters arising outside her workplace. She belonged to a single person reception committee as she welcomed MK cadres and other members of the ANC who were passing through Mbeya and in transit to Dar es Salaam. Most of them had no money, food or accommodation and she had to pay from her pocket for their needs. In one instance there were about thirty ANC refugees who came to her place, asking for help as she could not manage. Fortunately, she had the support of the Tanzanian Area Commissioner who was well versed with the ANC's struggle for liberation. He immediately arranged for a bus that took them directly to Dar es Salaam but would be paid for by Thunyiswa. Most of the cadres and others would arrive unannounced—all that they were told was to look for Edith Thunyiswa when they reached Mbeya. To a large extent she did not have a private or social life and a perfect example is what happened one day while she was at the local cinema, enjoying herself. Some local children came and called her to come out of the cinema because three chaps had arrived unannounced from South Africa. It was raining and they were wet, hungry and did not have anywhere to sleep. Edith Thunyiswa had to sacrifice her day at the movies and went home to make fire, cook and dry their clothes. She also offered them a place to sleep and paid for their transport to Dar es Salaam the following day. What kept her going was that Kholeka, her younger sister, was based at Iringa, not far away from Mbeya, and was stationed there with Hilda Bonqo; the three were in constant contact.

PROBLEMS IN EXILE

One of the declarations passed by the First Conference of African Independent States concerned its unwavering loyalty to the Universal Declaration of Human Rights. On racialism, the conference declared that it considered the practice of racial discrimination as evil and inhuman. It was deeply convinced that racialism negated of the basic principles of human rights and human dignity, to the extent that it was becoming an "element of such explosiveness which is spreading its poisonous influence more and more widely in some parts of Africa that it may well engulf our Continent in violence and bloodshed." Therefore, the conference condemned the practice of racial discrimination and segregation in all its aspects all over the world, especially in the Union of South Africa, in the Central African Federation, Kenya and other parts of Africa.[38]

The issue of racialism and prejudice would soon raise its ugly head at one of the regional hospitals where some of the South African nurses were based. The issue was finally resolved by the Tanzanian Minister of Health who was probably aware of the declaration of the First Conference of Independent African States, including the Tanzanian government's anti-racist policies. This was because in some hospitals where white expatriate nurses were in charge, the relationship between local nursing assistants and the nurses from South Africa was not amicable. Mary Jane Socenywa, who was based at Mwanza Hospital, had problems with the attitude of local nurse assistants. The latter were influenced by the expatriate white nurses to rebel against the South African nurses. These reactionary white nurses would inform the local nursing assistants from this rural area that the two professional nurses from South Africa had come to occupy their (local nurses) rightful positions. According to Socenywa, the question that these local nursing assistants could have asked themselves is, how could two foreign nurses achieve this? There was so much tension that this issue went as far as the Minister of Health for his immediate attention, because the two South African nurses wanted to resign and sought a transfer to another region. The Office of the Minister of Health carried out an investigation and the Minister was personally involved in trying to find a solution. He set up a small investigation team to probe and find out the root cause. Eventually the commission discovered that expatriate white nurses caused all the trouble by influencing the Tanzanian nursing assistants. The situation was resolved after the Minister of Health's personal visit to the Mwanza hospital, to address the problem personally. The results were that drastic action was taken against those who incited the Tanzanian nursing assistants. They were fired with immediate effect, (Interviews, Socenywa and Thunyiswa). Socenywa recollected the following about her arrival in Tanzania:

> We went straight to work. It was quite an experience. Although there were trained nurses (as nursing assistants), but they were not registered (as professionals). Some of them thought why we being blacks from South Africa could hold posts that belonged to them. They thought that we were of the same standard in terms of training. It did not take long before they could realise what was the difference . . . well this affected the system because it was a state of transition. Fortunately they got rid of all the people (white expatriate nurses who were against us) in terms of administration. *Abantu abamnyama kade bathi bemnyama benjena* they think they are better than us, *bafuna umuntu omhlophe, nalaba abamhlophe abafuni ukuba* under the black government *kodwa* otherwise they (Tanzanian public) were quite nice to us. (Interview, Socenywa)

Another problem mentioned by Socenywa was communication with the local populace in Tanzania. Never mind that the Tanzanian nursing assistants were not registered as professionals, they were quite experienced. The facilities at the rural hospitals were not bad, relatively speaking, as the nurses from South Africa did not expect to work in what Socenywa described as "flashy hospitals that were well equipped." Tanzanians used to refer xenophobically to the expatriate African nurses from South Africa as "waKimbizi," loosely translated by Socenywa as meaning, "'you are a refugee who ran away from your own country." The South Africans experienced language difficulties and therefore communication was a problem when they first arrived. This was because the majority of the population spoke kiSwahili and not English. The difficulty was that the South African nurses had to take into cognizance language issues which we face quite frequently inside the hospital ward when dealing with patients. Fearing marginalization, the nurses from South Africa had to learn and understand the everyday language, because if there was a communication breakdown between the nurse and the patient, the nurses would not be able to compile proper medical history and provide a correct diagnosis. It was crucial that the patient should understand the nurse and vice versa; even the expatriate white nurses made an effort to speak fluent kiSwahili. Hence the expatriate South African nurses had to learn and understand the dominant language of the people as quickly as possible so that they could provide medical doctors with proper medical histories. Apparently, the expatriate white male doctors were spoiled; they could not bother themselves to be fluent in kiSwahili, for they expected the nurses to compile medical histories of patients. Thus, according to Kholeka Thunyiswa: "We had to struggle very hard to know the language. The sooner we did, it was better for us, and the language business was the most difficult. In fact it also became part and parcel of our own language even when we were sitting together as South Africans, we held our conversations in Swahili. Also, Nyerere had proclaimed Swahili as official language so everybody was compelled to speak in Swahili . . . we had no other way but to understand the language because [otherwise] there would be no pay at the end of the month," (Interview, Socenywa).

Talking about pay at the end of the month, the nurses from South Africa were not satisfied. They were employed on the same conditions as they were in South Africa and given permanent posts, meaning that if you left South Africa as a nursing sister, you would be allocated the same post in Tanzania. But salaries in Tanzania were very low compared to those they were earning while they were still based in South Africa. When the nurses left for exile they did not request information about salaries and conditions of service. They raised such issues as employment packages immediately when they arrived in Tanzania, and to their disappointment discovered that they were expected to earn meager salaries when compared to other expatriates. They were now in a catch twenty-two situation and could not return to their country of origin; it was too late, and according to Socenywa, they were struggling. In terms of conditions of employment, the nurses thought they would be given the same conditions of employment as other expatriates where the country of origin contributes in terms of salary and other benefits. For example, salaries and benefit of white expatriate nurses from the United Kingdom were taken care of by both the UK and Tanzania according to an agreement reached by these countries. This was not the case with the African nurses from South Africa. Yes, they were appointed into senior positions, corresponding to the ones they held in South Africa, but Tanzanian authorities told them that they could not qualify in terms of conditions of employment offered to expatriates from other countries. Their argument was that Tanzania did not have diplomatic relations and bilateral agreements with apartheid South Africa. These nurses were then expected to wait for two to five years, and then they could be allocated the proper allowances. However, when the period of their contract expired, their new contracts were not revised but were drafted again according to existing original agreements reached in 1961. There were no benefits other than low salary and gratuity.

Frustration set in and hence came the idea that overseas countries such as England could offer better job prospects, salaries, benefits and opportunities to them as nursing professionals. That is why some of the nurses accepted job opportunities overseas. Some went to settle with their spouses in their countries of origin, (Interview, Thunyiswa, Thunyiswa, Miya and Socenywa). According to Kholeka Thunyiswa, she had never thought about leaving Tanzania and she is still living in Tanzania up to this day and enjoys her adopted country's culture. This highlights processes of acculturation, integration and assimilation as experienced by some of those who were in exile.

Regardless of these processes, Kholeka Thunyiswa, together with her sister and others, had to find a solution to persistent difficulties at the workplace. These were characterized by the problem of being underpaid with no prospect of vertical movement or promotion, regardless of professional qualifications and work experience. Most of the nurses resigned from the Department of Health because of differences with their employers. Kholeka Thunyiswa later resigned and joined the Dar es Salaam City Council's public health division. Edith Thunyiswa subsequently joined a non-governmental health organization in 1974. She recalled the following about unfair treatment in her place of employment:

> I worked in Tanzania for twenty years and in 1974 (after resigning from the Department of Health) I worked (in the public health sector) for a non- governmental organization. What made me take the decision was because when we arrived, we were told that we would be promoted but after a year it was announced that there were no promotions forthcoming. They took some of the Tanzanian junior nurses for training overseas, I do not know where, and when these junior nurses returned they were made seniors above us; they became matrons and we were never promoted since our arrival. So we thought there was no future.

Continuing about difficult work place experiences and other forms of discrimination, particularly salaries, Edith Thunyiswa noted:

> It was worse because of the money they were giving us we could not do anything. It was just like pocket money for everybody including Tanzanians. We were not regarded as expatriates because expatriates earned more because your home government pays a certain percentage of your salary and the Tanzanian government would also pay its fair share of your total salary. With us our government was not paying anything for us and the Tanzanians said they were not going to compensate us—they told us they would employ us on local terms. Yes, they took us on local terms but they were not promoting us, which was very strange (we were prepared to compete with local nurses for senior positions) . . . we had no problems working with our Tanzanian colleagues, there was simply no promotion for us . . . we were nursing sisters right through and no promotions . . . some of the 20 nurses decided to go on further study, some of them got married, but most of them went to England to further their studies . . . I went to work and stay in Dar es Salaam after I joined the non-governmental organisation.

Majodina identifies four distinct issues in order to understand the profound experience exiles have in a new culture:

- The honeymoon stage: this is the initial reaction of fascination, admiration of the new country and friendly relations with hosts.

- The crisis period: when the initial difficulties are experienced, difficulties in language, cultural values, leading to feelings of frustration, anger and anxiety.

- The recovery stage: when the crisis is resolved by a number of methods, for example, learning the language, forming social networks and so on.

- The adjustment stage when the newcomer begins to enjoy life and new culture. (Majodina, 1998, 52)

Most of the stages are relevant to the nurses' experiences in Tanzania, but differ in so far as the issue of cultural values is concerned. Most of the nurses did not express difficulties in this regard. It was the issue about the employment conditions—that is, contracts, salaries, and benefits—that led to feelings of frustration, anger and anxiety. Most of the nurses enjoyed life and culture by forming friendships and spending leisure time with Tanzanian professionals from different sectors.

FAMILY AND OTHER DIFFICULTIES WHILE IN EXILE

Communicating with the families that they left behind in South Africa was haphazard and quite difficult for the nurses. Different forms of communication were used in this regard. It included letter writing or sending a word of mouth through couriers and other measures. Kholeka and Edith Thunyiswa's strong-willed mother could not stand the pain of losing her two daughters and decided to follow them; she arrived unannounced for a visit in Tanzania in 1964. Such was her bravery that the first time that Kholeka Thunyiswa heard that her mother had come to visit only occurred upon the latter's arrival at the local bus station in the rural town of Iringa. She received a message through one of the male secretaries who worked at the local hospital. He came rushing into the hospital office and proclaimed that there was someone who resembled her at the local bus station and was asking about her whereabouts. He just said to Kholeka, "I think she is your mother." Kholeka instructed the male secretary to return to the local station keep her company and ask this stranger to wait for her while she tried to contact her boyfriend who was later to become her husband. She succeeded in doing so, and together with her boyfriend she drove to the local station. They had to return back home, after desperately searching for the two they had gone to pick up. On their arrival at Kholeka's home they were surprised to find this old woman, who turned out to be Kholeka's mother, and the local man waiting for them. She had welcomed herself and was comfortably seated and jokingly welcomed Kholeka and her future son-in-law into the house. She explained to them that she could not wait forever at the local station, for she was too excited to wait for her daughter. Apparently, when the male secretary returned to the station with the message, Kholeka's mother persuaded and convinced him to take her to Kholeka's house. As pedestrians, they walked all the way and did not use the motorway but took short cuts through the alleys; this is the main reason why Kholeka could not locate them.

Soon, Kholeka invited her sister, Edith, to come and visit, and their mother soon regaled them about her journey from Port Elizabeth, South Africa, to Tanzania. She had paid for the entire trip from her own pocket and confirmed the fact that she was helped by the ANC office in Dar es Salaam to learn her children's whereabouts. The ANC had built new communities in the various host countries. The diasporas of the late 20th century were more globalized than earlier ones, in the multiplicity of their destinations and networks. The liberation movement managed to build trans-national networks, while maintaining a fierce loyalty to its country of origin, South Africa, which it hoped to liberate. This fact notwithstanding, the ANC people failed to notify Kholeka Thunyiswa about her mother's arrival. All they did was confirm the areas where both her daughters were stationed.[39]

To Kholeka and Edith, this unexpected guest who happened to be their mother, was certainly welcome. Life was bliss while she was around and she certainly spoiled her two daughters. But, like any loving mother, she was very protective and concerned by what she saw on her arrival. Kholeka Thunyiswa recalled:

> While she was there I was coughing (from some allergy) and I had grown so thin, she was extremely worried and she said when you write us letters you tell us lies that you are alright which is not the case. So I told her I had this allergy, I am getting treatment . . . so Dr. Clark (who was also Superintendent of the hospital) invited her for coffee and during the process she discussed the problem with Dr. Clark . . . she thought it might be because of climatic conditions and asked Dr. Clark why don't they transfer me. . . . Personally, I had been forever asking for a transfer because things were getting complicated . . . Dr. Clark kept on saying No . . . I could tell he did not want me to leave that region. But with the presence of my mother the transfer was confirmed . . . it was 1, 2, 3, then I got a transfer to work in Dar es Salaam where I got further treatment at the national hospital and my life improved for the better. (Interview, Thunyiswa)

In 1980, Edith Thunyiswa's husband, a senior official of SACTU, was transferred to Lusaka and she had to go and settle in Zambia with him.

She worked for a local clinic in Lusaka. By then she had an adopted child, Nomthandazo, who attended school in Tanzania. When she was transferred to Lusaka, Edith Thunyiswa enrolled Nomthandazo at SOMAFCO.

Some of the nurses had children when they left South Africa. Only one of the nurses later managed to bring her child into exile, the child's name was Gloria. Hilda Bonqa left her two young children when she left South Africa. Georginah Masusu had a son, Sello, who last saw her mother when she left South Africa in 1961. Late in the 1980s or early in the 1990s, Sello Masusu, by then a grown man, had to go to Tanzania after his mother had passed away. His mother died in 1989/90, while raising another child whose name was Nana and whose father was Tanzanian. Georginah Masusu was not married to Nana's father and due to their differences; she had refused him permission to take responsibility for Nana's life. Sello Masusu had gone to Dar es Salaam to finalize pressing issues connected to his mother's death and also arrange for Nana to come and stay with him in South Africa.[40] According to Kholeka Thunyiswa, Sello Masusu had a tough upbringing and at one stage MaSisulu offered to make arrangements for Sello to join his mother in exile but Georginah turned down the offer. While in exile, Georginah lived an isolated life and was based in Dar es Salaam with both Kholeka Thunyiswa and Finess Luke. The three of them worked for the Dar es Salaam City Council's public health department after their resignation from the government Department of Health. Kholeka Thunyiswa was often worried by the manner in which Georginah tended to be secretive and kept her difficulties about her health to herself. Absenteeism had become Georginah's habit. Hence Kholeka took the responsibility of paying her surprise visits after she had been unofficially away from work for a long time. Usually, when there were no response Kholeka would forcefully open the door, barge into the room and would find Georginah inside the house sitting alone and would, as a concerned sister, ask, "why do you isolate yourself like this and why don't you go to the hospital because you do not look healthy and you are staying next to a big hospital-why do not inform us that you are sick?" Georginah would always answer that "I have been to the hospital and was given prescription and treatment." According to Thunyiswa, "the next day you will hear she was admitted at Morogoro Hospital, the next day at another hospital." She would not notify them about such demanding trips undertaken under trying conditions. Finally, Georginah Masusu decided to go to Zambia to seek medical help, again, without notifying her colleagues in Dar es Salaam. That is the reason why she ended up being admitted at a hospital in Lusaka, where she passed away, (Interview, Thunyiswa).

Finess Luke died of a heart attack during the early 1980s and was buried in Dar es Salaam. Apparently she died on the day when she was paid out her gratuity; money she never enjoyed. Both Luke and Masusu were not forthcoming about their health problems; they were careless about their health, quite a surprising behavior exhibited by qualified professional nurses. Some of the nurses drank alcohol heavily so as to deal with their difficulties. Whenever Kholeka Thunyiswa encouraged Luke to go and consult a doctor she would reply, "I do not want to, I do not want to know *into zenzekayo la phakathi.*" Though they were still best of friends and treated each other like sisters, Luke had defected and joined the PAC by the time she had passed away. The story is that she had a fallout with one of her male drinking partners who was also from South Africa. She had accused this character, nicknamed in a joking manner as Ntlifitlifi, of trying to kill her after she was stabbed whilst asleep in her bedroom. The assailant escaped through the window and no one was able to identify him. But Luke was convinced it was Ntlifitlifi who attempted to kill her because they were at loggerheads. She owed him money and at one stage Ntlifitlifi threatened to beat her up because she could not meet keep her promises to pay him back. Ntlifitlifi was later arrested and convicted. But Duma Nokwe questioned the merits of this sentence, appealed and represented the accused in court. The latter was subsequently released from jail because of Nokwe's legal acumen. Apparently, the accused, as his nickname aptly describes him, was too old and frail, and an alcoholic who could not harm a fly. He could not also jump through the window from the top of a tall building and escape without seriously hurting himself. But Luke was both unconvinced and dissatisfied with the outcome of the court case. She challenged Nokwe whom she accused of bias. The turn of events became a big issue that finally led to her resignation from the ANC. Ultimately, Luke joined the PAC and by coincidence she passed away on the day when she was appointed to become the leader of that organization's Women's Section/League, (Interview, Thunyiswa).

Both Masusu and Luke showed signs of stress, strain and sense of loss. Masusu might have felt the strain and stress due to the effort required to make necessary adjustments regarding her relationship with Nana's father, and might have shown a sense of loss through the fact that she left her son behind in South Africa. Masusu expressed her feelings of rejection by rejecting Nana's father, who was Tanzanian. Luke also showed signs of stress and strain as expressed by drinking heavily. She showed a sense of loss, confusion, impotence and feelings of rejection by the ANC after the incidents involving Ntlifitlifi. She joined the PAC due to not being able to cope.

BACK HOME AND OTHER CHALLENGES IN POST 1994 SOUTH AFRICA

When the nurses learned about the possibility of returning home during the early 1990s they were overjoyed. At last, South Africa became the last country to be politically liberated in terms of the Pan African struggle for liberation. These nurses had realized their dreams of freedom. After spending more than 30 years in exile it was quite an exhilarating yet ambiguous experience to return to their home country and to meet long lost family and friends. Because she missed home so much, on her return home in 1990, Kholeka Thunyiswa stayed in South Africa for two years, much against her husband's will. Her protesting husband had to return reluctantly and alone to Tanzania, to take care of the family.

To understand the reactions to the reparation of South Africans after 1990, it is necessary to place them in the political, social and economic context of that time. For some, returning home was excruciatingly painful because of unwarranted behavior from ignorant and unscrupulous family and community members, who were not familiar with the conditions in exile. The returning nurses came back into a very different world from the one they left behind in December 1961. For example, naïve relatives expected them to return with suitcases full of money and other rich trappings. Tension set in when this did not materialize—in fact most of the nurses had now officially retired from work because of their age. Such expectations from the nurses' families could be understood and contextualized as the result of an unstable economic environment in South Africa. Visible signs of economic stagnation, high unemployment and poverty bedeviling various African communities carried over from the 1980s were still visible even during the late 1990s. They were also not adequately prepared for the societal changes when compared to the relatively peaceful lifestyle in Tanzania and Zambia. They were taken by surprise when they encountered the vicious politics and violence perpetuated by an invisible 'third force' that engulfed South Africa during the CODESA negotiations'—including the high crime rate. The most disturbing trend in the progress of a new democratic dispensation in South Africa was the continuing spiral of violence that went hand in hand with major breakthroughs in the negotiation process. Violence rapidly became the principal method of resolving disputes in a country with a history of severe repression in which police were distrusted and feared. Acts of violence were compounded by the criminal aspect, mostly in black townships where there was a virtual breakdown of law and order resulting in a state of near anarchy.

The returnees also mentioned a different problem-the fact that people were now self-centered, greedy and operated as individuals. It was now a case of everybody for himself, unlike the times when they left for exile. There was now an obvious lack of communal lifestyle, *inhlonipho* and *ubuntu,* particularly amongst the younger generation. But both Edith and Kholeka Thunyiswa were very happy about the intact extended family network support and the warm welcome they received from their extended family that still believed in African communalism. It seems as if their mother's visit while they were still in exile helped in this regard. She prepared the extended family, for they were well informed about the nurses' lives in exile—including the conditions they were living under—hence the Thunyiswa family could not wait for the two of them to return to their country of origin. On their return, the family showered them with the love and tender care that they deserved for their bravery and commendable deed of offering their services to the Tanzanian people. In hindsight, and during one of her yearly visits and pilgrimages back to South Africa, Kholeka Thunyiswa was: "*very grateful* ngezi *relatives* zami . . . ngibona *how other families are-me and my sister were very lucky . . . that is why I went to pay respect to my mother's grave* ndathi *hey* Mama ndiyabulela ndifike ekhaya ilikhaya, abanye abayitholanga lenhlalo esiyifumeneyo . . . izinto zijike kakubi . . . babe ne *impression* ukuthi sizobuya nemali, imali siyitholaphi?. . . . ne *salaries* bezi *low. But what else can you do in a developing country* into emnandi phaya (in Tanzania) is that abantu phaya bano buntu," (Interview, Thunyiswa).

Majodina identified primary characteristics inherent and intrinsic to the process of return and refer to such factors:

- The decision to return.
- The need to re-adapt to a society that has changed profoundly during the period of absence.
- The fact that old points of reference and foci of physical, social and emotional identification have altered.
- The different experiences encountered in exile, whereby the returning person built emotional, social and professional ties.
- Lastly, the fact that returning is the result of a previous decision to return, taken directly by the returnee or a member of the family group, (Majodina, 1998).

Edna Miya, who returned to South Africa for good in 1992, was one of the nurses that Kholeka Thunyiswa believed was unlucky. She was not as lucky as the Thunyiswa sisters because the odds were stacked against her when she returned home. When coming back to a home country, the returning person does not anticipate differences between him/herself and fellow countrymen, especially when the physical environment is similar. What is more pertinent is the fact that friends/family also do not expect the returnee to have difficulties in re-entering the home country. One final difference in adaptation to a foreign culture and adaptation to home concerns the element of change and awareness of change. When adapting to a foreign environment, there is of necessity a change in the physical and social surroundings, but the newcomer does not change within him/herself from the onset, (Majodina, 1998).

On her return, Miya realized that she was resented and ill treated by the majority of her immediate and extended family. She stayed with one of her sisters under difficult conditions and believed that what made matters worse was the "suitcase full of money" matter. The money she had at her disposal was enough just for her survival and part of it was the stipend provided to each returnee by the UNHCR. Conditions at home became so unbearable that she had to leave and look for her own accommodation after being rejected by her own family. Miya was helped in this regard by one woman who happened to be an ANC courier who used to visit her home in Zambia. She had subsequently moved from Tanzania to Zambia around 1965 when her husband was relocated by the ANC to the SACTU office in Lusaka.

It soon became noticeable to Miya that the pervasive fractious family relationship was fanned by divisive national politics engulfing South Africa during the early 1990s. Most of her family members were staunch supporters and members of the IFP and she was a stalwart of the ANC. This was exacerbated and complicated by the volatile relationship between the ANC and the IFP during the early 1990s including the political violence perpetuated by those who were against the political settlement. The official explanation was that these were incidents of political rivalry among different political formations, notably the IFP and ANC, and they were portrayed as 'black on black' violence. Initially, this kind of violence was largely confined to Natal. As the violence spread to other parts of the country, especially to African urban townships in the then southern Transvaal, it had the overall effect of maintaining a climate of fear in the country.

Miya had no options but to leave her sister's house and eventually found accommodation at a multi-racial old age home where she has stayed since 1996. Life was now very interesting for her. For the first time, she shared accommodation with die-hard supporters of the old dispensation who were not used to an African woman talking back to them on equal terms. Moreover, they had never shared accommodation with an ANC loyalist—their nemesis during the dark days of apartheid.

Luckily for Miya things fell into place as time went on; first, as a member of the ANC, she benefited from the special pension allocated by the South African Treasury to those who were members of liberation movements who had retuned from exile. This was part of the new dispensation agreed upon during the negotiations for a democratic political settlement. Second, she astutely planned her life while she was in exile. She had sold her house in Lusaka for substantial cash before she returned to South Africa and invested her money at Barclays Bank. In hindsight, Miya was grateful that she invested the money and did not bring it with her back to South Africa. She believed that if this did not happen, and opted to bring a suitcase full of money with her in 1992, her family and relatives would have taken advantage of her and abused her money. Probably they would have disowned her immediately after running out of cash, and revealed their true political colors. Fortunately again for Miya, the Chairman of Barclay's Bank in Zambia was Dr. Nalumango, a medical doctor who used to work with Miya at the Lusaka Hospital. After staying for four years at the old age home, Miya contacted Nalumango and explained her plight to him and asked him to transfer her savings into her bank account in South Africa. Her wise investment afforded her an opportunity to buy herself a well-kept flat in the Durban beachfront area where she still lives comfortably, (Interview, Miya). This is where oral history interviews were conducted with her. Miya paid cash for the flat and only pays her levies, which she could afford because she qualifies for the monthly senior citizen pension paid by the state. Because she could afford it, she therefore decided to leave the old age home so her room could be allocated to another needy senior citizen—just like her during the hard times when she returned from exile and was disowned by her own family. Edna Miya had this to say about her experiences- including reasons why she moved out from the old age home:

> Into eyenze ukuthi ngihambe e old age home kwafika ukuthi ugovernment wethu uyasinika imadlana encane (pension money), and kukhona abahluphekayo kakhulu *and* ngivale indawo yabanye abahluphekayo abanganayo le *luck* enginayo, uma ngiloku ngihlezi phezukwemali ngizoyenzani, angiyishiyele abanye lendawo abasenkingeni ephezu kwalena engikuyo, well noma bangathuka. *I mean* kumele ngilikhuluma iqiniso, kusizani ukuvala indawo ngoba kukhona umuntu oyidingayo indawo, uhlupheka ngaphezu kwami, nami ngiyahlupheka kodwa angihlupheki

> njengabanye—angishiyele lona ohlupheka ngaphezu kwami, ngayishiya lokho indawo ngoba ngangicabangela abantu ngendlela engangibona bahlupheka ngayo, also nokuba *independent* nje . . . ngihleli kahle kakhulu, *I have no problem*, ngoba ngathenga *cash (the flat)*, angina sikweletu- ngikhokhela i *levy. I think our government has been very fair to us, some of us are unemployable, I am quite happy here* (in her own flat), angikhali ngalutho. . . . (Interview, Miya)

But Edna Miya also became a victim of corruption and crime syndicates operating within government bodies. This also formed part of her painful experience on her return to South Africa. While in exile, Miya and her husband were also members of the MK underground. Many MK cadres and couriers—including members of the ANC and SACTU leadership—used their home in Lusaka as a safe house. This meant that, together with her husband, they were listed by the ANC as members of MK who qualified for South African National Defence Force (SANDF) benefits—again this was part of the deal struck during the negotiations for a democratic South Africa. Miya was one those demobilized militarily and was accordingly paid her benefits by the newly formed SANDF. She collected her payment in a form of a check from the Durban headquarters of the SANDF and went to deposit it at local bank in the city of Durban. It was early in the morning and the bank was not yet open when she arrived and had to wait outside the vicinity for the bank to open at 9 o'clock. Unknown to Miya, a criminal syndicate had an insider working for them at the SANDF headquarters. This person supplied information to this group of thugs about those who would come to collect large sums of money due to them. They had followed Miya, now a very old woman, in her seventies, to the bank, hijacked, blindfolded her, and put her in the boot of their car. They took her to a secluded spot where the criminals dumped her. This area was around the vicinity of the city of Durban. They robbed Edna Miya of her belongings—including the check from the SANDF. It was quite a substantial amount of money since her services (and those of her late husband) in the MK dated back to the 1960s. She survived this horrible ordeal that traumatized her. But through sheer luck she had not by then cashed the check and reported the incident to both the authorities and the bank. The check was cancelled and a new one was made out in her name, and she was subsequently paid what was due to her. This was quite a traumatic experience to her and it was definitely not what she went out to fight for. Edna Miya had first hand experiences of the challenges facing post-apartheid South Africa and recalled the following about the hijacking and attempted robbery—including the possible identity of the female SANDF insider:

> Labantu (the criminals) bangithole eBank ngisalindile *outside* ukuthi kuvulwe e *bank* kodwa kukhona lo owawumbona ukuthi nguye owayethumele labantu ngoba she is the only one owayezi ukuthi ngiyothatha icheque e Natal Command akekho omunye enjalo ke ebuwumungane walo obekunguyena who deals ne Natali nama *cheques* ase *Demobilisation office* eku *army* ePretoria. *So she knew I was going to get this cheque, she knew* . . . hayi bandla ngaya emaphoyiseni. *I was doing the right thing, the Defence Department replaced the cheque* ngase sengithi hayi ayiyekwe lento ngoba abantu bahluphekile, base beyi yeka amaphoyisa . . . angithi nakhu bangifaka emontweni, sangena emotweni, omunye ngapha, omunye ngale, bangivala amehlo safika kwenye indawo la ekwajoina khona inkosikazi engu number 3, ila engangena khona *in the boot of the car, it was a very good experience* ngokuthi sihlala sizwa abantu ukuthi *they are kidnapped* singazi ukuthi kanjani, namhlanje *I know*, ngoba mhlawumbe kuyokwenzeka okukhulu ngowenzeka kimi. . . . (Interview, Miya)

CONCLUSION

The most painful challenge for the nurses who returned from exile is the declining standard of nursing amongst the professionals. According to them, what they had experienced, particularly the professional conduct of some of the newly trained nursing professionals, leaves much to be desired and is a disgrace to their profession. Nevertheless, Edna Miya is forever positive and thinks the standards will improve in time:

> *Nursing standards in South Africa have gone down, it has gone down to zero. It is very sad to see nurses doing embarrassing things in the name of the profession, what I saw on Tuesday was worse, a nurse* uphikisana ne *patient, in uniform* ngahlala ngathula, kuthe sengihamba ngathi *your behaviour is an embarrassment to the nursing profession*, ngisho kathathu. I *also said to her, I think you bought your nursing certificate , a well trained nurse would not behave like this,* ngasho ngabaleka *before she could shout at me/scorn me*, ngathi mina ngenhliziyo sengimutshelilile uzwile, futhi ngimutshele phambi kwabanye abantu, ngathi *you are a disgrace to the nursing profession*, ngesikhathi *when she planned to respond I ran away.* Esibhedlela you expect to get help, uzoxolela ukuthi bekugcono usahleli ekhaya, *unless of course they know who you are (they treat you better), that is*

no longer nursing anyway. I think as time goes on things will change, I am sure about this. . . . (Interview, Miya)

NOTES

1. Interview with Edna Miya, conducted by Brown Maaba, 19 July 2002, Durban, SADET Oral History Project.
2. 'The First Conference of Independent African States,' Accra, April 15–22, 1958, J. A. Langley, *Ideologies of Liberation in Black Africa 1856–1970*, London, Rex Collings, 1979, 765–775.
3. Brown Maaba on behalf of the SADET Oral History Project conducted interviews of Kholeka Thunyiswa, Edna Miya and Mary Jane Socenywa and Sifiso Ndlovu interviewed Edith Thunyiswa. Maaba interviewed Kholeka Thunyiswa in new Brighton-Port Elizabeth on 1/10/2002, whilst she was on holidays in South Africa. He interviewed Socenywa on 14/9/2002. I interviewed Edith Thunyiswa on the 8th of August 2002 at the ANC headquarters in Johannesburg.
4. See Jane McLarty Papers, A2197, B1.1, 'Baragwanath College of Nursing: History of Nursing, Lecture 6,' University of Witwatersrand Department of Historical Papers; C. Searle, *The History of the Development of Nursing in South Africa, 1652–1960: A Socio-Historical Survey*, Struik, Cape Town, 1965.
5. In the case of South African indigenous medicine and practitioners, see for example, five volumes of the James Stuart Archives in C. Webb and J. Wright, *The James Stuart Archive of Recorded Oral Evidence Relating to the History of the Zulu and Neighbouring Peoples*, Durban and Pietermaritzburg, 1976–1986, 5 vols., proceedings; Harriet Ngubane, *Body and Mind in Zulu Medicine: An Ethnography of Health and Disease in Nyuswa-Zulul and Thought and Practice,* London and New York, Academic Press, 1977; A.T. Bryant, *Zulu Medicine and Medicine Men, Cape Town, Struik, 1966;* About the African Continent see M. Last and G.L Chavunduka, *The Professionalisation of African Medicine*, Manchester, Manchester University Press, 1986.
6. See S. Marks, *Divided Sisterhood: Race Class and Gender in the South African Nursing Profession*, St Martin's Press, New York, 1994, Chapter 4. James B. McCord and John Scott Douglass, *My Patients were Zulus*, Muller, 1946. The first African to train as a medical practitioner was John Nembula and he received his degree in Chicago in 1891, see S. Zondi's PhD thesis about Nembula, University of Cambridge; C. Bourquin, *The Story of Masana Hospital*; see also the publication *Elim* Hospita[l]; both hospitals were set up by the Swiss Mission (both publications are available at UNISA). See also Searle, 1965; Last and Chavunduka, 1986.
7. Archaic, ideological and racist terms such as non-European, non-white abound in the text and have similar meanings as in the past.
8. See Jane McLarty Papers, A2197, B1.1, 'Baragwanath College of Nursing: History of Nursing, Lecture 6,' University of Witwatersrand Department of Historical Papers; Marks, 1994. C. Searle, 1965.

9. Interview with Edna Miya, conducted by Brown Maaba, 19/7/2002, SADET Oral History Project.
10. Interview with Henry Makgothi, conducted by Sifiso Ndlovu, Johannesburg, 7/4/2002, SADET Oral History Project; Marks, 1994.
11. See B. Pogrund, *How Can Man Die Better: The Life of Robert Sobukwe*, Jonathan Ball, Johannesburg, 1990, 32.
12. Union of South Africa House of Assembly Debates, 18th January to 22nd June 1957; hereafter cited in text as Assembly Debates, 1957.
13. J. McLarty, "Amendment to the Nursing Act and its effect on Non-European Representation," *South African Nursing Journal*, March, 1956; hereafter cited in text as Amendment to the Nursing Act; Searle, 1965.
14. Assembly Debates, 1957; Marks, 1994; M. Jarrett-Kerr, *African Pulse: Scenes from an African Hospital Window*, London, The Faith Press, 1960, Chapter 4; Searle, 1965.
15. M. Jarrett-Kerr, 1960; Marks, 1994; Union of South Africa House of Assembly Debates, 18th January to 22nd June 1957; C. Searle, *The History of the Development of Nursing in South Africa, 1652–1960.*
16. FEDSAW Papers, Memorandum for submission to the Board of the South African Nursing Association, approved by the members of the non-European Group of the Witwatersrand branch present at a general meeting on 9/12/1954, held at the non-European Hospital, Johannesburg, AD 1137/Cb2-Db, University of the Witwatersrand Department of Historical Papers.
17. FEDSAW Papers, Letter from the African National Congress Women's league and the Federation of South African Women, signed by Mary Ranta-the national secretary of the Women's League and Helen Joseph the national secretary of FEDSAW on 8/5/1957, AD 1137/Cb 2-Db, University of the Witwatersrand Department of Historical Papers.
18. South African Nursing Act, No 69, of 1957; hereafter cited in text as Nursing Act, 1957.
19. FEDSAW Papers, Circular No 1 issued by the Organising Committee for National Conference of Nurses, 8/8/1957, AD 1137/Cc 1–3, University of the Witwatersrand Department of Historical Papers.
20. See memorandum and statement on incident at Boksburg-Benoni Hospital' issued and signed by V. Peteni and N.J. Ramusi of the Rand Nurses' Professional Club, FEDSAW Papers, AD 1137/Cc6, University of the Witwatersrand Department of Historical papers; hereafter cited in text as FEDSAW papers, 1137/Cc6.
21. FEDSAW Papers, Memorandum submitted to the Federation of South African Nurses and Midwives and to the Rand Nurses Professional Club by the FEDSAW, 9/2/1958; See also pamphlets titled 'Nationalist government piles insult on injuries,' "Nurses beware!"; "Why should nurses carry passes?" AD 1137/Cc 4.1–4.7; Cc 1–3 and Cc 5, University of the Witwatersrand Department of Historical Papers.
22. *The Star*, 22/3/1958.
23. FEDSAW Papers, Memorandum to the Matron of Baragwanath Hospital and the Principal of the training College for Non-European Nurses, AD

1137/Cc 4.1–4.7, Cc 5, University of the Witwatersrand Department of Historical Papers.

24. "Pretoria Gang: New Plot to Degrade Others," *South African Nursing Journal*, April 1959, pp.4–5. The editors of this Journal published these documents in order to highlight the dangers posed by those they referred to as agitators. The editors believed that "for some time now our Non-White Members have been subjected to pamphleteering and in some instances victimisation and reprisals have resulted." See also Searle, *The History of the Development of Nursing in South Africa, 1652–1960*.
25. "United We Stand, Divided . . . !," *South African Nursing Journal*, April 1959, 5–6; hereafter cited in text as United We Stand.
26. "Nurses' Grievance at King George V Hospital," *Natal Mercury*, 10/8/1961; K. Luckhardt and B. Wall, *Organise . . . or Starve!: The History of the South African Congress of Trade Unions*, Lawrence and Wishart, London, 1980, 312.
27. "300 Non-White Nurses in protest March," *Natal Mercury*, 11/8/1961, "Nurse Complaints Were Politically Inspired-Elston," "Man Arrested near Hospital," *Natal Mercury*, 12/8/1961; Marks, 1994; Luckhardt and Wall, 1980.
28. Interview with Edna Miya. IsiZulu not translated-note how she uses both isiZulu and English during the interview.
29. Interview with Edna Miya, conducted by Brown Maaba. Luckhardt and Wall have a slightly different interpretation of events mentioned above. They also claim that professional nurses were involved in the burning of the linen room whilst Miya eyewitness account note that it was nurse aids.
30. Z. Majodina, "Home at Last: The Re-entry Adaptation of Returned South African Exiles," PhD thesis, University of Cape Town, 1998, Chapter 3.
31. Bechualand is a former British protectorate now referred to as Botswana.
32. See M. Gunther, 'The National Committee of Liberation (NCL)/African Resistance Movement (ARM),' in SADET, *The Road to Democracy in South Africa: Volume 1 (1960–1970)*, Zebra Press, Cape Town, 2004, Chapter 5.
33. On Fish Keitsing role and the routes into exile see S.M. Ndlovu, "The ANC in Exile," in SADET, *The Road to Democracy in South Africa*, Chapter 11.
34. About these MK cadres journeys into exile in June 1962 see S. M. Ndlovu, "The ANC in Exile," SADET, *The Road to Democracy*, Chapter 11.
35. L. Bucheret, *Education in the Development of Tanzania: 1919–1990*, Athens, Dar es Salaam and London, Ohio University Press, Mkuki na Nyota and James Curry, 1994.
36. A. Beck, *Medicine, Tradition, and Development in Kenya and Tanzania: 1920–1970*, Massachusetts, Crossroads Press, 1981. See also R. Aikhtar (ed), *Health and Disease in Tropical Africa: Geographical and Medical Viewpoints*, London, 1987; Last and Chavunduka, 1986.
37. Interview with Edna Miya; See also Beck, 1981; O. Jakobsen, "Economic and Geographical Factors Influencing Child Malnutrition in the Southern

Highlands, Tanzania" in R. Aikhtar (ed), *Health and Disease in Tropical Africa*, Chapter 9.

38. "The First Conference of Independent African States," Langley, *Ideologies of Liberation in Black Africa.*
39. Interview with Kholeka Thunyiswa. Kholeka's mother visited them again during the 1970s, but passed away during the 1980s whilst she was making arrangements to visit her exiled daughters for the third time.
40. He subsequently adopted his sister and is staying with her in South Africa.

Part II

Human Trafficking and Exploitation

Chapter Seven

Trafficking of Young Women and Girls: A Case of "Au Pair" and Domestic Laborers in Tanzania

Elinami Veraeli Swai

INTRODUCTION

A huge number of women are currently participating in labor, inside and outside their countries. This has attracted world community and scholars in various fields and has been constructed as a social issue in need of immediate solution. Women's movement and their participation in various activities has been identified as immoral and linked with illegal activity of transaction of human beings. This linkage cannot be separated from a recent manifestation of the North/South, East/West divide. Thus virtually anything that disturbs this divide is seen as illegal. Thus, women's movements and participation in global economy has been constructed as a threat to national and global security, a construction that has created moral panic.

This chapter explores the diverse ways that house girls and au pairs negotiate their identities as women and construct their life course trajectories. I situate them within the debate of trafficking of human beings and exploitation of women in a global economy. Based on critical ethnographic research with two house girls in Tanzania and one Tanzanian au pair in the United States, I present these women's narratives of their experiences before and after engaging themselves in house girl and au pair activities. Based on representations of "informal labor" and "women's movement," I critique the discourses about human traffic that immortalize women's movement and their activities, specifically those which are considered "informal" such as paid domestic activities and au pairing. Using the notion of habitus, I analyze and describe how social, historical and political context in Tanzania have shaped women's lives and experiences and how women have actively configure their identity in participating in "not so formal" domestic and au pair activities.

THE MORAL PANIC AND ITS CONSEQUENCES ON WOMEN'S LIVES

It is important in this chapter to stress that African women have for a long time been portrayed as victims of male partners, relatives or neighbors. Some scholars have identified them as victims of social and political processes. These representations imply that African women are incapable of safeguarding their rights as women. Their voices and actions within such a framework become muted and criminalized. For example, given that working "informally" is either illegal or not fully decriminalized, a woman who decides to engage in such activities is made to admit her guilt or the decision is understood as not of her own volition. Only by claiming to have been kidnapped, lured, or misled into moving and engage in certain activities can she expect any help from most women's organizations or the State.

Criminalization of women's behavior can be traced back to the Puritan vision of a "godly community," in seventeenth Century, during the time that Western society created the idea of virtuous female identity centered on chastity. Young girls and women were expected to be obedient, humble, and modest and to assume domestic responsibilities. Their movement from inside the house and their homes to outside were linked with immorality. Those who failed to adhere to female virtues were punished.

Politicians, scholars and researchers have attempted to incite people into emotional acceptance of female virtuous and failure from this standard has created moral panic. Now, no doubt, certain movements of women, particularly those not permitted by male relatives such as a husband, father, brother or uncle, are associated with immorality.

Stanley Cohen's (1972) *Folk Devils and Moral Panics* defines the moral panic as when "[a] condition, episode, person, or group of persons emerges to become defined as a threat to societal values and interests; its nature is presented in a stylized and stereotypical fashion by the mass media; the moral barricades are manned by . . . right-thinking people; socially accredited experts pronounce their diagnoses and solutions; ways of coping are evolved or (more often) resorted to; the condition then disappears, submerges or deteriorates and becomes more visible."[1]

A moral panic, as expanded upon in Stuart Hall et al.'s (1978) *Policing the Crisis*, is also distinguished by its "ability to connote a whole complex of social themes."[2] The moral is discursively drawn as a symptom or symbol of larger social, cultural, political, and economic issues. As the prominence of particular individual issues shifts, the message can be redrawn. But for whom is the moral drawn and re-drawn? The focus of the discourse about trafficking of women intends to achieve two goals: to instill and enforce a moral order by criminalizing women's activities outside their homes and communities. This discourse fails to account for women who loiter aimlessly in rural areas, engaged in other illicit activities or live their lives on other people especially men.

The discourse of trafficking of women discursively naturalizes activities that dehumanize women by linking activities that women perform with the traditional discourse on the role and position of women in society. This discourse, which persistently invokes the images of women outside of their homes as being under attack—being raped and sexually exploited—draws in the support of scholars, both feminists and non-feminists alike. While many feminists often object to unequal allocation of resources to men and women, they paradoxically support the policing of women's decisions to appropriate alternatives to end their oppression and exploitation. In an uneasy alliance with the views of the Right, this support from the Left lends an air of common sense to the strengthening of women's protection: law and morality are enforced; vulnerable women in the global economy are protected.

The literature of trafficking of women has been written by feminists, human rights activists, religious groups and other social and cultural activists since 1980s.[3] While it is difficult to synthesize all what has been written, an essential aspect of this debate especially about African women is carried out to create public sympathy for the exploitation and oppression of African women in global economy. The rhetoric about exploitation of African women was established through a variety of debates: by stressing that African women are illiterate, poor and are confined in the home. Their movement outside their confined homes may attract men who may take advantage of their ignorance.

A study on trafficking in women in East Africa by GTZ, a German organization in East Africa for instance, combined women and children in their analysis. This study reports trafficking in children as to be facilitated by a "family friend"' or acquaintance and people in a position of trust, and these trafficked children " . . . find themselves living on the street or in slum areas and are at this stage vulnerable to abuse, especially commercial sexual exploitation."[4] The analysis continues to identify African women as been trafficked to Saudi Arabia and United Arab Emirates for domestic labor and for prostitution. These women, the study reports, are " . . . deceived as to the amount of money they will earn, the working conditions and sometimes even as to the type of job they will do (for example, promised work as nurses, nannies). These women, the author continues are forced to work 18 hour days, have no rest day, are underpaid or not paid at all, are raped, beaten, threatened and locked in the house . . . such women suffer gross human rights violations in complete isolation; they are forbidden from communicating with anyone, including their families . . ." (Weedon, 1999, 4).

There is no doubt that the issues addressed by anti-trafficking campaigns are in urgent need of attention, including unprecedented levels of movement of women from rural to urban areas, movement of unqualified people from one country to another, particularly from developing countries to developed ones, unwanted aliens in developed nations, the exploitation of informal and illegal migrants, and the growing use of migrants as indentured or even slave labor.

However, anti-trafficking campaigns are unable to separate women from children, identify the real 'informal employment' and to remedy the oppression and exploitation within this sector. This is in part because the framing of these grave problems as "trafficking" or criminal "smuggling" assumes that the affected trafficked women are moved, without their knowledge and against their will. The "trafficker" in this transaction becomes the lure and main culprit in women's exploitation. Such a framing of the problem leaves many crucial questions unasked and unanswered, questions such as: What are the conditions from which women are moving? Why are most women able to move with the assistance of smuggling operations? What are the global market options currently available for women? How are socio-cultural and historical processes and practices implicated in this?

I would argue that the myth of construction of African women by sexual harassment and rape, has gained resonance as it has followed the pattern of a moral panic. Not only does the construction of this particular moral panic about women's participation in the global economy serve conservative interests vis-à-vis women's sexual regulation and the marginalization of their agency, but it also casts any woman who does not participate in "womanhood" activities, such as being at home, being an obedient daughter or a married woman, as an outcast, one that needs to be punished or even excommunicated. Thus, the panic undermines the production of counter-narratives as well as any debate on the broader and more complex reasons that women make decisions to participate in the global economy as house girls and au pairs. This situation calls for research on the structural, cultural and psychological factors that prompt women in making decisions to become a house girl or an au pair. I suggest that the politics of identifying African women as unique kind of women, who cannot understand whether they are been trafficked or not, represent them as victims. The construction of African women as illiterates, poor and invisible in public sphere serves as a perfect alibi for their illegal trafficker and exploiting employer to lure and exploit them. In this situation, African women become victims in need of rescue from traffickers and exploiting employers. I argue that rather than identifying women as victims and their behavior as immoral, it is more useful to situate them in a specific historical, economic and social context in which their subjectivities are developed.

This study takes issue with two presumptions in particular: first, that there is an ideal woman and second, that all women interpret the world in the same way. The imagined woman and the imagined relationship between women and global processes are virtually never idly constructed, but typical codes are embedded in certain meanings with certain implications. This chapter proposes an alternative way of understanding African women and house girls and au pairs as highly differentiated group of people with differences of sexual orientation, class, ethnicity and age; each with different ways to interpret her world and different goals in life. The decisions that these women make—to be or not to be a house girl—may be shaped by socio-cultural and historical conditions in their homes and communities, but these conditions are not in themselves a cause their marginalization or their decision to become house girls.

One of the common arguments on issues pertaining to women who work in not so 'formal' employment, such as house girl or au pair, has been the growing interest in showing how social systems, processes and practices work to oppress women. With an emphasis on cultural analysis, most scholarship demonstrates that the decision to become a house girl or au pair is a part of a larger global process. This articulation is thus a form of direct connection between what ahouse girl and au pair are and can do, and the impact of global processes upon them. I argue that the linkage between global processes and what a house girl and au pair do is not necessarily determined, absolute and essential for all women. To understand the reason one decides to engage in a particular activity like house girl or au pair, we have first, to identify each house girl and au pair not as a generic group with a fixed experience, but as complex individuals each embodying concrete experiences that shape the way they interpret social processes. In understanding these varying and contradictory experiences we need to ask, under what circumstances can the global processes work to create a condition, which may work to shape how women think and act? Asking this question prior to making connections between a house girl or au pair with the social processes, will help in moving away from any essentializing, objectifying, and further dehumanizing women. It will allow for identifying women as individuals with different dispositions, habits and preferences who interpret social forces in different ways.

Furthermore, linking women's movement and their involvement in various 'informal' activities is to marginalize their agency and valorize prostitution, sexual harassment, and women's dependency in the homes and communities. There are two significant pernicious effects associated with such rhetoric and the actions based upon it. The first is the essentialization of women as victims or as a threat to societal health and the global economy, a debate that has an effect in disempowering those who are engaged in employment outside the home and formal employment sector.

Secondly, such regulation of women's movements and activities, the marginalization of their agency, and attendant constructions of their roles and positions in society and in global economy, chip away at the gains made in the liberation of women over the last thirty years. In essence, this moralizing control represents an outright disparaging of several other feminist concerns. The debate is centered on moral limits regarding the persistent inequalities of gender, race, class, and sexuality. This focus hinders the discussion of broader structural problems. The contexts of such differences in economic, political, social, and cultural power are lost, as any argument that does not reference the hot button or the main issues and simplified morals is accused of "missing the point." Feminists and other advocates of women's experiences in the global economy must work actively to return the discussion to these inequalities and their sources, as well as the potential for change.

Third, demonizing women's movements and their engagement in informal employment further complicates the process of finding solutions to their concerns and problems. Exploitation "away from home" is conceptualized as a separate problem from exploitative and/or untenable economic relations "at home." This sanitizes and helps to hide the domestic issues of exploitation by focusing on external/international exploitation. Women's oppression and exploitation come to be identified with their movements within national boundaries and abroad and loses its moorings from the organization and expansion of capitalist social relationships wherein women and their labor are alienated. In the process, exploitation at home is left naturalized and therefore depoliticized as a safe site for women. As a result, the fact that capital is accrued and accumulated through employers' appropriation of a portion of women's labor power is concealed. Moreover, the fact that people often move because they have been dislocated from their homes is left unaddressed by the romanticization of being "at home." By making women's movement the problem, it is assumed that women's movement and engagement in 'informal' employment is something that is inherently damaging. Informal sector has of recent been identified as a space for women to pull away from the constraints of poverty, dependency, and gender conflict. At the same time, women's engagement in the informal sector, in activities such as domestic service and au pairing, is seen as exploitative and "dehumanizing."[5] Yet, despite public perceptions of house girls and au pairs as exploited and ignorant, with narratives that they are duped and lied about the horrendous condition of their employment.

THEORETICAL FRAMEWORK

House girls and au pairs appear to appropriate their social capital to access available alternatives—being house girls or au pairs—that lie within their reach. Pierre Bourdieu argues that for one to make a decision is not entirely dependent on individuals or social structures (patriarchy, the state or the global economy), but in "the relation between two realizations of historical action, in bodies and in things."[6] "House girling" and "au pairing" are activities that have been developed within the global context, and many women, especially those who are restricted from formal education, skills training, and capital, may identify themselves with these activities more than with other jobs available in the world. This identification shape their thinking and behavior not for adaptability as evolution theorists may want us to believe, but for sheer life survival and development.

Bourdieu's concept of habitus provides a useful way of theorizing ways and reasons women make the decision to become house girls and/or au pairs.[7] Habitus, like social capital, refers to the framework within which individuals make decisions and act, based on their needs, interests, and preferences; together with the specific social position one inhabits. Here he argues one's experiences and actions within a specific situation act as a background to perception, cognition and a basis for intentions. The objective conditions of the habitus give individuals a sense of what is possible and what is not possible to do. Different habitus and, therefore, different practices emerge from different needs, interests and social positions.

Because women differ by habitus and resources (including level of education, social position, material resources, needs and interests), their decisions also differ. Others may despair due to life conditions at home and decide to become beggars or a prostitutes regardless of abuse and mistreatment; others may be faced with the same situation and decide to look for a job in town or abroad. Others just acquiesce.

Feminist researchers on women's identity and experience, together with adult education researchers, are increasingly exploring the context in which people's experience is formed and how that experience shapes one's thinking and behavior. These scholars have shifted from looking into individual's perception and attitude into looking at one's context, including her history, social, economic, political and location.

This chapter is based on empirical research with two house girls in Tanzania and one au pair in the US, I analyze the intersection of their gendered, class, ethnicity, age and location and how these have produced these women's subjectivity and how they negotiate their identities despite all odds.

First, the concept of identity and African womanhood identity is discussed, which inform the chapter as a whole. This is followed by discussion of socio-cultural and historical conditions in rural Tanzania, which intersect with cultural ideas about Tanzanian womanhood. This frame is used to identify the current condition of Tanzanian women and the roles and position of house girls and au pairs in the global economy, which underpin the three substantive sections of the chapter.

IDENTITY

Women all over the world have engaged themselves in various roles in society. Like other women, African women, and Tanzanian women in particular, do not all share the same interests, desires, roles and positions, (Weedon, 1999). But socio-cultural and historical processes produced various policies, practices and institutions, which support their ideologies that stereotype women as ignorant, backward and easily subject to exploitation. These ideologies effect the identification of women as different from men and a possibility for assigning them certain roles and positions different from those of men. Womanhood, as an identity different from manhood, has come to be seen as imposing on women certain standards that categorize them as normal or abnormal.

Feminists have used the politics of identification as method to understand the process(es) of identification. In other words, rather than focusing on women as "women," the end product of their identification, they examine the processes in which "women" comes to be and behave like "women." This has proved to be more useful because it points to the dynamic processes in which and individual comes to be a 'woman,' the process one she undergoes to negotiate and struggle to achieve self-actualization.

Many feminist researchers have recognized that "'womanhood," and African womanhood in particular, is a social identity for African women imposed on them, from Western idea of middle class women morality.[8] These ideas erroneously represent African women as extensions of men and systematically plot them inside the house to assume roles that have not, and do not fit their socio-cultural and political realities.

African feminists suggest that to understand African women's real experiences (including their reasons for doing what they do as women), we need to identify the role and impact of the West in the production of ideas about African womanhood, and the continued dominance of Western institutions in the production and manipulation of knowledge. They further argue that understanding African women's realities is a useful analytical device for moving away from identifying African women as abstract entities and to pay attention instead on individual women's experiences, based on local or regional cultural epistemologies.[9]

This concept has its origins in Mudimbe's idea of exploiting African philosophy in order to understand traditional African systems of thought and experiences.[10] Many African feminists have started to identify African women from an African perspective and have pointed to the complex position of women in African societies and describe it as fluid and situational.[11] Unlike in the West, women's roles and position in many African societies have been found not to depend on their gender, but on a myriad of interconnection and interdependence of relationships and positions. In other words, many African women's roles and position are produced through a multiple interconnected relations and positions within and beyond the continent. Throughout this chapter, an understanding of the process of identifying African womanhood is useful to illustrate the processes by which house girls and au pairs in Tanzania have been constructed and their struggle to negotiate their identity in the current global economy.

METHODOLOGY

This chapter is based on findings from critical ethnographic research conducted with two house girls in Dar-es-Salaam, Tanzania, and one au pair in North America in June to September 2004, followed by a further three months in June to September 2005. During the time of my research, I encountered a lot of resistance to the framework I was employing. My aim was to capture and document narratives of domestic workers who had worked both in Tanzania and those who had involved themselves in au pair program in the US. "Au pair" is a French phrase meaning "at the par" or "at the peer" level, and is used to describe someone who boards temporarily in someone else's home. Both a house girl and au pair do the same kind of a job, which is termed "informal employment," only that an au pair works abroad.

In this research, I utilized several research methods, including document analysis, interviews and participant observation. The women were identified through purposive sampling emanating from my personal contact with the women in question. I engaged in an analysis of documents about the socio-cultural and historical conditions of rural Tanzania and looked into policies and practices on education for girls and women. I also analyzed the policy on land in relation to women in rural Tanzania. Most interviews were conducted in women's workplaces, although on several occasions we talked over lunch or afternoon tea in restaurants. Sometimes we would decide to change a venue and meet outside in the park due to the noise of restaurant talk, people's staring or music, which interfered with our taped conversations. But even in those places, noise interference was often unavoidable as wind and car horns often drowned out dialogue, despite my use of modern recording devices.

I considered women as active participants in the knowledge system I was constructing. Therefore, I found participatory methods such as sharing our life stories particularly appropriate in engaging women in the knowledge that we were constructing together. Participatory methods are considered particularly useful in enabling research participants to have more control of their lives.[12] Interviews touched on the women's activities in their jobs as house girls and au pair, but added questions about the condition of their lives in the past and in the present, and how they visualize their future. Participant observation captured the actual activities that the house girls and au pair were engaged in. In this case, my observation was focused on these women's cooking, cleaning, arranging the house and any other household chores they were performing. After completing the interviews, I read to each woman her transcript for checking, editing, and validation. None of the women asked to make changes to their transcripts.

RESOURCE ALLOCATION AND CONSTRUCTION OF TANZANIAN WOMANHOOD

Before examining the allocation of resources to women in rural Tanzania, it is important to understand the historical context from which they emerged. Social and economic policies that have been implemented in Tanzania were developed during the German and British colonial regimes. In the re-organization of society and re-allocation of resources, colonialists identified women as extensions of men, and it was seen as legitimate to allocate resources to men with the idea that women would benefit from their relationship with men. Colonial administrators were worried that if women accessed resources on equal terms with men, this would offset the fabric of society where women were supposed to take care of home and children, while men went outside the home for employment.

In the education sector, education for women was geared towards being good wives and mothers, with a curriculum that insisted on cookery, sewing, crocheting, knitting, and literacy for bible study.[13] The curriculum also incorporated issues of morals and values. For example, women were taught "how to behave like women," what to wear, and the virtues of hard labor. Christian values insisted on leaving behind traditional beliefs and practices, as well as beliefs and practices of "witchcraft and sorcery." In this way, local knowledge that women possessed and used to solve their perceived problems were marginalized and demonized.

On the issues of access to land and use, the colonial powers introduced a land tenure system in which land was transformed from communally owned, where women could access and utilize it freely to plant food crops, to formal land tenure with legal rights. Land tenure alienated women from free access to land through the institutionalization of monetary terms and other means as compensation for land access. This apart, land as a public resource was to be used primarily for cash crop plantation. Women as food crop producers were automatically alienated from the land, and their accessing it demanded exploitation of their labor or even their humanity.

During and after political independence in 1961, not much was changed in terms of content and structure from the inherited colonial policies and practices, especially with regard to the empowerment of women. To concretize this system, the government embarked on a project to expand basic education and launch literacy programs to ensure that every child and adult obtained at least basic education and literacy skills. The policy of "Education for Self Reliance" aimed at equipping all citizens with the skills and knowledge to enable them to be effective in terms of economic production. Nyerere's argument was that people are generally served better when the state takes a strongly interventionist stance and that this intervention would act as a form of delegitimizing failure by expanding basic education to tertiary and university levels.[14] As correctly observes, literacy became "a necessary means of reaching the people at various sites to explain the objectives of [socialism] and the means by which they could be realized," (Mushi, 118). The curriculum focused on attaining reading, writing and simple arithmetic, and national awareness with particular emphasis on agriculture, national ideology, nutrition, animal husbandry and home economics, (Mushi).

Thus the rapid expansion of basic education and literacy programs, which culminated in the introduction of Universal Primary Education in 1977 and literacy campaigns in 1979, secondary and tertiary education was introduced in the country within the framework of the Manpower

Requirement Approach (MRA).[15] This approach focused on human capital philosophy—an approach to education geared towards expansion of people's capabilities to meet perceived social needs, including an individual's command of resources.[16] For example, the fundamental question of what type of education should be provided was debated from the time the government attained political independence. Such a question entailed that the provision of education was to reflect the government and political elites' conceptions of the purpose of knowledge and education in the society.

Education in this conception is geared towards inculcating knowledge and skills to solve perceived problems. In this way, the provision of education created a condition that devalued certain knowledge systems that were not perceived as necessary by the political elite, and which could be tapped to widen people's needs and interests. It can be argued that these educational policies and practices institutionalized exclusion and marginalization of women and other groups; that they prevented these people not only from accessing formal employment but also from developing their full professional potentials and capacities. The land tenure and employment policies were not re-aligned to cope with educational change. This change could have had a significant impact on the empowerment of women in the society.

WOMEN AND INEQUALITY IN ACCESSING RESOURCES IN TANZANIA

As literature in Tanzania shows, women in Tanzania are overrepresented among the underprivileged, although their disadvantages vary with age, income, wealth, ethnicity, and region.[17] Compared to men, they have a higher rate of illiteracy, unemployment and poverty. Women in Tanzania also have unequal access to property, credit and employment opportunities. Most of them are engaged in the informal sector and unpaid work, without benefits such as social security or unemployment compensation. Women are also underrepresented in domestic politics and labor unions. They suffer from limited bargaining power both inside and outside the household, and many are victims of domestic violence.

Thus, in Tanzania, women were curtailed around a common identity through the provision of education and allocation of land, both of which developed policies and practices that excluded them with the consequences of silencing and pauperizing them. I argue that the process of silencing and pauperize women on the one hand, and their inability to participate in formal employment on the other, effects the linking of their participation in informal employment and the contemporary debate about trafficking of human being. Political elites fear that women's movement and participation in remunerated activities would increase their autonomy and threaten social cohesion. These fears are mirrored in the debate of women movement and their participation in informal employment in the form of "trafficking" leads to the construction of women as "already victims" of global processes, exploited and oppressed, rather than informed individuals who can exercise their agency and make choices to achieve their individual self-actualization.

The following section provides a brief description of three women in this study, who in the midst of their structural marginalization and exploitation, as well as in the cultural identification as women, made a conscious decision to improve their lives through various means.

WENI

Weni is a 35-year-old woman working as a house girl in a suburb of Dar-Es-Salaam. She hailed from Iringa where she had been living with her seven siblings; she is the first born in the family. When she completed standard seven, like many other children in her rural village, Weni was not selected to go for further education because her parents could not afford the fee. Usually, in a society where there are many children to send to school, a family would decide who gets the priority, and the boys tend to be the chosen ones. Girls are normally remanded at home to learn about domestic economy. After completing her basic education, Weni lived with her parents working in their potato farm and helping to sell them in the nearby market. Sometimes she helped her mother with selling other items such as cookies and cooked potatoes at the bus station and to the bus passengers bound for Dar-es-Salaam. As she narrated her story Weni recalled: "Life was very hard for all of us because though we tried very hard to till the land, plant, weed and harvest on time, we did not realize much from selling because everybody else was doing the same thing. Not many people bought potatoes from others in the neighborhood, and we did not have a large farm, which could produce enough to sell in bulk to other places such as Morogoro, Dodoma or Dar-es-Salaam. In such a situation, we did not have other materials such as cloth, shoes or even a bed to sleep on."

Weni recalls how she dreamt of ending her poverty and that of her parents and siblings. She could not get any paying job in her rural village, and she had not acquired job training to give her options in life. The only thing she dreamt of doing was to work as a house girl in a rich family, where she could use the skills she had from assuming family chores. This resonates with Bourdieu's (1990) concepts of habitus and field, in which individuals use their habitus to understand what is possible and what is not possible to do, given their position in a particular field. Weni possessed skills (habitus) in household chores, and becoming ahouse girl (field) was the only alternative for her to pursue. At the beginning, Weni recalls:

> I did not know where to start. I did not know who to ask, or how to get information of who would want to hire me as a house girl. But one day, Mungu sio Athumani—meaning God has no partiality as men do—I was selling potatoes as usual, and one woman from the bus asked where she could find a girl to look after her children in Dar-es-Salaam. I told her I was interested and was ready to go with her. She said she was going to Mbeya and after one week she would pick me up on her way back to Dar-Es-Salaam. I knew that was the only chance for me to engage in a paying job. It did not matter how much she would pay me, I was earning nothing at home and the life was not that enjoyable at home.

When Weni asked permission from her parents she was met with a very negative response. Her father threatened to curse her if she left without permission from him. Weni realized that her parents were not considering her as a person, but as free labor. She decided to go ahead with her plan and that was her beginning, leaving her rural village to what she considered her freedom as an independent individual.

In her role as a house girl, Weni acknowledged that though she works very hard and for long hours, and although she knows that what she is being paid does not measure up to her labor, her life in her employer's home is much better than that of her own home. In her job she has a guarantee of food, better shelter, clothing and some money to send home and to pay the school fees for her two youngest siblings.

TINA

Growing up in rural Songea in the southern part of Tanzania, Tina describes herself as the best house girl any employer would want. She stated, "I just know I am the best house girl in the vicinity because I enjoy what I do and many people have approached me to work for them. I like my employer and we get along very fine."

Tina narrated her story of growing up in rural Songea as a bad dream that she will not forget for her whole life, and which she does not want to dream ever again. She was raised by her single mother who gave birth to her before marriage, but who married later when Tina was about age 4.

While trying to fit in with her half sister and half brother, who came immediately after her mother's marriage, Tina realized very early in life that she was not accepted as one of the family. Tina recalled vividly how her stepfather did not like her from the beginning and how together with her mother he treated her cruelly, differently from her half sister and brother. As she narrated:

> My parents (meaning her stepfather) was not a poor man, he was a primary school teacher and we were not a large family as many others in the neighborhood. But I always did not have enough to eat, nice cloth like my younger sister, or as nice bed sheets as she had. Worse still, when I was about 14 my stepfather started raping me. He did this many times, and whenever I complained to my mother she reprimand me saying I am trying to break her marriage with my lies. When I remember this, I always think my mother thought I was the worst thing to happen to her life, a curse or something, I suppose.

After completing standard seven and enduring several rapes, Tina decided to elope with her secret boyfriend, whom she had met at school. But life did not go as smoothly as she had envisaged and later she begged her aunt who lived in Dar-es-Salaam to take her in and let her live at her house. It did not take long before Tina got a job as a house girl in the neighboring house, where she had worked for more than ten years at the time of the interview.

KUMBWA

After completing form six at Jangwani Girls' High school in the city of Dar-Es-Salaam, Kumbwa stumbled onto an organization that was involved in recruiting girls for au pair jobs in America. By the time I conducted this interview, Kumbwa was 21 and had been working as an au pair for five years. I was curious to know how she came to be an au pair after she had studied in the most prestigious girls' school in the country. Here is her story:

> I am the last born of the family of six children. I have two sisters and three brothers, all of whom had finished high school and two of them undergraduate education. When I completed my form six, my elder sister, who had an undergraduate degree of more than four years, was still looking for a job and was so desperate to take any job she could get. This was very depressing for the whole family because there was no

> office that she had not visited. It is not that she had no good grades, for she has upper second. So when I finished school I did not want to follow her footsteps, but to look for a job that could take me out of the country. That is why I agreed to enroll for au pair and I have not regretted my decision.

The only challenge that Kumbwa identifies in her job as an au pair was to fit in American culture, but as days passed and with her motivation to learn she was able to cope. At the time I interviewed her, she was in her second year of undergraduate education, while still working with her employer who had two teenage girls, she said: "I love kids. When you are with a family, you learn a lot of things, their food, their language expression, their jokes and the like. We live together like one family. I love it here. I sometimes miss home, but I think I am far happier than if I remained at home. If I were still at home I might still be searching for a job or a college like many of my schoolmates. I will never regret my decision to become an au pair."

CONCLUSION

In this chapter, I attempted to illustrate some of the ways in which contemporary discourses on trafficking of human beings in a global economy sanitize 'home' oppression and exploitation while demonizing women's agency in the global economy. I suggest that women should not be identified as victims of the global economy prior to listening to their stories. Furthermore, I argue that criminalizing women's agency and their activities will neither deter employers' exploitative practices nor end women's movements. Sensitizing people with wild ideas about women in the global economy does not address the structural context that operates to shape people's behavior towards women, let alone resolve the issue of reallocation of resources between men and women on equal terms. Yet these measures are in place because moral entrepreneurs define women's movement as a threat to public health and moral values, link those activities to women's oppression and exploitation, and use statistics to bolster their claims. This primary construction of the threat is circulated and stylized by the media, an institution that depends on others for information and on sensation for profit. Policymakers, eager to claim credit, responded to calls for action with new laws and the reinvigoration of old ones to reinforce a monolithic view of women as "victims" and/or to curtail women's movement. While the panic of "trafficking" and "informal" employment seems to fade away, its implementation goes on quietly, perhaps with bribery—giving opportunity to those with more social capital and denying it to those who are weaker.

NOTES

1. S. Cohen, *Folk Devils and Moral Panics*, (London: MacGibbon and Kee Foucault, 1972), 9.
2. S. Hall, C. Chas, J. Tony, John, C., and R. Brian, *Policing the Crisis: Mugging, the State, and Law and Order*, (New York: Holmes and Meier, 1978), 19.
3. J. Doezema, "Loose Women or Lost Women? The Re-emergence of the Myth of 'White Slavery' in Contemporary Discourses of 'Trafficking in Women.'" In Gender Issues, 18 no, 1 (2000): 23–50.
4. C. Weedon, Feminism, Theory and Politics of Difference, (Oxford: Blackwell, 1999).
5. Global Alliance Against Trafficking in Women (GAATW) 1999. "Human Rights Standards for the Treatment of Trafficked Persons." Available at http://www.inet.-co.th/org/gaatw/.
6. P. Bourdieu, *In Other Words: Essays Toward a Reflexive Sociology*, M. Adamson, Trans. (Stanford, CA: Stanford University Press 1990); P. Bourdieu, *The Logic of Practice*, R. Nice, Trans. (Stanford, CA: Stanford University Press, 1990); P. Bourdieu and L. Wacquant, An Invitation to Reflexive Sociology, (Chicago: University of Chicago Press, 1992), 126.
7. P. Bourdieu, Outline of a Theory of Practice, R. Nice, Trans. (New York, Cambridge: Cambridge University Press, 1977).
8. O. Oyewumi, *The Invention of Women*, (California: University of California Press, 1997); A Mama, "Challenging Subjects: Gender and Power in African Contexts." Paper Presented at the Conference of Nordic African Institute: "Beyond Identity: Rethinking Power in Africa." Uppsala, October 4–7th 2001. A. Mama, "Women's Studies and Studies of Women in Africa during the 1990s," In, CODESRIA, (Dakar, 1997).
9. O. Oyewumi, forthcoming; Mama, "Challenging Subjects: Gender and Power in African Contexts."
10. Y. Mudimbe, "African Philosophy as an Ideological Practice: The Case of French-Speaking Africa," *African Studies Review*, Vol. 26 (1983): 3–4.
11. Oyewumi, *The Invention of Women*; Mama, 1997; T. Dangarembga, *Nervous Conditions*. (London: Seal Press, 2004); I. Amadiume, *Male Daughters, Female Husbands: Gender and Sex in an African Society*. (London: Zed Books, 1987); I. Young, "Is Male Gender Identity the Cause of Male Domination?" In D. Meyers, *Feminist Social Thought: A Reader*, (New York and London: Routledge, 1997).
12. P. Christensen, and A. James, (Eds.) Research with Children: Perspectives and Practices, (Routledge Falmer, 2000).
13. A. Kweka, "Emerging Forms of Non-Formal Education in Tanzania," *Papers in Education and Development*, No. 16, (1995): 129–138; P.A.K. Mushi, "The Fortunes and Demise of Literacy Drive in Tanzania," Papers in Education and Development, No. 16, (1995): 117–128.

14. S. Yahya-Othman, "Tanzania Engendering Academic Freedom," In Sall Ebrima (Ed.) *Women in Academia: Gender and Academic Freedom in Africa*, (Dakar Senegal: CODESRIA, 2000), 24–46.
15. N. Alphonce, "Trends and Strategies in the Tide of the Transformation of Higher Education in Tanzania," *Papers in Education and Development (PED)* No 22. (2002): 117–129; J. Galabawa, "Funding: Selected Issues and Trends in Tanzanian Higher Education," Higher Education Vol. 21, (1991): 49–61.
16. A. Sen, *Poverty and Feminines: An Essay on Entitlement and Deprivation*, (Oxford: Clarendon Press, 1982).
17. Yahya-Othman, 2000; R. Meena, "Adult Education," Meena Ruth Mbughuni, Patricia Olekambaine, (Eds.) *Education in Tanzania with Gender Perspective*, Dar-es-Salaam: SIDA, (1990): 68–82.; M. Mbilinyi, "Secondary and Higher Education." Marjorie P. Mbilinyi, Meena Ruth Mbughuni, Patricia Olekambaine, (Eds.), Education in Tanzania with Gender Perspective, (Dar-Es-Salaam: SIDA, 1990): 49–67.

REFERENCES

Alphonce, N. "Trends and Strategies in the Tide of the Transformation of Higher Education in Tanzania." *Papers in Education and Development (PED)* No 22, (2002); 117–129.

Amadiume, I. *Male Daughters, Female Husbands: Gender and Sex in an African Society*. London: Zed Books, 1987.

Bourdieu, P. *In Other Words: Essays Toward a Reflexive Sociology*. M. Adamson, Trans. Stanford, CA: Stanford University Press, 1990.

———. *The Logic of Practice*. R. Nice, Trans. Stanford, CA: Stanford University Press, 1990.

———. Outline of a Theory of Practice.Cambridge: Cambridge University Press, 1977.

Bourdieu, P., & Wacquant, L. An Invitation to Reflexive Sociology. Chicago: University of Chicago Press, 1992.

Christensen, P. and James, A. (Eds.) Research with Children: Perspectives and Practices, Routledge Falmer, 2000.

Cohen, S. Folk Devils and Moral Panics. London: MacGibbon and Kee Foucault, 1972.

Dangarembga, T. Nervous Conditions. London: Seal Press, 2004.

Gagnon, M. *Other Conundrums: Race, Culture and Canadian Art*. Vancouver: Arsenal Pulp Press, 2000.

Galabawa, J. "Funding: Selected Issues and Trends in Tanzanian Higher Education." Higher Education Vol. 21, (1991): 49–61.

Global Alliance Against Trafficking in Women (GAATW) "Human Rights Standards for the Treatment of Trafficked Persons," 1999. Available at http://www.inet.-co.th/org/gaatw/

Hall, S., Chas C., Tony, J., John, C., and Brian, R. Policing the Crisis: Mugging, the State, and Law and Order. New York: Holmes and Meier, 1978.

Iliffe, J. A Modern History of Tanganyika. New York: Cambridge University Press, 1979.

Kweka, A. "Emerging Forms of Non-Formal Education in Tanzania." Papers in Education and Development, No. 16, (1995): 129–138.

Lin, N. "Building a network Theory of Social Capital." Connections. Vol. 22, (1999): 28–51.

———. Social Capital: A Theory of Structure and Action. Cambridge. Cambridge: University Press, 2000.

———. "Inequality in Social Capital." Contemporary Sociology. Vol. 6, (2000): 785–795.

Mama, A. "Women's Studies and Studies of Women in Africa during the 1990s." In, CODESRIA. Dakar, 1997.

———. "Challenging Subjects: Gender and Power in African Contexts." Paper Presented at the Conference of Nordic African Institute: "Beyond Identity: Rethinking Power in Africa." Uppsala, October 4–7th, 2001.

Masika, R. Gender, Trafficking and Slavery. Oxford: Oxfarm, 2002.

Mbilinyi, M. "Secondary and Higher Education." Mbilinyi Marjorie, P. Mbughuni, Meena Ruth, Olekambaine, Patricia. (Eds.). Education in Tanzania with Gender Perspective. Dar-Es-Salaam: SIDA, (1990): 49–67.

Meena, R. "Adult Education." Mbughuni, Meena Ruth, Olekambaine, Patricia. (Eds.). Education in Tanzania with Gender Perspective. Dar-es-Salaam: SIDA, (1990): 68–82.

Mudimbe, Y. "African Philosophy as an Ideological Practice. The Case of French-Speaking Africa." African Studies Review, Vol. 26, (1983): 3–4.

Mushi, P.A.K. "TheFortunes and Demise of Literacy Drive in Tanzania." Papers in Education and Development, No. 16, (1995): 117–128.

Nazroo, J. and Karlsen, S. "Pattern of Identity Among Ethnic Minority People:
Diversity and Commonality." Ethnic and Racial Studies, Vol. 26 no. 1, (2003): 902–930.

Oyewumi, O. The Invention of Women. California: University of California Press, 1997.

Sen, A. Poverty and Feminines: An Essay on Entitlement and Deprivation. Oxford: Clarendon Press, 1982.

Swai, E. "Construction of Identity as a Learning Activity: Embodiment and Culture. Unpublished PhD Thesis. The Pennsylvania State University, 2006.

Weedon, C. Feminism, Theory and Politics of Difference. Oxford: Blackwell, 1999.

Yahya-Othman, S. "Tanzania Engendering Academic Freedom." In Sall Ebrima (Ed.) Women in Academia: Gender and Academic Freedom in Africa. Dakar Senegal: CODESRIA, (2000): 24–46.

Young, I. "*Is Male Gender Identity the Cause of Male Domination?*" In Meyers, D. *Feminist Social Thought: A Reader*. New York & London: Routledge, 1997.

Chapter Eight

Emerging Issues in the Trafficking of African Women for Prostitution

Victor Nnamdi Opara

SYNOPSIS

This chapter explores crucial issues that impact the trafficking of women in Africa. It begins by locating the origin of trafficking in Africa, and proceeds to bring to the fore various social, political, economic, religious and cultural problems that African women so co-opted and burdened undergo in their home and destination countries. The chapter argues that these factors underpin trafficking in Africa, increase the vulnerability of African women to trafficking, and also make the ugly and dehumanizing trade an attractive business for criminal syndicates. The chapter posits that the African and international community cannot treat the symptoms of trafficking without first diagnosing the disease. A diagnosis will assist in locating the underlying factors that trigger as well as exacerbate trafficking in Africa. Trafficking should be tackled from the roots. A holistic response to the call for eradication of trafficking in Africa requires an engagement of these root factors because they are the breeding grounds for trafficking. In an attempt to fill this gap, the chapter offers both a descriptive and prescriptive analysis of the root causes of trafficking in Africa. Structurally it comprises two parts. Part I embodies the introduction, gives the general dimensions of trafficking, outlines the history of trafficking in Africa, lays down a compendium of trafficking statistics, gives an overview of the factors influencing trafficking in Africa, and describes the operative mechanisms of trafficking syndicates. Part II contains a close-contextual analysis of African and international approaches to the eradication of trafficking, including the effects of the structural adjustment program on trafficking in Africa. It also appraises the U.S. Trafficking Victims Protection Act and the Nigerian Trafficking Act. Finally, it delineates the responsibility of states in the provision of grass-root solutions to human trafficking.

PART I: TRAFFICKING IN AFRICA, DIMENSIONS, NUANCES, AND UNDERPINNINGS

Introduction

> *One area of particular urgency is the eradication of extreme poverty.* The latest report of the World Bank indicates that the recent financial and economic crisis has driven large parts of populations into poverty—measured by the World Bank as income of less than US$1 per day. *The victims of poverty are in fact denied almost all rights. . . . These conditions are compounded for the most vulnerable, in particular children and women, who in some parts of the world are being increasingly exploited through trafficking, forced labor and prostitution.* The Bank's report speaks about the failure of existing economic strategies to combat poverty and calls for new, socially oriented approaches.[1]

Human trafficking has increasingly become the order of the day in Africa. Trafficking in Africa is indeed a national, regional, and international problem that has engaged the whole African continent and the global community, international crime detectives and law enforcement agencies including the Interpol, and a broad array of practitioners and advocates of human rights. The fight against human trafficking is a complex international problem that requires the cooperation of government agencies and nations at large.[2] The continuous increase of trafficking in Africa indicates the failure of the international community as a whole to address this universal problem, though it does now have a more concrete definition. The phrase *trafficking in people* or *trafficking in persons* was first used in global vocabulary to describe the exportation of women and children, especially for prostitution.[3]

The general economic restructuring mandated by the International Monetary Fund (IMF) and the World Bank through the structural adjustment program (SAP) and privatization as preconditions for financial aid to Africa, have had a tremendous impact on the economic and political conditions in Africa, which now encourage trafficking in persons. SAP remains one of the strongest foundations of Africa's economic problems this century. SAP has arguably left many Southern states much poorer than they were when they signed on for financial assistance.[4] This unfortunate situation has been soberly lamented by some scholars.[5] Broad cuts to the public sector had a disproportionate impact on lower cadre public sector jobs. Unemployment made people more desperate for financial help.[6] As such, many crime syndicates sprung up in Africa. While trying to better their financial status, these syndicates saw the need to take advantage of the growing regional poverty through recruitment of desperate Africans into their networks, first for drug trafficking purposes and now for human trafficking, mainly into the sex industry. As will be demonstrated in this chapter, poverty remains a major reason why Africans fall prey to trafficking syndicates. Poverty also underpins the political instability and corruption in Africa, as everyone is eager to rule in order to embezzle public funds and secure better economic prospects for himself and his family, including generations yet unborn. This situation leads to political disruption in almost all parts of the African continent. The resultant effect is that people, especially women and children, flee conflict or the aftermath of conflict, or migrate for personal security in order to escape abuse and violence. This makes Africans, especially African women, easy targets for trafficking syndicates. As has been observed: "Trafficking in women is fuelled by poverty, sexism, and racism, all of which combine to create a situation of unequal bargaining power and vulnerability. In developing countries or countries with economies in transition, conditions of poverty—which are aggravated for women because of their traditionally lower economic status in these countries—can lead women to accompany traffickers. These conditions can also compel families to sell their female relatives to traffickers in the hope that they will have an opportunity to earn money for themselves or their families."[7]Other social and cultural factors also underpin trafficking in Africa, thereby forming a surge in the trajectory of human trafficking on the continent.

African women undergo various social and cultural problems in their home countries, including androcentric cultural practices which make women unequal to men;[8] unequal access to education, employment, and social benefits;[9] illiteracy or inadequate education; harmful traditional stereotypes that depict women as property, commodities, servants, and sexual objects; criminal justice systems that ignore and even perpetuate violence and discrimination against women;[10] religious doctrines and practices that are lopsidedly gendered; (see Amina Lawal in section C) political insecurity and crushing economic depressions in Africa,[11] among others. At the other end of the spectrum, trafficked African women also face several social and cultural problems in their destination countries, including insecurity, exploitation and exposure to disease, racial discrimination and language barriers, among others. These problems increase the vulnerability of African women to trafficking while at the same time making trafficking in women an attractive business for syndicates. This chapter posits the need to address these root factors.[12]

Using a human rights framework, this chapter argues that African states and destination states in Western Europe have a responsibility under international law (1) to act with due diligence to prevent human trafficking; (2) to investigate and prosecute traffickers; and (3) to assist and protect trafficked persons.[13] Unfortunately, the first prong of the international responsibility does not appear to be receiving any attention at present. This responsibility "to prevent human trafficking" can be fulfilled when states "address the factors that increase vulnerability to trafficking," (U.N. Principles,) which means addressing the root causes of trafficking in Africa and their transnational implications for trafficking victims. The analysis draws on existing human rights instruments, and is intended to contribute to the efforts of human rights practitioners and advocates in the fight against trafficking. Viewed through this lens, the analysis uses existing trafficking conventions to address the somewhat neglected fundamental factors that underpin trafficking in Africa, with a view to assessing their degree of impact on the continuous increase in trafficking on the continent. The analysis posits that the international community does not pay particular attention to most of these factors. Rather, all the energy of the international community has been channeled to the effects of trafficking on victims, with particular emphasis on preventing exploitation of victims by traffickers and pimps. While this is a good development, it only serves as an *ex post facto* solution, which limits the inquiry to the peripherals. Unfortunately, such a limitation means that only a modicum of the problem has been addressed so far. The chapter argues that there is a need to fight trafficking in Africa from its roots. This will provide a holistic response to the trafficking pandemic in the African continent. Such a holistic approach might also assist in fashioning a viable solution to the endemic human rights violations that trafficking has generated in Africa. Furthermore, the chapter argues that the international community cannot treat the symptoms of trafficking without diagnosing the disease. In an attempt to fill this lacuna, the study offers both a descriptive and prescriptive analysis of the root causes of trafficking in Africa. In view of the criticisms that most trafficking instruments have generated in recent times, this analysis uses as an interpretive tool, the principles and guidelines on human rights and human trafficking as released by the U.N. High Commissioner for Human Rights. The general thrust of this study is to advance scholarly considerations of human rights by illustrating that close engagement of some blatant factors in social, economic, political, religious, and cultural practices can assist in preventing trafficking, and equally provide the normative clarity which society requires to appreciate fully the intersections between those impugned practices and trafficking.

Trafficking in Africa encompasses transactions in three dimensions: small arms and light weapons, drugs, and human beings. In a broader perspective, it also involves illegal money flows that result from such transactions. Each of these dimensions of trafficking has had its toll on the African continent—a continent that is facing a plethora of urgent and complex issues, including inadequate infrastructure, endemic corruption and embezzlement, the HIV/AIDS pandemic, low gross domestic product (GDP), and the world's highest level of poverty, among others. It follows that a discourse that encompasses all dimensions of trafficking in Africa will surely be engaging and broad. In an attempt to delineate the discussion in this chapter, the analysis focuses on human trafficking, although passive references are made to other forms of trafficking where necessary. Human trafficking generally involves coerced recruitment and transportation of people for a variety of forced labor and slavery-like practices, including forced domestic labor, manual or industrial labor, commercial marriages,[14] and the sex trade or prostitution. That means that even human trafficking, although just one dimension of trafficking, is still a broad topic. Accordingly, on a narrower dimension, this study focuses on trafficking in African women for prostitution, using Nigeria as a model for other African countries. The study further limits its geographical inquiry (respecting the destination of trafficked African women) to Western Europe. In other words, the study uses as a model for other African countries, Nigerian women trafficked to Western Europe for prostitution.

This choice was not made without careful consideration of relevant factors. First, I chose 'human trafficking for prostitution' in light of the fact that this particular branch of human trafficking raises pressing and complex human rights issues, including human (in)security, the rule of law, social well-being, personal and public health concerns, etc., that ought to shock the sensibilities of the international community. The paper does not however engage all of these nuanced episodic details, although the reader should continually bear them in mind. According to the United Nations Development Fund for Women (UNIFEM), trafficking in women for prostitution is one of the fastest growing organized criminal activities in the world, following in frequency only the trades in narcotics and weapons, (Trafficking to Italy, 17). Second, the choice of Nigeria as a model for other African countries is made for the following reasons: (1) Nigeria is the worst hit African country in the trafficking pandemic and as such poses the strongest challenge to the continent as well as the international community;[15] (2) Nigeria is the most populous country in Africa, which could translate to traffickers having a wide variety of women to choose from; (3) As a result of Nigeria's oil resources, it is more economically viable than most African countries. Since poverty is a major reason why African women fall prey to trafficking, if an oil-rich country like Nigeria is unable to fend for its residents, it logically follows that most African countries would not be able to stop trafficking on their own without international assistance; (4) Nigeria is considered to be a regional power within the African continent. This means that Nigeria wields both political and military power in Africa. As such, if Nigeria is unable to rescue itself from the hands of traffickers, it unequivocally illustrates the inability of most African countries to fight traffickers; (5) Nigeria offers a perfect example of religious diversity within the African continent with its 50–50 Christian to Muslim ratio. It is indisputable that Nigeria has recorded the highest number of fatal religious conflicts, and these have claimed the lives of thousands. These religious conflicts are joined by others, such as ethnic conflicts and conflicts arising from communities' assertions of their rights to self-determination, which are fuelled by the activities of oil companies in their bid to explore for resources at the detriment and expense of the environment and human rights. All of these conflicts have rendered Nigeria somewhat of a "jungle." Since trafficking thrives in atmospheres of conflict, it follows that a war-torn country like Nigeria offers attractive recruitment incentives to traffickers; and (6) Nigeria equally offers a good illustration of all other features of trafficking in Africa and across the world.

TRAFFICKING STATISTICS IN AFRICA AND THE WORLD

The most current international statistics on human trafficking appear in the Fifth Annual Trafficking in Persons Report, released in June 2005 by the U.S. State Department. The Report, authored by John Miller, states that about 600,000 to 800,000 people are trafficked across international borders every year, of which about 80 percent are women and children.[16] This is not significantly different from the amount of global trafficking reported by the U.S. State Department in 2004, where it is estimated that between 700,000 to four million persons were trafficked annually around the globe, with 50,000 women and children trafficked annually for sexual exploitation into the U.S.[17] Reports confirm that thousands of African women are trafficked every year to Western Europe and North America,[18] with Canada serving as a conduit for trafficking to the United States.[19] According to a Reuter's news report in December 2000, figures given by governments and non-governmental organizations suggest that between 700,000 and two million women and children are victims of trafficking annually.[20] Anti-Slavery, an NGO concerned with the eradication of trafficking and related slavery-like practices, has observed that "[i]t is impossible to know [how many people that are trafficked] and statistics are difficult to obtain because trafficking is an underground activity."[21] This observation appears to be correct because a great deal of trafficking is undocumented due largely to its underground nature.[22] The effect of this revelation is that the reported cases are likely to be below the real trafficking figures. The extent of human trafficking cannot be ascertained with great precision, but it is usually proxied by multiplying the figures for border apprehensions. According to the United Nations Office on Drugs and Crime, in the past 21 years there has been a rise in trafficking in persons, caused by a large number of factors, including the end of the Cold War, which led to opening of borders and a rise in the movement of people, the debut of organized crime in the international arena, and the increased demand for sex tourism. There are about 200,000 to 500,000 illegal sex workers in the European Union, and Eastern Europe accounts for two-thirds of them.[23] They are illegal because they are not officially registered as sex workers. In fact, the U.N. Office on Drugs and Crime emphasized the contagious nature of the global criminal network: "Over the past decade, trafficking in human beings has reached epidemic proportions. No country is immune. The search for work abroad has been fuelled by economic disparity, high unemployment and the disruption of traditional livelihoods."[24] It is estimated that Nigerian and Albanian women constitute the largest proportion of the approximately 20,000 prostitutes in Italy.[25] The Organization for Migration reports that in 1997 alone, 500,000 women of Russian and Ukrainian origin were trafficked into Western Europe.[26]

On the African scene, Nigeria presents the biggest challenge to the African continent and the international community at large. Although trafficking for prostitution is a more recent phenomenon in Nigeria, it has climaxed in the last decade. The major obstacle in the assessment of human trafficking in Nigeria is lack of statistical data.[27] This problem is compounded by the clandestine nature of human trafficking. Moreover, most Nigerians find it difficult to disclose their traveling plans to friends and neighbors due to fears that the information recipient may foil the plans or impose herself on the person facilitating the movement.[28] Notwithstanding these statistical shortfalls, figures of deported trafficking victims exist, which could be used as a basis for statistical inquiry.[29] Between March 1999 and December 2000, 1,178 Nigerians were deported from five countries for trafficking related reasons, and the most were from Rome, Italy. Of this number, only 12 were men, (Nightingale, Labor Migration 3–4). This remained substantially the same in 2001 as revealed in a homegrown Nigerian trafficking study, (*Trafficking to Italy,* 20) which indicated that more than 1,116 Nigerian women were repatriated in 2001. The Nigeria

Police Desk Office on Human Trafficking reported that between 1999 and 2001, over 8,633 trafficked persons were deported back to Nigeria, (Ume-Ezeokeke, Desk Review, 4). In 2001, the Nigerian Ambassador to Italy reported that there were about 10,000 Nigerian prostitutes in Italy, (Ume-Ezeokeke, Desk Review, 4). This figure doubled in 2002 as the number of Nigerian women involved in Italian sex trade rose to 20,000.[30] To sum up the figures of deportations so far, between 1999 and 2003, 19,774 Nigerians had been deported from Europe for human trafficking offences relating to prostitution.[31] Thereafter, in 2004, many Nigerians were deported from Italy and Saudi Arabia. Between January and March 2004, over 1000 Nigerians were deported from Saudi Arabia, and an additional 386 Nigerians were also deported from Saudi Arabia in April 2004, all for trafficking offences;[32] while between April and May 2004, 371 Nigerian women were deported from Italy, (Joint Report on Human Rights, 45, 5.7.2). A combination of these deportation figures, and the dead and maimed trafficking victims, as well as those that have either legalized their stay or are still working illegally or are stranded abroad will give some indication of the huge number of Nigerian women who have been trafficked to Europe for prostitution. Against this backdrop, it appears that the estimates of the U.S. Diplomatic Mission to Nigeria that as of May 2003, "as many as 300,000 [Nigerian women] have been trafficked since 1997" is a correct assumption of facts, (Mohammed, 2003). It is also estimated that over 500,000 African women and children have been trafficked, (Ume-Ezeokeke, Desk Review). A synthesis of these two estimates reveals that Nigerian women constitute more than 50% of all Africans who have been trafficked, anywhere in the world. While it is an established fact that most trafficked African women agreed to migrate for the sake of better economic prospects, some of them are just kidnapped and trafficked for prostitution against their wishes. In Sussex, England, more than 40 African teenage girls, some as young as 14, who were seeking asylum in the United Kingdom were taken away from children's homes and sold as prostitutes in Italy.[33]

It is worthy of note that on the national level, Edo State in Southern Nigeria presents the biggest challenge within the Nigerian trafficking menace. The Nigerian Ambassador to Italy has advised the Speaker of Edo State legislature, that, of all the prostitutes in Italy, Edo women constitute 80 percent.[34] In fact, the most influential cultural organization in the state, the Edo Cultural Association, wrote to the traditional Monarch of the State, Oba Erediauwa, advising him that, "prostitution had become a ravaging fire spreading from city to city, village to village and house to house in Edo State. 'There is practically no home in Edoland without a girl being sent to Belgium, Holland, Spain, England and especially this country, Italy,'"

(Chigbo, Igbinedion Versus Prostitutes). [35] In fact the wind of trafficking in Edo State is so infectious that married women desert their matrimonial homes with infants and toddlers to join trafficking rings, some men deliberately give up their wives to traffickers, high school children are lured away from school to join the trade, and parents sign up for their daughters to join the rings, (Chigbo, Igbinedion versus Prostitutes).

This statistical inquiry will not be complete without mentioning the ill profits that traffickers make from this transnational trade in women. In 2000, human traffickers realized estimated profits of $7 billion from prostitution alone, (Reuters, Mafia Makes Millions). The profit margin in human trafficking increased in 2004 as the industry earned more than $10 billion from human trafficking.[36] The realizable profit has further risen to $11.8 billion in 2005, (Jiméenez, 2005 and U.S. Trafficking Report). This trend of constant increase in profit reveals that the penalties for the crime are meager; as such, traffickers seem better off defaulting than stopping their nefarious trade.[37] It further illustrates that there are incentives in the industry despite attempts by the international community to stem its tide. That means that the international community needs to increase the punishment for trafficking, including an increase in fines and prison terms.

OVERVIEW OF ROOT FACTORS INFLUENCING TRAFFICKING IN AFRICA

The most significant reason why African women are vulnerable to traffickers seems to be socio-economic hardship.[38] There are, however, other social factors.[39] From an analytical point of view, trafficking of African women for the sex trade is underpinned by a plethora of socio-economic, religious, and political factors. For any state discourse or policy initiative to be successful in tackling sex trafficking in Africa, it has to re-examine these factors. At the outset, it must be noted that in traditional African inheritance discourse, there are both patriarchal and matrilineal inheritance systems, depending on the country and community in question. Patriarchy is a form of inheritance where children inherit from their father's lineage whereas in matrilineal societies, children inherit from their mother's lineage. For example, Nigeria predominantly practices patriarchy whereas Ghana practices matriarchy. Patriarchy appears to be the dominant mode, though it appears that the form of inheritance that a country practices has little or no impact on the social constructs that set the stage for human trafficking. What counts most is social construct and not inheritance structure. The way a society views women matters a lot, and goes a long way in determining how other factors merge to make or mar women.

Accordingly, all African societies have identical social, economic, religious, and political factors that trigger and exacerbate trafficking in women; the difference (if at all) may only be a question of degree. Some of these factors are discussed below. First, the present cultural preference for boys impacts on trafficking.[40] Traffickers and complicit family members view women as cheap and less treasured commodities that can be shipped away to foreign lands in order to better the family's prospects, whether or not the woman consents to assume that role.[41] This practice appears to empower traffickers to take undue advantage of unsuspecting women. Ironically, the mother of a trafficked woman is more likely to have a hand in the general arrangement, although genuinely ignorant of the horrendous nature of the deal.[42] Yet the same mother is much more likely to hesitate in entering into that deal when it comes to shipping away her son. This is where gender and social constructs play crucial roles. Generally, under most African customs, before a son undertakes any journey, even if it is just a temporary relocation from countryside to the city, consultation of family members is required. A mother does not have any power to send her son on such journeys without permission. However, such family consultation does not apply where a daughter is to travel, presumably because society does not care about what happens to her. This reflects the androcentricism of some African cultures.[43] Unfortunately, this is one of the practices that statutes cannot change, and the only solution lies in persuading Africans to re-examine their values. This re-examination strategy could work better if targeted at the working population and children. The aged people (senior citizens) are more likely to resist such persuasive gestures, since most of them are too deep into "the tradition of our forefathers."

Second, social values are also responsible for gender inequity in other necessities of life. As a result of poverty, most African families are unable to afford good education for all their children. Hence scale of preference is usually drawn in families to determine who gets what level of education. The African girl child is more likely to lose out in this scale.[44] This loss throws her into a vicious cycle of poverty. Without education, her economic potential is significantly minimized. This in turn affects her career opportunities.[45] Unfortunately, her brothers, for whose benefits her education was sacrificed or disrupted, may not assist her financially when they start working. This leaves her financially desperate. As such, she becomes more vulnerable to traffickers, ever ready to accept any offers that are capable of improving her financial status.[46] In essence, social values assist in fuelling trafficking. That said, culture could be positively re-defined. This goal can be achieved through creation of public awareness of the negative impacts of some cultural values in society.[47]

Third, throughout the transformative stages of the female child's life, African social values instill in her a feeling of inferiority compared to her brothers and male counterparts. This stereotypical feeling of worthlessness appears to force young women to take their future into their own hands, in the belief that no matter what happens to them, their families would not have much to lose. This superiority–inferiority dynamic forces a lot of African women to accept debasement and subordination. It is not surprising that 60 percent of trafficked African women are lured by promises of attractive remunerations, (Nightingale, Labor Migration, 4) which, when compared to the multifaceted problems at home, makes acceptance of the offer an attractive, acceptable, or even the most viable option.[48] Of course, article 5 of the Convention on the Elimination of All Forms of Discrimination Against Women[49] calls on states to modify the social and cultural patterns of conduct of men and women, with a view to achieving the elimination of prejudices and customs, and all other practices which are based on the idea of the inferiority or superiority of either of the sexes or on stereotyped roles for men and women. Although laudable, the objectives of this provision can be achieved mainly through social re-orientation, rather than legislation alone. Most African countries do not have gender equality clauses in their constitutions. At best, the equality clauses are restricted to birth, and are hardly given any practical efficacy. They only exist in the books. For example, although the Nigerian Constitution expressly prohibits discrimination on grounds of circumstances of birth,[50] in practice, Nigerian culture regards as illegitimate children born outside marital union.[51] The conflict between Nigerian traditional culture and the Constitution should have been resolved in favor of the Constitution since it is the supreme law of the land.[52] Unfortunately, tradition does not fade easily. Notwithstanding this quagmire, it appears that a combination of social re-orientation and legislation will achieve a better result in the call for elimination of discrimination on grounds of gender. No society is static. Cultural values should be dynamic in order to keep pace with development. While it is obvious that enforcement of gender equality legislation against private actors will be difficult to achieve, it would be easy to enforce it against public institutions and agencies.[53] Moreover, inclusion of gender-equality education in the curriculum of kindergarten, primary schools, and high schools will go a long way in re-orientating the minds of children and young people, who basically are the leaders of tomorrow.

The fourth factor that has promoted the trafficking of African women is the constant political instability and internal unrest in Africa. While political instabilities are triggered by public actors or politicians, most internal conflicts emanate from individuals and constantly take the form of religious disagreements or ethnic clashes. On the one hand, some of the very concrete problems in particular regimes in the African social and political context that call for immediate resolution include government-directed or government-assisted assassinations,[54] flagrant abuse of women and ethnic minorities,[55] and general human rights violations and insecurity.[56] At the other end of the insecurity spectrum are incessant religious conflicts that have resulted in the killing or displacement of hundreds of thousands of Africans. In particular, Nigeria has become the hub of ethno-religious conflicts. Nigeria has encountered several fatal religious conflicts between the Christian and Muslim faiths in the last three decades. Usually religion and ethnicity seem to merge once a conflict ensues between individuals. It appears that members of affected communities are more interested in knowing the ethnicity and religion of the parties than the merits of the dispute. The merging of religious and ethnic sentiments was demonstrated in various conflicts in Nigeria: Zangon-Kataf (1992), Tafawa-Balewa (1991, 1995, and 2001), Jos (2001), as well as the Sharia crisis that commenced in Kaduna in 2000 and has become somewhat of an annual or bi-annual exercise.

The genesis of Nigerian ethno-religious crisis was the Maitatsine religious riot which started as an intra-religious or sectarian conflict in Kano State in the 1980s.[57] The *Zangon Kataf* crisis of 1992 occurred in the Zangon Kataf municipality in Kaduna State, and was triggered by the relocation of a market that was hitherto dominated by the Hausa-Fulani ethnic group. The ownership of the land is not known with historical certainty. This relocation that started as an economic crisis diverged into ethnic and religious dimensions, leaving many people dislocated and displaced from their homes.[58]

The *Tafawa-Balewa* crises of 1991, 95 and 2001 all occurred in the Tafawa-Balewa municipality in Bauchi State. The historical ownership of this land is disputed among the Sayawa and the Hausa-Fulani. While the Sayawa are Christians, The Hausa-Fulani are Muslims. The 1991 *Tafawa-Balewa* crisis was triggered by a disagreement between a Fulani and a Sayawa meat seller who allegedly sold pork meat to the Fulani, pork being meat that is forbidden in Islam. The Fulani protested and a fight ensued, which spread to the entire municipality and other parts of the state. This resulted in the deaths of several people as well as destruction of property.[59] The 1995 *Tafawa-Balewa* crisis was triggered by the protest of Christian women against a planned reception in honor of Alhaji Ibrahim Musa, a Hausa Muslim who had been appointed as Commissioner to replace a Sayawa man, Mr. J.K. Manzo, in the Bauchi State Executive Cabinet. An attempt by the Mayor of the municipality to impose levies on all staff for the reception was resisted by Christian women, especially the Sayawa whose son had been removed. The Hausa-Fulani countered the protest and this resulted in severe conflict and anarchy. Many villages were razed and people were displaced. The 2001 *Tafawa-Balewa* crisis was triggered by the imposition of sharia on Tafawa Balewa municipality. Christians opposed this imposition and Muslims once again countered them. This also led to a conflict which left many people dead and several properties destroyed, (Je'adayibe, 2002).

The effect of the expansion of sharia (from religious law *simpliciter* to state law) in the Northern states of Nigeria climaxed in the Kaduna crisis of 2000. Christians resisted this expansion and Muslims countered. This led to open war and mass killings. The official records of the Kaduna state government report that "a total of 1,295 persons died, unspecified numbers were buried, while some others were declared missing."[60] This sharia crisis in Kaduna spread to most cities in Northern Nigeria. As the Christians constitute a minority in the North, they were arguably the most vulnerable in the drastic carnage. The Christians in the Southern part of Nigeria (South-East in particular) retaliated against local Muslims in reprisal killings, (Report of Judicial Commission). The entire country was in turmoil. During and after the war, some Christians left Kaduna and other Northern states and returned to the Southern part of Nigeria, while some Muslims also left the Southern states and returned to the North.

The *Jos* crisis of 2001 appears to have broader layers than the purely ethno-religious dimension, although the primary triggers have been linked to religion. The two recorded immediate causes are (a) the appointment of a Hausa Muslim, Mallam Usman Mukhtar Mohammed, as the coordinator of the poverty alleviation project of Jos municipality in Plateau state, which was opposed by the indigenous people; and (b) an attempt by a Christian woman to walk through a road block on a Muslim Jummat prayer ground. In addition to these religious anecdotes, historical, political, ethnic as well as economic interests added color to the conflict. Once again this led to a lot of casualties, loss of lives and property, and individual displacements, (Je'adayibe, 2002). The *Jos* crisis had lots of spillover effects on the entire Plateau state. Several reprisal attacks occurred in other cities, unabated until the recent massive killings in the *Yelwa-Shendam* crisis of 2004. The crisis was politicized by the Plateau state government. It was during this period that some "uniformed men" went to a Church and attacked Christians who were worshipping. 50 people were killed in that attack. This forced several others to flee their homes. Some weeks later Christians retaliated in a reprisal attack, and as usual, several lives and property were lost. Muslims in Kano state retaliated against local Christians, which led to the Kano reprisal killings, (Je'adayibe, 2002). All the above conflicts arose in and were confined to the Northern part of Nigeria,[61] which is predominantly Muslim, with the Christians being in the minority. On the other hand, in the Southern part of Nigeria, where the Christians are in the majority and the Muslims in the minority, there has been religious harmony and cooperation, except for the one isolated incident of reprisal killing in the South-East following the drastic carnage against Christians in Kaduna state in 2000.

Indeed, traffickers have been capitalizing on these unfortunate situations.[62] Intuitively, it might even appear better for a woman to be trafficked than face the aftermath of these ethno-religious conflicts. During these conflicts, although men are usually killed by opposing factions, women are not spared. Women are usually targeted for a variety of reasons, including the use of rape as a weapon of war: "Rape is one kind of war booty, women are raped because war intensifies men's sense of entitlement, superiority, avidity, and social license to rape . . . rape is a weapon of war used to spread political terror, rape can destabilize a society and break its resistance, rape is a form of torture, gang rapes in public terrorize and humiliate women, rape is used to terrorize and silence women and force them to flee homes . . . rape is used in ethnic cleansing."[63] Women who find themselves in these conflict ridden communities are usually forced to flee from their homes and seek refuge elsewhere in order to remain alive. This ugly situation results in such women either becoming internally displaced persons or refugees. This vulnerable state gives expression to the plight of women during ethno-religious conflict in Africa. A woman in such a situation, when confronted by a trafficker, has little or no option than to succumb. As she is hungry, homeless, stressed, insecure, afraid, helpless and desperate, a trafficker's offer might seem to her manna from heaven. Ethno-religious conflicts and political instability deserve immediate resolution in Africa. Indeed, Africa is not alone in this menace. Political instability and ethnic acrimony affect other developing and transition economies as well, in Asian, Latin American, and Eastern and Central European countries, which have to battle with internal strife, civil war, and economic depression.[64] It is reported that hundreds of thousands of women from these regions are trafficked into prostitution in Western European countries such as Germany, the Netherlands, Italy, and Austria.[65]

Fifth, the travel plans of most Nigerians, as could be true of other African societies, are kept secret from friends and neighbors due to fears of opportunistic behavior. The prospective traveler is usually afraid of many things: the information recipient may impose herself on the person facilitating the movement, or may collude with thieves to rob the traveler. Moreover, as trafficking is unlawful in Nigeria, there is also the fear that the information recipient might alert the police. However, in reality, the possibility of police intrusion is rare because usually the prospective traveler will not call the arrangement trafficking but will rather use other benign words to describe the deal, thus avoiding public condemnation. Although this appears to be a minor problem that exists within families, in reality, its negative effects on the community are enormous. It increases the "lemons problem." Since traffickers know that the woman or family they are dealing with is unlikely to reveal their identity, they would take advantage of the opportunity to perpetuate their deceptions. In view of the information asymmetry that already exists between the trafficker and the woman, disclosing the trafficker's identity and the trafficking arrangements generally would have assisted in several ways. Some people who have material non-public information about the trafficker may be willing to speak out once they become aware of the deal. As such, a trafficker's reputation within the community would play a crucial role in determining whether accosted women will eventually agree to undertake the trafficking voyage. That is, the rate of success that previous women had in the trafficker's deals would matter a lot. Moreover, because of the communal nature of Nigerian communities, which is equally true of all African societies, people will surely speak out once they become aware of such arrangements even when their advice is not sought. Unfortunately, all these assessment tools are lost as a result of the secrecy that surrounds trafficking transactions in Nigeria and other African communities. The downside is that this "don't ask don't tell" attitude positively conditions the market for traffickers to the detriment of trafficked women. It is therefore possible for two cousins or neighbors to be trafficked by the same syndicate at different periods but within a short interval, without each knowing that the other is negotiating or has negotiated a deal with the trafficker. In that case, presumably the first woman to be trafficked would have gotten some material non-public information about the trafficker that would be very useful to her cousin or neighbor in making a decision respecting the trafficking offer. Unfortunately, because her cousin or neighbor has not made any disclosures about her plans, it becomes difficult for the first woman or her family to reveal her plight to the cousin or neighbor. As a result, the cousin or neighbor has to suffer the same tragedy that the first woman passed (or is passing) through in the hands of the trafficker. This trend goes on and on in a vicious cycle that keeps empowering traffickers.

Sixth, lopsided religious doctrines and practices, as well as criminal justice systems that ignore and even perpetuate gender violence and discrimination may indirectly encourage trafficking in women. One remarkable example of such abhorrent criminal justice cum religious systems was the horrifying story of a Nigerian woman, Amina Lawal, who was found guilty of adultery and sentenced to death by stoning at the age of 31 by a Sharia court at Bakori in Katsina State of Nigeria on March 22, 2002. Her alleged offense was that she had a child outside marriage. The only evidence against Amina was her pregnancy or baby, which under the applicable Sharia penal law in several states of Northern Nigeria was enough evidence to convict her of adultery. On the other hand, the man named as the father of Amina's baby girl reportedly denied having sex with her and the charges against him were discontinued. The lopsidedness of this religious penal law is reflected in the differing standards of evidence required from a man and a woman: to convict a man of the same crime, he must either confess directly to the court or at least four men must attest to witnessing the physical act of sexual intercourse. This shows that while it is very easy to convict a woman under the law (through her pregnancy or child), it is extremely difficult to convict a man for the same offence (four males must witness the intercourse). Except in the pornography industry, adult video shoots, or gang rape cases, it is rare for four men to be present while two other people are having sex. Moreover, even the more recent sexual revolution of the "threesome" only involves three consenting adult participants. In addition to the above lopsidedness, in the event that four women witness the intercourse and testify against the man, their evidence is not valid under this law. This translates to the virtual impossibility of convicting male offenders. Amina's conviction was appealed to the Sharia Court of Appeal, Katsina State. Her conviction provoked strong opposition from several human rights organizations around the world, most of which were represented at the Appeal Court hearings. Fortunately, on September 25, 2003, the Katsina Sharia Court of Appeal quashed Amina's death sentence.[66] While the Court of Appeal's decision is a welcome relief, it must be pointed out that the impugned Sharia law remains valid in Northern Nigeria. Amina Lawal's case did not challenge the validity of the law; rather the holding of the case distinguished the facts of Amina's circumstances as an exception to the law.

OPERATIVE MECHANISMS OF TRAFFICKING SYNDICATES

Trafficking generally involves a chain of persons working in different countries, including origin/source, transit, and destination countries. Trafficking syndicates have a network of associates working all over the globe with one common objective: to successfully transport their human goods from a source country to a destination country for profit. Traffickers use several strategies to achieve this nefarious objective. The first step is to woo their victims with elaborate stories of better lives abroad. This they accomplish through job advertisements in local media and then target their victims.[67] Some unsuspecting African women respond to such local advertisements with the hope of discovering greener pastures abroad, only to end up as prostitutes. Upon arrival in Europe, their job descriptions change drastically.[68] Once trafficked women arrive in a destination country, traffickers utilize a variety of strategies to make them subservient and dependent. Instilling fear in a woman is the most potent psychological strategy that traffickers have used in gaining control over most of their African victims. Other psychological coercive strategies include threatened harm to the victim or her family at home, humiliation, threats of deportation, and at times openly killing the most uncooperative as a deterrent to others.[69] Physical coercion is another strategy that has proved potent for traffickers, and this includes rape, torture, beatings, starving, forced abortions, imprisonment, and confiscation of victim's passports and other travel documents.[70] Psychological coercion has proved most productive for traffickers of African women, due largely to the traditional belief in ancestral spirits or the supernatural held by some African families and communities.[71] Traffickers often subject the women to some juju ritual before leaving the source country. At the ritual, the woman is made to take oaths of allegiance, secrecy, confidentiality, and repayment of the costs of her journey and other incidental expenses, as solely determined by the trafficker. Traditional priests in the community frequently administer these oaths at a shrine. The entire scenario generates its own aura of fear, coupled with the ritual rites and the presence of the priest. Thereafter, the woman feels obligated to the trafficker, and would not disclose her sufferings to any other person.[72] A vivid description of the procedure is provided below:

> A contract is made with the woman and she has to swear an oath to a shrine. The woman swears the oath in the presence of a priest, the madam and the parents (mostly the mother) usually a number of rituals are a part of the oath swearing—a goat or chicken is slaughtered, "nonsense words" are said and wine spilled on the ground. The woman subjects herself to the bidding of the madam and is obliged to pay back money to her. The oath to the shrine is not an unusual phenomenon but a part of ordinary life and the social system in parts of Nigeria . . . Even if the mother and the girl or young woman are not fully aware of the implications of the contract and believe that the woman is going abroad to work as a housemaid, in the cleaning business or even to receive an education the woman is obliged to the oath and to the bidding of the madam . . . the sworn oath given by the victims and

> their sense of obligations towards the shrine make them fear of reprisals even before they are sent off to a foreign country, (Joint Report on Human Rights, 40–41, 5.2.1–2).

The thought of a juju ritual instills fear of reprisal on trafficked African women, thereby compelling them to endure their sufferings in silence. They automatically become afraid of testifying against the traffickers.[73] This has had the adverse consequence of complicating the task of law enforcement agencies and criminal investigators who obviously require both the evidence and tips of trafficked women for thorough investigation and successful prosecution of traffickers.[74] In one reported incident, a Nigerian woman who was trafficked to the U.K. refused to give evidence to the U.K. police because of the fear of the oath she had sworn.[75] To illustrate the immense impact of juju rituals on trafficking in Africa, the Edo State of Nigeria (the state notorious for having the highest number of women trafficked to Europe for prostitution), in 2000 enacted the Edo State "Criminal Code (Amendment Law)."[76] Section 233A of the law categorically criminalizes the administration of any form of oath on a woman or girl or the performance of any fetish ritual aimed at facilitating or enabling a woman or girl to travel out of Nigeria for the purpose of prostitution. In addition, the law also prohibits any person from sponsoring a woman or girl by giving her financial, physical, or material assistance to facilitate her traveling out of Nigeria for the purpose of prostitution or any immoral act, (Edo Criminal Code). The law was strongly opposed by organized crime syndicates who resorted to several vilifying strategies against the Edo State government and legislature, thus throwing the state into a pandemonium.[77]

Despite the good intentions of the Edo State legislature in tackling the juju ritual element of trafficking, most trafficked African women are still not willing to volunteer information to their state police because of the implications it would have on their safety and on the safety of their families at home. The Nigerian police, for example, are known to collaborate with criminals, and in some cases high profile confidential tips given to the police with the aim of facilitating criminal investigations have leaked to the criminals, who then retaliate against the whistle-blower.[78] Hence, the continued reluctance of deported trafficking victims to give evidence against their traffickers appears justifiable. African governments should map out adequate protective mechanisms for those who testify.[79] Until such state-oriented institutional measures are enacted, trafficking victims may remain lukewarm in assisting trafficking crime investigators.[80] In reality, it must be admitted that mapping out such adequate protective mechanisms in order to obtain the testimony of trafficking victims involves extensive and comprehensive reform of the police force and other law enforcement agencies. If this remains the case, such a police reform in the context of Africa is at best unachievable at present.

Another psychological coercion which traffickers utilize in controlling their victims is to place them in debt bondage. This appearance of indebtedness makes a trafficked woman feel bound to her traffickers. Through this mechanism, traffickers are able to control all the earnings of their victims. Since only traffickers know the amount of expenses incurred in effecting a woman's migration, the general assessment is unduly lopsided. A trafficked woman takes whatever figure traffickers quote as the amount to be repaid. In addition, upon arriving at the destination country, there is a simulated change of control all in an attempt to further exploit trafficked women: the trafficker sells the woman to a Madam or pimp. The Madam owns the apartment that accommodates the trafficked woman, and also sets the conditions of sexual services and remittance of proceeds. The Madam is also in charge of receiving payments from clients. The amount that a trafficked African woman is expected to repay to the Madam usually ranges from $20,000 to $45,000; (Ume-Ezeokeke, Desk Review, 16) sometimes extending to as much as $48,000.[81] Unfortunately, because the Madam is in control of the proceeds, coupled with the fact that a trafficked woman does not keep a record of her income, there is no accountability. Suffice it to say that notwithstanding the huge profits that a trafficked woman generates, she still remains indebted to the Madam because payments made by clients disappear into the Madam's coffers. As such, a trafficked woman is thrown into a vicious cycle of debt repayment. This strategy assists the Madam in ensuring that trafficked women do not leave the brothel.[82] This strategy has been most effective for syndicates who traffic African women, as they have been able to use it as a mechanism of controlling their victim's conscience. The juju ritual mentioned earlier correlates with this model to compel the woman to remain in the brothel, as she believes that she is indebted to the Madam until the debts are repaid. In order to facilitate the efficiency of this strategy, the Madam and trafficker confiscate the travel documents of trafficked women, (Ume-Ezeokeke, Desk Review). The above analysis provides some insight into the lives and predicaments of trafficked African women.

PART II: INTERNATIONAL, REGIONAL, AND NATIONAL APPROACHES TO THE ERADICATION OF GLOBAL TRAFFICKING

International Response

All the trafficking mechanisms mentioned in Part I of this chapter contravene existing international human rights conventions. Trafficking women for prostitution leads to loss of human dignity. Pioneering efforts of the international community to address trafficking of women started during the trade in white slaves, and were limited to suppression of sex trafficking, as opposed to prostitution. Prostitution was treated as a matter strictly within the internal jurisdiction of states.[83] In 1904, the League of Nations enacted the International Agreement for the Suppression of the White Slave Traffic to regulate procurement of women for "immoral purposes."[84] Its principal aim was to put an end to the sale of women into prostitution in Europe, in a period of economic adversity. In 1910, the League of Nations came up with the International Convention for the Suppression of the White Slave Traffic, which punished any person who "hired, abducted, or enticed for immoral purposes any woman under the age of twenty-one, or used violence, threats, fraud or any compulsion on a woman over twenty-one, notwithstanding that the various acts which constituted the offense were committed in different countries."[85] In 1933, the International Convention for the Suppression of the Traffic in Women of Full Age was enacted.[86] It punished acts of procuring, enticing, or leading away a woman, even with her consent, for "immoral purposes" to be carried out in another country, (Lawson 1988). In 1949 the United Nations (UN) consolidated all previous international efforts on this subject in one instrument: the 1949 Convention for the Suppression of the Traffic in Persons and of the Exploitation of the Prostitution of Others.[87] The Convention characterized prostitution as being incompatible with the dignity and worth of the human person, and obligated state parties to punish any person who exploited the prostitution of another person, even with that person's consent, (Convention for Suppression of Exploitation, art. 1). It further obligated states to punish any person who kept or managed or knowingly financed or took part in financing a brothel or knowingly let or rented a building or any other place or part for the purpose of prostitution of others, (Convention for Suppression of Exploitation, art 2). This convention has had a porous enforcement mechanism and as such has not been of much help to human rights advocates and practitioners. The failure of the Convention appears to be due to its over-ambitiousness. Instead of focusing on trafficking, it delved into both trafficking and prostitution. It required states to take all the necessary measures to repeal or abolish any existing law, regulation, or administrative provision by virtue of which persons who engage in or are suspected of engaging in prostitution are subject either to special registration or to the possession of a special document or to any exceptional requirements for supervision or notification, (Convention for Suppression of Exploitation, art 2). Arguably, the Convention's bidding that states should not criminalize the prostitute herself is a welcome development, yet it failed to draw a distinction between trafficking and prostitution *per se*. While the prohibition of trafficking may gather momentum in many respects, an extension of that prohibition to prostitution is likely to encounter some difficulties. Prostitution *per se* is a matter purely within the national boundaries and jurisdiction of individual states. Hence it appears necessary to draw a distinction between the two concepts. The distinction between prostitution and trafficking is embodied by the 1979 Convention on the Elimination of All Forms of Discrimination Against Women (CEDAW) which focuses on trafficking and exploitative prostitution. It prohibits "all forms of traffic in women," and obligates states to "take all appropriate measures, including legislation to suppress all forms of traffic in women and exploitation of prostitution of women," (CEDAW, preamble). Hence a distinction is drawn somewhat between trafficking and prostitution. Trafficking is generally prohibited, but prostitution is only prohibited when it is "exploitative." As such, prostitution by choice appears permissible.[88]

Due to the failure of the above conventions to tackle the mounting problems of human trafficking, the international community proceeded to consider other legal options. The foundation of the most current U.N. Convention on trafficking was laid in 1998 at the Seventh Session of the Commission on Crime Prevention and Criminal Justice, where Argentina proposed the drafting of a new convention to prohibit trafficking in minors due to the increasing evidence of the activities of organized criminal networks in the trafficking of minors. This welcome initiative was expanded to include trafficking in all persons. The international community specifically noted the increased vulnerability of women and children and the need to protect and support them.[89] States agreed that the best way of achieving the desired objective was to introduce a Protocol to the U.N. Convention against Transnational Organized Crime.[90] This decision led to the Protocol to Prevent, Suppress and Punish Trafficking in Persons, Especially Women and Children, Supplementing the U.N. Convention against Transnational Organized Crime,[91] (UN Trafficking Protocol) which was passed in 2000. This Protocol outlines three main purposes: (a) to prevent and combat trafficking in persons, with special emphasis on women and children; (b) to protect and assist victims of trafficking; and (c) to promote cooperation among states in order to meet the objectives of the Protocol, (UN Trafficking Protocol,. art. 1, 2 & 4). One remarkable achievement of the Protocol so far is its attempt to define human trafficking. Thus for the first time in human history, the international community reached a consensus on what the definition of trafficking should be. Trafficking is defined in article 3 of the Protocol as:

> (a) The recruitment, transportation, transfer, harboring or receipt of persons by means of threat or use of force, of deception, of abuse of power or of a position of vulnerability or of giving or receiving of payments or benefits to achieve the consent of a person having control over another person for the purpose of exploitation. Exploitation shall include, at a minimum, the exploitation or the prostitution of others or other forms of sexual exploitation, forced labor or service, slavery or practices similar to slavery, servitude or the removal of organs.
>
> (b)The consent of a victim of trafficking in persons to the intended exploitation set forth . . . shall be irrelevant where any of the means set forth in sub-paragraph (a) has been used.

This definition appears to focus on coercion and exploitation. The operative mechanisms of traffickers mentioned in Part I of this paper are all implicated in this definition. It follows that this instrument prohibits them all. Moreover, any inquiry into what should be the appropriate legal parameters where the trafficked woman consented to be trafficked should equally end because this instrument places a strict liability on trafficking. As such, the consent of the victim is immaterial to the offence of the trafficker. Overall, the existence of these conventions suggests that the international community acknowledges that trafficking for prostitution is harmful. Unfortunately, since its commencement in 2000, this UN Trafficking Protocol has not been successful in eradicating human trafficking. This inefficiency has led to its criticism in several quarters. As a result, in 2002 the UN High Commissioner for Human Rights came up with the UN Principles and Guidelines on Human Rights and Human Trafficking, (UN Principles) which serves as an interpretive tool in the enforcement of the UN Trafficking Protocol.

INTERSECTIONS BETWEEN STRUCTURAL ADJUSTMENT PROGRAM AND TRAFFICKING

Africa's trafficking pandemic is largely fuelled by poverty. Africa's poverty level has become somewhat institutionalized. Africa remains the most backward region in the world today in terms of gross domestic product (GDP), technology, and attraction of foreign investments, among others.

It is also the region most cited for economic stagnation and retrogression. The defunct Organization of African Unity (now African Union) noted that "at the close of the 20th century . . . of all the regions of the world, Africa is indeed the most backward in terms of development from whatever angle it is viewed and the most vulnerable as far as peace, security and stability are concerned. . . ."[92] The high rate of poverty in Africa is exacerbated by corruption and embezzlement, which have infiltrated almost all sectors of African governments, institutions, and agencies.[93] Unfortunately, there does not appear to be any public accountability; as such, impunity is the norm. One notable model of abbreviated development that the World Bank and the International Monetary Fund (IMF) applied to most African states is the controversial structural adjustment program (SAP), which has arguably left many African states much poorer than they were when they signed on for financial assistance. This unfortunate situation has been soberly lamented[94] and critiqued[95] by some scholars. SAP was adopted by the World Bank and IMF in the 1980s. SAP was designed to achieve the objectives of neo-liberal economics. Neo-liberal economics is largely geared towards a less interventionist state which minimally participates in the market, and integration of national economies into the international market economy. Africa responded to SAP through the African Alternative Framework to Structural Adjustment Program for Socio-Economic Recovery and Transformation,[96] which advocated for an alternative approach that emphasized self-reliance, human development, and economic transformation. It must be noted that although SAP turned out to be a dismal failure in Africa and other Southern states, that doesn't mean that the policy is inherently ineffective. In fact, the lesson learned from the project is that economic policies should not be applied to all countries as part of a random straight-jacket formula, but should rather be tailored to the needs of the targeted countries, taking into consideration their historical background, political structure, geographical locale, and role of public institutions.[97]

SAP has resulted in the accumulation of debts of about $40 billion by African and other Southern economies,[98] which in turn limits the ability of these countries to fend for their citizens.[99] In very recent times the meetings of the G8 have resurrected further issues respecting the role of globalization in the world order and the need to cancel old debts owed by some impoverished Southern countries. The impact of external debt has been a focus for activist campaigns for more than two decades. Debt has long been a grave concern for people in the South because it is the reason given by their governments for adopting harsh austerity measures that curtail public services and restructuring of economies in harmful ways. The global debt crisis has triggered issues pertaining to the logic of development assistance. For every dollar that wealthy countries provide in aid to impoverished countries, thirteen dollars flow back in debt service payments. Developing countries pay back well in excess of one hundred million dollars every day.[100] For over two decades, Southern states have been caught in this cyclical web of taking out loans to pay off old debts, with the attendant effects of their governments agreeing to new sets of harsh rules on each occasion. Since the beginning of SAP in the early 1980s, African countries have continued to wallow in debt and the treadmill of loans, conditions, rescheduling, and more loans while poverty intensifies in the African continent in particular, and the South in general. External debts typically amount to multiples of most Southern countries' GDP, and it is impossible to service those debts without dipping into scarce foreign exchange and government revenues, which would have been used to support economic, social, and educational projects. It is therefore necessary that the international community should consider the effects of mounting debt repayments and servicing of interest on African countries, and indeed all affected Southern countries. These measures have contrary effects on residents of Southern states, especially women. As governments reduce their spending on viable national projects, the economic power and educational opportunities of the people decrease. This trend increases illiteracy and financial desperation. As women are the worst hit, they become easy targets for traffickers. There is a need to change this model if the international community truly desires to fight human trafficking from the roots.

U.S. APPROACHES TO HUMAN TRAFFICKING

As a result of the ubiquity of the United States in global issues, an inquiry into international responses to trafficking will not be complete without mentioning the efforts of the U.S. This move is made more necessary due to the fact that the domestic trafficking law of the United States requires it to perform a global peer review function through a global monitoring and assessment of state actions in trafficking matters. In October 2000, the U.S. Congress enacted the Trafficking Victims Protection Act of 2000.[101] The Act has three purposes, namely (1) to prevent trafficking; (2) to punish traffickers; and (3) to protect victims, (U.S. Trafficking Act, 7101a). Accordingly, the first purpose of the Act could be interpreted as revealing the U.S. Congress's intent of tackling trafficking from the roots. The Act created an Interagency Task Force (the "Task Force"), charged with the task of studying and combating trafficking in the U.S. and other countries, (U.S. Trafficking Act, 7103). The Task Force is also charged with the duty of monitoring anti-trafficking measures in other countries. The U.S. President is endowed with the discretion to withhold non-humanitarian, non-trade assistance to countries that fail to meet the minimum standards established by the Task Force, (U.S. Trafficking Act, 7107). The Act makes provisions for economic assistance through programs that are aimed at benefiting both trafficking victims and the public, (U.S. Trafficking Act, 7104). The Act also provides for educational programs, lending programs and other assistance geared towards the reduction of power disparity between potential trafficking victims and traffickers, (U.S. Trafficking Act, 7104a). In line with its statutory mandate of studying and combating trafficking, the Task Force produced its first report on July 12, 2001,[102] which listed countries that have a significant number of trafficking victims. The listed countries were subdivided into three tiers, with each tier depicting the Task Force's assessment of a listed country's efforts at meeting the U.S. Trafficking Act's minimum standards for the prevention and elimination of human trafficking, (First U.S. Trafficking Report, 8). This U.S. approach in monitoring global trafficking is called peer review. Peer review is the systematic examination and assessment of the performance of a state by its peers or by a designated institution. In most cases, it is a non-adversarial process, and aims to gather data from the country under review. Such data is then used to assess the country's compliance with particular policies, principles, and practices. From a legal perspective, peer reviews are traditionally used to gauge compliance with international norms such as the U.N. Trafficking Protocol.[103] This documented reporting of global trafficking measures which have been undertaken by listed countries has continued on an annual basis culminating in the most recent report released on June 3, 2005, (U.S. Trafficking Report).

Although the U.S. Trafficking Act has made a profound impact on the fight against human trafficking, its enforcement agenda appears to overlook the root causes of trafficking. Indeed, as the title of the Act connotes, the entire focus of the Act's enforcement is on the protection of victims. While it is good to protect victims, neglecting the root causes of what led victims to their predicament appears to be a misplacement of priorities which is akin to pouring honey into a leaking container. Some of the resources channeled towards the protection of victims could as well be redirected toward projects that make potential victims "untraffickable." That way the arsenal of traffickers would be destroyed. At present, notwithstanding the resources spent on victims' protection on a yearly basis, the number of trafficked victims continues to escalate. This casts doubt on the efficacy of the Act's enforcement agenda. Moreover, financial assistance to affected trafficking countries are made strictly on their acceptance of U.S. policies respecting issues incidental to trafficking. For instance, the U.S. government adopted a strong position against legalized prostitution in its December 2002 National Security Presidential Directive, as a result of U.S. policy on prostitution, which it sees as "inherently harmful and dehumanizing, and fuels trafficking in persons, a form of modern-day slavery."[104] While the U.S. policy on prostitution is sound, it would have been better to limit its application within the U.S. Requiring that U.S. trafficking grants be made strictly on a country's prohibition or statutory renunciation of prostitution amounts to imposition of U.S. domestic policies on other countries. This is hegemonic. After all, the U.N. Trafficking Protocol doesn't draw such a connection between trafficking and domestic prostitution. It only prohibits international trafficking for prostitution, not domestic prostitution, (First U.S. Trafficking Report, art. 3a). It seems that it would have been sound policy for the U.S. to concentrate on trafficking, which is an international issue, rather than delving into prostitution, which is purely a domestic affair.[105] All these distractions appear to prevent the Task Force from addressing the root factors that underlie human trafficking. It is therefore not surprising that the rate of human trafficking is constantly on the increase.

REGIONAL RESPONSE

On the African scene, the Economic Community of West African States (ECOWAS) has taken some steps to address the trafficking pandemic in the continent. Through the efforts of President S.E. Mathieu Kerekou of the Republic of Benin, an action on trafficking in West Africa was initiated and presented to the Authority of Heads of State and Government in its 25th Ordinary Session held in Dakar, Senegal, on Dec. 20–21, 2001. At this session, ECOWAS made a Declaration on the Fight against Trafficking in Persons.[106] The Declaration recognized that "poverty, lack of education and lack of equal opportunity make persons, especially women and children, vulnerable to becoming victims of trafficking; [and] that perpetrators of trafficking in persons, using coercion, abduction, fraud, or deception are taking advantage of the social or economic vulnerabilities of men, women, and children, in order to exploit them," (ECOWAS Declaration, preamble). The Declaration commended member states who have signed and ratified the U.N. Convention against Transnational Organized Crime and the U.N. Protocol to Prevent, Suppress and Punish Trafficking in Persons, Especially Women and Children, and urged those who have not done so to sign or ratify the instruments at the earliest possible date, (ECOWAS Declaration, Proclamation 3). It also urged member states to adopt legislative and other legal frameworks to fight human trafficking, (ECOWAS Declaration, Proclamation 5). Of particular relevance to this analysis is the responsibility placed on member states to "[e]stablish comprehensive policies, programs, and other measures to prevent and combat trafficking in persons," (ECOWAS Declaration, Proclamation 8). This provision expressly obligates states to implement policies and programs that aim to prevent trafficking, and by implication requires states to fight trafficking from the roots. This is a clear recognition that human trafficking is generated by preventable internal factors. The next move of ECOWAS was the ECOWAS Initial Plan of Action against Trafficking in Persons (2002–2003),[107] which was a legal framework that outlined the most urgent actions against human trafficking that ECOWAS member states were required to implement in 2002–2003. Unfortunately, the success of these regional measures in the eradication of human trafficking in Africa is yet to be seen.

NATIONAL RESPONSE

In Nigeria, prior to July 2003, trafficking of women could only be punished through legislation aimed at punishing components of the offense, such as some isolated provisions of the Nigerian Constitution, the Nigerian Criminal Code, as well as the Penal Code of Northern Nigeria.[108] Prosecutions of traffickers were only possible through the creativity of prosecutors. Unfortunately, this mechanism always involved circuitous processes and available penalties under these schemes were not sufficiently proportionate to the severity of the offense. These varied strategies also had the potential of again victimizing the victims of trafficking. Moreover, the applicable scope of the provisions in trafficking cases was somewhat vague. This had the potential of letting some trafficking offenses go unpunished no matter how egregious. These difficulties in trafficking prosecutions were alleviated in July 2003, when the Nigerian National Assembly enacted the Trafficking in Persons (Prohibition) Law Enforcement and Administration Act 2003 (Nigerian Trafficking Act).[109] This move is seminal. It marks the first time in the history of Nigeria that the National Assembly passed a measure that holistically addresses the problem of human trafficking. As will be illustrated below, Nigeria's government outlined an appropriate legal framework in compliance with relevant international instruments such as the U.N. Trafficking Protocol and the U.N. Guidelines on Human Rights and Human Trafficking, (UN Trafficking Protocol and U.N. Principles). This is a step in the right direction. It literally means that Nigeria has laid a foundation in the fight against human trafficking, and shows Nigeria's determination to prevent human trafficking. By enacting this legislation,

Nigeria became the first and only country in West Africa to have a trafficking law. The Nigerian Trafficking Act should inspire and motivate human rights practitioners and advocates, as well as serve as a guide and stimulant to institutional frameworks built to fight against trafficking. The definition of *trafficking* in the Nigerian Trafficking Act is substantially drawn from the U.N. Trafficking Protocol. According to the Nigerian Act, "trafficking includes all acts and attempted acts involved in the recruitment, transportation within or across Nigerian borders, purchases, sales, transfer, receipt or harboring of a person involving the use of deception, coercion or debt bondage for the purpose of placing or holding the person whether for or not in involuntary servitude (domestic, sexual or reproductive) in force or bonded labor, or in slavery-like conditions."[110]

The Nigerian Trafficking Act established the National Agency for the Prohibition of Traffic in Persons and Other Related Matters (NAPTIP), (Nigerian Trafficking Act, section 1, 1) for the purpose of monitoring and enforcement. The legislation highlights as two functions of NAPTIP the "adoption of measures to increase the effectiveness of eradication of traffic in persons" (Nigerian Trafficking Act, section 4c) and the "taking of such measures and or in collaboration with other agencies or bodies that may ensure the elimination and prevention of the root causes of the problem of traffic in any person," (Nigerian Trafficking Act, section 4h). These mandates are essential to the fight against human trafficking. It means that interpreters, law enforcement agencies, and anti-trafficking government agencies have a duty to tackle trafficking from the roots if the aims of the act are to be achieved. The Nigerian Trafficking Act has succeeded in removing the stigmatization of trafficked women by mandating the "taking charge [by the Agency, in] supervising, controlling and coordinating the rehabilitation of trafficked persons and participation [on of trafficked persons] in proceedings relating to traffic in persons," (Nigerian Trafficking Act, section 4k). This is a welcome development in view of the fact that due to the heightened corruption that pervades the Nigerian police, any provision that casts a gory specter on trafficked women could be utilized by corrupt Nigerian police as an avenue to extort and further violate the human rights of deported trafficked women. The act's gestures in this regard are laudable because it supports the proposition that the primary purpose is to protect trafficked women and would-be trafficking victims from the horrendous trafficking net of syndicates, pimps, or Madams. Moreover, the provision complies with the objective of the UN Trafficking Protocol and the interpretive framework established by the U.N. Guidelines on Human Rights and Human Trafficking.

Another advantage inhering from the Act is that the removal of any criminal charges for trafficked women is likely to eliminate fear of adverse domestic legal consequences. As such, those who fall prey to the trafficking snares may not be bothered about deportation threats, which is one of the fear factors that syndicates and Madams strategically adopt in gagging and taming trafficked women. In fact, if the home front offers better legal protections, some courageous women may willfully turn themselves over to the police of the destination country rather than risk the bondage of syndicates.

That said, the Nigerian government should engage in international, multilateral and bilateral co-operation with other countries in order to achieve success in its bid to eradicate human trafficking. Trafficking is a transnational menace. Through bilateral agreements, Nigeria could achieve substantial success in this direction. Moreover, such transnational cooperative measures will be complying with U.N. Principles and Guidelines on Human Trafficking, the Economic Community of West African States' (ECOWAS) Declaration on the Fight Against Trafficking in Persons,[111] as well as the Nigerian Trafficking Act. One of the provisions of the Nigerian Trafficking Act recognizes that "the Agency [NAPTIP] shall be responsible for strengthening and enhancing effective legal means for international co-operation in criminal matters for suppressing the international activities of traffic in persons," (Nigerian Trafficking Act, section 4i). In line with this bidding, the present accord between Nigeria and the U.K. to trap human trafficking gangs and help their victims is commendable. The Attorney General of Nigeria, Akinlolu Olujinmi, and the Solicitor General of the U.K., Harriet Harman, in London on November 17, 2004, signed a Memorandum of Understanding in which they agreed to share intelligence on criminals and make it easier to extradite suspects.[112] The present bilateral agreement between Nigeria and Italy is also noteworthy. At present, it seems too early to assess the efficacy of the bilateral agreements. Considering the fact that NAPTIP was formed in August 2003 and commenced full operations from its Abuja corporate headquarters in February 2004, it seems reasonable to suggest that NAPTIP needs time to document the events that have transpired so far. Nevertheless, more bilateral treaties are needed with other destination countries.[113] Nigeria should equally take advantage of the robust trafficking instruments within the United Nations body. Intuitively, Nigeria's attempt to fully adhere to the UN Trafficking Protocol is commendable. So long as Nigeria uses the U.N. Principles and Guidelines on Human Trafficking to interpret the Nigerian Trafficking Act, and make requisite amendments in the future to reflect human rights dynamics, its efforts are likely to receive the support of the international community.

Under the UN Trafficking Protocol, states are required to protect victims of trafficking. This obligation falls upon whichever state the victim is in at any given time. Some states appear not to be complying with this protocol.[114] On the other hand, the present warm reception that Nigeria gives to trafficked persons meets the mandate of this Protocol, which requires states to "facilitate and accept" the return of victims who are their nationals or had residency rights during their trafficking. In fact, the Nigerian Trafficking Act expressly mandates NAPTIP to carry out this function: "The Counseling and Rehabilitation Unit [of NAPTIP] shall . . . be responsible for counseling, after care rehabilitation, social re-reintegration and education of trafficked persons; and counseling and the promotion of the welfare of convicts," (Nigerian Trafficking Act, section 9,3). However, the present Nigerian police attitude of parading repatriated trafficked persons on national network news of the Nigerian Television Authority[115] runs counter to the UN Trafficking Protocol and the U.N. Principles and Guidelines on Human Trafficking.[116] This police show-off and self-congratulation may turn out to be fatal to the victims: first, their families may be humiliated by such gestures; second, their traffickers may be apprehensive. Any of these two affected groups may arrange to kill the victim in order to protect their image, also called 'honor killing' in some countries. Moreover, considering the rampancy of extra-judicial killings and summary executions in Nigeria,[117] a trafficker could easily take advantage of the incessant ethnic and religious riots in Nigeria to harm his deported victim. At present, it does not appear that Nigeria is capable of curtailing summary executions; as such there is no public interest served in further exposing victims to danger. When the Nigerian trafficking wave finally subsides, the international community would know those that contributed to its eradication. There is no need for the police to jubilate over insignificant "achievements" of being instrumental to the deportation of trafficked victims to Nigeria.

As protective of victims and would-be victims, and as deterrent to traffickers as the Act may be, its substantive usefulness in achieving these objectives lies in its enforcement mechanisms. Substantive law without procedural mechanism is not worth the paper on which it is written.[118] Part of the institutional measures undertaken by Nigeria in compliance with the UN Trafficking Protocol is the establishment of NAPTIP. NAPTIP is charged with the responsibility of investigating and prosecuting offenders, rehabilitating and counseling victims, as well as providing public awareness on human trafficking, (Nigerian Trafficking Act, preamble and section 4). This makes Nigeria the first state in West Africa to establish an agency to monitor trafficking in conformity with the U.N. Trafficking Protocol and the U.N. Principles and Guidelines for Human Trafficking, as well as the ECOWAS Declaration Against Human Trafficking.[119] NAPTIP is in its infancy and regulations have just recently been effected. It is therefore too early to carry out an assessment of the Act.

Notwithstanding that it is still too early to assess the achievements of the Act and of NAPTIP, deported women should be given adequate support for proper reintegration into Nigerian society. They should be able to access protection programs capable of helping them in dealing with their traumatic experiences. Unfortunately, there are presently no long-term shelters for returned or deported victims of trafficking in Nigeria. Presently existing shelters only offer protection and rehabilitation for a maximum of two weeks, after which victims are expected to be independent, (Joint Report on Human Rights, 43–44, 5.4.6 and 5.6.2). This is grossly inadequate. This has the potential of forcing victims back into the cycle of want and re-victimization. Under the UN Trafficking Protocol, states are required to take all necessary measures to prevent "re-victimization" of trafficked persons.[120] Moreover under the ECOWAS Declaration Against Trafficking in Persons, states are required to "protect victims of trafficking from further victimization," (ECOWAS Declaration, at Proclamation 8). Re-victimization usually occurs in situations where deported victims cannot properly reintegrate into their home country as a result of lack of employment opportunities and finances to meet their needs. In situations of this nature, victims stand the risk of being trafficked out again, and usually to another destination country or a different location in their last destination country where the environment and people will be completely new, and accessing assistance is rarely feasible. Re-victimized people are likely to be subjected to harsher terms than their previous trafficking experience. This would render victims more vulnerable as traffickers will beef up monitoring and surveillance of the victims to block all possible avenues of assistance and escape. This problem is critical because it is one of the root factors that has the potential of encouraging trafficking in Africa. If deported victims are re-victimized, it logically follows that all the efforts of the origin and destination countries, as well as other members of the international community, in bringing the victim back to her home country are in vain. Again, it is like pouring honey into a leaking container. Arguably, it is also paradoxical because instead of protecting the victims, the institutional measures would in reality worsen the victims' predicaments. This problem can only be addressed if NAPTIP and other African anti-trafficking agencies adopt necessary measures to counter the possibility of re-victimization of returned victims.

However, the positive role of Nigerian NGOs in this regard must be emphasized. The Italian government and a Nigerian faith-based NGO, the

Catholic Society, entered into an agreement respecting the reception and support of victims of trafficking who are returned to Nigeria. The Catholic Secretariat has been acclaimed as having a "'holistic attitude' regarding return and reintegration" of trafficking victims, (Joint Report on Human Rights, 47, 5.7.15). Generally, African NGOs deserve to be applauded on their contributions toward the eradication of human trafficking in Africa. The present Nigerian Trafficking Act under review was pioneered by the Women Trafficking and Child Labor Eradication Foundation (WOTCLEF), an NGO founded by the wife of the Vice-President of Nigeria, Titi Abubakar. WOTCLEF submitted the draft bill to the Nigerian National Assembly and followed it up to the point of enactment through the assistance of the Deputy Speaker of the House, Hon. Chibudom Nwuche, who became the sponsor of the bill. However, a lot still needs to be done by African NGOs. There is no room for complacency. Nigerian NGOs' intervention in trafficking is not an isolated experience within the international community,[121] but all NGOs should co-operate in all possible ways to ensure complete eradication of trafficking networks in Africa.[122]

On a critical note, the Nigerian Trafficking Act appears to suffer from unskillful drafting and structural pitfalls. First, the preamble of the Act gives the undisputed impression that the Act is about the establishment of NAPTIP. This could rightly be interpreted as the legislative intent because in addition to the preamble, the first ten sections of the Act are devoted to the establishment of NAPTIP. This is an unfortunate misplacement of priority. It amounts to placing the cart before the horse. NAPTIP was formed to enforce and monitor the Act. It follows that without the Act there wouldn't be any need for NAPTIP. Second, Part I of the Act entitled "Establishment of the National Agency for Traffic in Persons Law Enforcement and Administration," does not draw any boundary between the sections that are geared towards the establishment of NAPTIP and those that are meant to prohibit trafficking in persons. For instance, sections 1 to 10 make provisions for NAPTIP, and immediately after section 10, there is section 11, which begins the prohibition for traffic in persons. Unfortunately, there is nothing like a new subheading (for e.g. Part II) to alert the reader about the transition. Third, in legislative drafting, citation sections or notes (which direct the reader on how to cite the Act) usually appear at the beginning of the Act it governs. In the Nigerian Trafficking Act under review, ironically the citation is the very last section.[123] Fourth, in a similar vein, in legislative drafting, interpretive sections are usually found at the beginning of an Act. Common wisdom supplies the logic behind such practice: the interpretations are meant to serve as a guide to the reader in deciphering the contours of the terms that are used in the Act in question.

This is necessary because the statutory interpretation of a word, phrase, or term may be different from its conventional connotations. Unfortunately, the interpretive section of the Nigerian Trafficking Act is section 50, the penultimate section. This is regrettable. It complicates the task of the reader and becomes somewhat otiose. Fifth, contextually, the Act generally limits its protection to persons "under the age of eighteen years."[124] This limitation of protection to persons less than eighteen years appears to give the impression that the legislative intent is to protect minors. As such, it could be argued that the policy behind the Act envisions that adults can protect themselves. This raises the issue of *consent*. In other words, the drafters of the Act seem to conclude that an adult who consents to be trafficked doesn't require the protection of the law. But in reality, this line of policy is myopic. Empirical data on trafficking reveals that there are lots of information asymmetries, and that majority of those who consent to trafficking (both adults and minors) encounter obstacles that were never anticipated when their consent was given. In other words, women who consent to trafficking face both the "lemons" problem (as a result of information asymmetry), and the "moral hazard" problem (as a result of the opportunistic behavior of the trafficker after the consent is given). The United Nations Office on Drugs and Crime succinctly captured the social attitude towards consent in the following words:

> Every year hundreds of men, women and children are trafficked illegally all over the world. Most of us assume that these people are willing participants in a criminal transaction. *We believe that they are simply looking for an escape from poverty. Rarely do we pause to think about the specific problems they encounter when they are being smuggled or what happens to them afterwards. The reality reflects a very different picture, namely that these people are often economically, sexually and physically exploited.* They pay large sums of money in order to be transported under harsh conditions to another country, often unknowingly under a false pretext. They end up forced to work in prostitution or engaged in other criminal activities in the country of destination.[125]

This observation locates the social context of the problems that consenting trafficked women face after the facts.[126] Unfortunately the Nigerian Trafficking Act appears to overlook this.

On the whole, notwithstanding lapses in the Nigerian Trafficking Act and NAPTIP's enforcement shortfalls, compared to other African countries Nigeria's efforts appear to have far-reaching potential of impacting the problem of trafficking in Africa. It is therefore commendable and should serve as a model for other African countries that have yet to comply with the Trafficking Protocol.

STATE RESPONSIBILITY IN THE CREATION OF GRASSROOTS SOLUTIONS TO TRAFFICKING

States have a responsibility to "ensure that their interventions address the factors that increase vulnerability to trafficking, including inequality, poverty and all forms of discrimination," (U.N. Principles, principle 5). There is a need for cultural reorientation with the aim of eliminating gender-based discrimination and related factors. Fighting trafficking from the roots requires that states devise effective prevention strategies based on the existing experiences of the people, (U.N. Principles, principle 5, guideline 7). There should be increased access to educational opportunities for children and youths. This would mean that governments have to fund education. As a result of gender imbalance in the educational sector due to poverty, which forces parents to draw a scale of preference between their sons and daughters, governments might consider reducing tuition for girls so that parents would have no reason to keep their daughters at home when their age-mates are in school. It must also be mentioned that although there is free primary education in some African countries, such as Nigeria, most parents still prefer to take their children to private schools, which are comparatively more expensive than public schools. All private schools in Nigeria are expensive, though some are more expensive than others. The reason for the massive boycott of public schools is due to inadequate funding from the government. Most public schools lack adequate infrastructure and dedicated teachers. Of course, teachers are not to blame because their salaries are left unpaid for months if not years. Like every human being, public school teachers have to pay their bills as well as meet their family responsibilities. Basically, the only way to achieve this appears to be by shirking their responsibilities and pursuing other ventures during official hours. As such, the government's free primary education only exists on paper. This attitude should change. It is the poor masses who cannot afford private education for their kids that suffer the effects of this government under-funding of the public schools, as they rely solely on public schools to meet their children's educational needs. Generally, the whole problem of trafficking haunts the poor because their children are usually the first to be approached by traffickers, since they are usually desperately in need. Unfortunately, social, economic and educational rights are not enforceable rights in Africa. At the international level, they are at best regarded as third generation rights. This is regrettable.

There should be information campaigns for the public with the aim of promoting awareness to the dangers of trafficking. This is a good way of sensitizing youths. At present, African youths hold the belief that in western countries there are lots of opportunities to make easy money with little or no effort. This is the myth that traffickers adopt in deceiving youths.[127] There is a need to debunk this myth and to create awareness in African youths that there is no free lunch in the West. In fact, it is more possible to have a free lunch in Africa than in the West. Experience has shown that Africans in Western countries have become so westernized that they will never offer a free lunch to anyone. Thus, there is the need to fill the gap that information asymmetry creates in the minds of African youths. The Nigerian Trafficking Act recognizes this fact: "The Public Enlightenment Unit [of NAPTIP] shall . . . be responsible for campaigns, seminars and workshops aimed at educating the public on the problem of trafficking in any person, thereby stimulating interest in and awareness about the problem," (Nigerian Trafficking Act, section 9, 2).

The government should fund youth-oriented projects that offer livelihood options. This would assist in creating more jobs. There is no need to draw any gender distinction in the project, because statistics presently indicate that crime and violence are rampant among young men. This is largely due to unemployment. Hence, while young women are being trafficked for prostitution, young men are being lured into gangs for stealing, becoming thugs for politicians who rig elections and assassinate their opponents, and turning into vandals for community leaders who wish to extort money from oil companies. They serve as a rallying point for youth organizations legitimately fighting for their community's rights to self-determination, but are also easily accessible tools for extremists who perpetrate ethnic and religious violence. Some if not all of these agendas, that unemployed young males are exposed to, are inimical to societal development and unity. As such, government-funded youth-oriented projects should cater for the needs of both male and female youths in order to avoid lopsided development.

States should develop national plans of action aimed at eradicating trafficking. One way of achieving this is by creating a partnership between NGOs and government institutions charged with the responsibility of combating trafficking.[128] NGOs are visibly fighting against trafficking. It is therefore necessary for governments to partner with them. A good example would be a partnership between NAPTIP and various anti-trafficking NGOs in Nigeria. This would be a practical way of recognizing that NGOs can play central role in improving the law enforcement response to trafficking by providing useful information on the incidents and patterns of trafficking. Some may argue that destination states should consider reducing some procedural difficulties that make it difficult for immigrants to migrate. If people can migrate on their own, then they would shun third party involvement. Although free mobility ought to be one of the benefits of globalization, it does not appear that destination countries are ready to open their borders for free flow of immigrants, especially those from developing countries. Yet the problem seems to lie with origin/source countries: if the home front is good, people may not want to move to another country.

CONCLUSION

This chapter has traced the problem of trafficking in Africa to its root causes. These root causes of trafficking are predominantly social, cultural, religious, and political factors that are internally generated in Africa. These factors appear to be completely neglected by both the African continent and the international community. The study therefore argued that any national, regional, or international measures that aim to tackle human trafficking cannot achieve significant progress unless these root causes of trafficking are first recognized and addressed. The study proceeded to highlight the modus operandi of trafficking networks in Africa, pointing out that these networks have been given a safe harbor in their operations, as a result of legal loopholes that ignore the root causes of this illegal trade. There is therefore the need for states to go back to the drawing board and map out strategies of eliminating the internal factors that trigger and exacerbate trafficking in Africa. It is not enough to fight trafficking from the surface.

NOTES

1. Report of the United Nations High Commissioner for Human Rights to the Economic and Social Council, UN Doc. E/1999/96 (emphasis added). Moreover, the Report of the Secretary General (E/CN.4/2002/80, 25 Jan. 2002) unequivocally pointed out that "the lack of human security and gross inequalities within and between countries are still the main reasons why people take dangerous migration decisions and why so many women and children end up being trafficked." See U.N. Human Rights System, Trafficking in Persons—Commission on Human Rights (2002), available at http://www.hri.ca/fortherecord2002/engtext/vol1eng/traffickingchr.htm (last visited Jan. 8 2006) [hereinafter Commission on Human Rights].
2. See Report, "Transatlantic Workshop on Human Smuggling," 15 (2000) *Geo. Immigr. L.J.* 167, 176–82.
3. See Kelly E. Hyland, "The Impact of the Protocol to Prevent, Suppress and Punish Trafficking in Persons, Especially Women and Children"8 (2001) *Hum. Rights Br.* 30, 30.

4. For a series of state studies documenting the shortcomings of this program vis-à-vis developing states, see Michael Chossudovsky, *The Globalization of Poverty* (1997). See also Enrique Carrasco & M. Ayhan Kose, "Income Distribution and the Bretton-Woods Institutions: Promoting an Enabling Environment for Social Development" 6 (1996) *Transnat'l L. & Contemp. Probs.* 1; J. Oloka-Onyango, "Beyond the Rhetoric: Reinvigorating the Struggle for Economic and Social Rights in Africa" 26 (1995) *Cal. W. Int'l L.J.* 1, 20–29; Bharati Sadasivam, "The Impact of Structural Adjustment on Women: A Governance and Health Rights Agenda" (1997) *Hum. Rights Quarterly* 630, 641–43. The structural adjustment program has been aptly described thus: "Structural adjustment consists of reforms aimed at stabilizing developing countries' external and internal balances and promoting their growth by devaluation, producer price increases, trade liberalization, privatization and supporting institutional changes. Its adoption has usually (but not always) occurred in a context of economic crisis and on the basis of promises of resources from donors, led by the two foremost international financial institutions, the IMF and the World Bank. The latter are also largely responsible for the design of adjustment programmes." See *Limits of Adjustment in Africa*, (Poul Engberg-Pedersen et al., eds., 1996): ix.
5. Francis Stewart, *Adjustment and Poverty: Options and Choices* (1995): 213 (lamenting that the exogenous developments that led to adjustment were not tackled by the World Bank and IMF. These developments include falling price of commodities and exorbitant debt servicing. These events were accepted rather than attacked. The policies of the World Bank and IMF arguably worsened these developments. The encouragement given to adjusting countries in order to facilitate expanded production of primary commodities actively assisted in worsening the commodity price situation.).
6. See E.E. Okojie, Obehi Okojie, Kokure Eghafona, Gloria Vincent-Osaghae & Victoria Kalu, *Trafficking of Nigerian Girls to Italy,* (July 2003): 17 (A study commissioned by U.N. Interregional Crime and Justice Research Institute), available at http://www.unicri.it/wwd/trafficking/nigeria/docs/rr_okojie_eng.pdf (last visited Oct. 26, 2005); hereinafter cited in text as *Trafficking to Italy* (observing that "some experts trace the beginning of trafficking in Nigerian women and girls for prostitution in Italy to the second half of the 1980s as a result of economic depression in Nigeria and the adoption of the Structural Adjustment Program. The resulting economic deprivations forced many Nigerians to leave the country in search of better economic opportunities in Europe, Saudi Arabia, the United States, and other countries. This marked the beginning or escalation of the brain drain out of Nigeria. Persistent unemployment among the youth and rising poverty led to the young desiring to go out of the country in search of greener pastures.")
7. See Janie Chuang, *Redirecting the Debate over Trafficking in Women: Definitions, Paradigms, and Contexts,* 11 (1998) *Harv. Hum Rts. J.* 65, 68.
8. See *Trafficking to Italy*, 26. (Noting: "Male children are more highly valued than female children, as the male continue with the family name, while the female children marry out of the family.")

9. Statistics from Nigeria's last census indicates that the number of women in the labor market is very few. Notwithstanding that the male-female population ratio was 50–50, out of the 26.6 million people in employed labor, only 9.8 million (36.8 percent) were females. See Florence Nightingale, "Nigeria: An Assessment of the International Labor Migration Situation." *GENPROM Working Paper No. 7*, at 3 (Gender Promotion Program of International Labor Office, Geneva), available at http://www.ilo.org/public/english/employment/gems/download/swmnig.pdf (last visited June 5, 2005); hereafter cited in text as Labor Migration. See also *Trafficking to Italy*, at 7.(Observed that "In Nigeria, women . . . have no direct access to credit facilities because of low income and lack of collateral. Their lack of formal training means that they are not able to access other opportunities available in the better paying employment sectors of the economy. Consequently, women have become prime targets for recruiters involved in trafficking for sexual exploitation.")
10. For e.g., see the horrifying story of a Nigerian woman Amina Lawal in section C of this Part I, 'Overview of Root Factors Influencing Trafficking in Nigeria.'
11. See The Joint British-Danish Fact-Finding Mission, *Report on Human Rights Issues in Nigeria,* (Jan. 2005) at 45, available at The Danish Immigration Service website: www.udlst.dk (last visited June 5, 2005); hereafter cited in text as Joint Report on Human Rights. Copies could also be obtained by e-mail: dok@udlst.dk. (Observing that "a recent survey conducted by IOM showed that it is mostly victims of internal conflicts that are being trafficked and that internally displaced children also are victims of trafficking. Internal conflicts in Nigeria are conducive to establishing illegal trafficking and also for recruiting children.") Another example is the Democratic Republic of Congo (the "Congo"). Following the independence of the Congo from Belgium in 1960, Congo has suffered from heightened corruption, authoritarianism, ethnic divide, to military administration and mismanagement of national economy. For more than 40 years, Congo has gone through vicious-cyclic coups, rebellions, unconstitutional regimes and a despicable political and constitutional history, which altogether have reduced human dignity to the lowest ebb. See generally W. Breytenbach et al, "Conflicts in the Congo: From Kivu to Kabila" 8 African Security Rev. 33 (1998). See also "Extract from the Report of the UN Secretary-General on UN Deployment in the DRC" 7 *South African J. Int'l Affairs* 183, (2000); hereafter Report on UN Deployment.
12. Commission on Human Rights; (The Commission on Human Rights adopted by consensus a resolution on traffic in women and girls in which it urged governments "to take appropriate measures to address the root factors, including external factors, that encourage trafficking in women and children").
13. See U.N. High Commissioner For Human Rights Principles and Guidelines on Human Rights and Trafficking, E/2002/68/Add.1 (2002), at Principle

2, available at http://www1.umn.edu/humanrts/instree/traffickingGuide-linesHCHR.html (last visited Sep 28, 2005); hereinafter cited in text as U.N. Principles.

14. Report of the Special Rapporteur on Violence Against Women, its Causes and Consequences, U.N. ESCOR, Commission on Human Rights 53rd Sess., Provisional Agenda Item 9(a), at 19, U.N. Doc. E/CN.4/1997/47 (1997).
15. Empirical data reveals that Nigerian women constitute more than 50% of all Africans who have been trafficked any where in the world. See Sani Mohammed, "Gaudy Promises Lure Children, Women into Slavery" *Crossroads* Vol. 10, No. 4 (May 2003), available at http://nigeria.usembassy.gov/wwwhxmay)3.html (observing that the U.S. Diplomatic Mission to Nigeria estimates that as at May 2003, "as many as 300,000 [Nigerian women] have been trafficked since 1997") (last visited May 2, 2005); See also Juliet Ume-Ezeokeke, "Desk Review for the Program of Action against Trafficking in Minors and Young Women from Nigeria into Italy for the Purpose of Sexual Exploitation," 28; hereafter cited in text as Desk Review. (A joint trafficking project by the UN Interregional Crime and Justice Research Institute and the UN Office on Drugs and Crime) (observing that an estimate of over 500,00 African women and children have been trafficked), available at http://www.unicri.it/wwd/trafficking/nigeria/docs/dr_nigeria_eng.pdf (last visited Oct. 26, 2005). A juxtaposition of the two studies supports the premise that Nigerians constitute more than one-half of all trafficked Africans.
16. U.S. Department of State, "The 2005 Trafficking in Persons Report" available at http://www.state.gov/g/tip/rls/tiprpt/2005/46903.htm (last visited Nov. 20, 2005); hereinafter cited in text as U.S. Trafficking Report. See also Marina Jiméenez, "B.C. is a Hub for Human Trafficking, Report Says," *The Globe and Mail,* (Thursday, June 9, 2005) which carried the highlights of the Report.
17. U.S. Department of State, "Office to Monitor and Combat Trafficking in Persons," available at http://www.state.gov/g/tip/, (last visited June 15, 2004). For a confirmation of this figure see the United Nations Office on Drugs and Crime, *Fact Sheet on Human Trafficking,* available at http://www.unodc.org/unodc/en/trafficking_victims_consents.html (last visited Oct. 26, 2005) (observing that, "a recent CIA report estimated that between 45,000 to 50,000 women and children are brought to the United States every year under false pretences and are forced to work as prostitutes, abused laborers or servants.").
18. http://europe.cnn.com/2001/WORLD/europe/02/04/immigration/index.html (last visited Dec. 10 2005). See also Chuang, 1998.
19. Jiméenez, 2005, which carried the highlights of a U.S. State Department's Fifth Annual Trafficking in Persons Report. The Report noted that "[t]he RCMP [Royal Canadian Mountain Police] estimates that about 800 people are trafficked into Canada annually and an additional 1,500–2000 are trafficked through Canada to the United States." See also "Trade in Humans Targeted" *Metro News,* Toronto, (Tuesday, March 9, 2004)

where Canadian Minister of Justice Irwin Cotler, observed that "Canada serves not only as a country of destination but also a country of transit for criminals flooding men, women and children into the United States."

20. Reuters Ltd, "Mafia Makes Billions from Trafficking People—UN" (Dec. 15, 2000), available at http://www.vachss.com/help_text/styles/archive-print.php, (last visited June 15, 2005); hereafter cited in text as Mafia Makes Billions.
21. Anti-Slavery "Human Trafficking Q&A" available at http:www.anti-slavery.org/homepage/antislavery/trafficking.htm (last visited June 10, 2005).
22. *Trafficking to Italy*, 17 (observing: "There is generally a paucity of data on the scale and trends in human trafficking around the world largely because of the criminal and underground nature of trafficking. Thus most available data are estimates by various researchers and NGOs working on the subject.").
23. United Nations Office on Drug and Crime, "Analysis and Statistics," available at http://www.unodc.org/unodc/trafficking_protocol_background.html (last visited June 15, 2005).
24. U.N. Office on Drugs and Crime, "Fact Sheet on Human Trafficking," available at http://www.unodc.org/unodc/en/trafficking_victim_consents.html (last visited Oct. 26, 2005).
25. *Trafficking to Italy*, 5; (the Study further reveals the history of human trafficking in Italy: "Trafficking of women to Italy dates back to the end of the 1980s when the fear of AIDS rendered drug-addicted Italian girls unattractive on the prostitution market, and the first Nigerian girls began to appear on the streets, especially in the central and northern Italy. Nigerians thus constituted Italy's first cohort of 'forced prostitutes' . . .").
26. Michael Specter, "Traffickers' New Cargo: Naïve Slavic Women," *N.Y. Times* (Jan. 15, 1998), 6.
27. *Trafficking to Italy*, 14 (noting that "[g]iven the poor state of record keeping in Nigeria, most of them [respondents in a trafficking sudy] had no data to fall back on. As a result, many of the answers were left blank as the respondents said they don't know much about the details of human trafficking although they are aware the problem exists . . . Most of the answers were the impressions or guesses of the respondents based on hearsay . . . In general, obtaining hard data was very difficult, and most of what was obtained represents personal estimates by respondents to the questionnaires. Some of the agencies which had data were very secretive, and reluctant to divulge them. Very little published data by these agencies are available, mainly because there have been no coordinated efforts to keep good records of human trafficking. Most of the available data are records of those repatriated, not of those who had been trafficked.")
28. This secrecy on the part of prospective trafficking undertakers exacerbates the problem of trafficking in that it positively conditions the market

for traffickers. For further analysis on this, see section E of this Part I below: 'Overview of Root Factors Influencing Trafficking in Africa.'

29. At the outset, it should be noted that on a general level it is not all deportations that are trafficking related. However, in this analysis, unless otherwise indicated, all the references to deportations are trafficking related. This brief explanatory note is meant to serve as a backgrounder to the reader in assessing the figures.
30. Osita Agbu, "Corruption and Human Trafficking: The Nigerian Case" *West Africa Review* (2003), available at http://www.westafricareview.com/vol4.1/agbu.html (last visited June 15, 2005) (Observing that "[a]t a March 2002 seminar organized in Lagos by the International Federation of Women Lawyers (FIDA), WOTCLEF [Women Trafficking and Child Labor Eradication Foundation] reported that there are about 20,000 Nigerian women involved in the sex industry in Italy. The *Daily Champion* of 12 July 2002 reported that 80% of foreign prostitutes in Italy were Nigerian women.") (emphasis in original).
31. Warm Africa, "Traffickers hold thousands of children, women in bondage" (12 Nov. 2003), available at http://www.warmafrica.com/index/geo/4/cat/3/a/a/artid/382 (last visited May 2, 2005).
32. Women's Rights Watch—Nigeria, "2004 Report on the State of Women's Rights in Nigeria" available at http://www.rufarm.kabissa.org/articles/2004report.htm (last visited May 24, 2005).
33. BBC News Online, "Child Asylum Seekers Sold for Sex" (Thursday, March 8, 2001), available at http://news.bbc.co.uk/1/hi/uk/1208611.stm (last visited May 26, 2005); hereafter BBC Child Asylum Seekers.
34. Maureen Chigbo, "Igbinedion Versus Prostitutes" *Online Nigeria Portal,* available at http://www.onlinenigeria.com/aids/edo_prosti.asp (last visited June 3, 2005). This figure was confirmed in a homegrown trafficking study conducted in 2003 in Edo State of Nigeria, see *Trafficking to Italy*, 7; (observing that "about 80% of girls and women trafficked into Italy from Nigeria are from Edo State.")
35. Ibid. (emphasis in original). In addition, Oba Erediauwa also received a letter from T.S.O. Olumoko, the Nigerian charge d' affires in Italy, which stated: "Any black woman [in Italy] is seen as a Nigerian prostitute. Many respectable women, including wives of diplomatic personnel have been propositioned and embarrassed in this manner."
36. "Trade in Humans Targeted" Toronto *Metro News* (Tuesday, March 9, 2004) (Quoting Canadian Justice Minister Irwin Cotler).
37. United Nations Office on Drugs and Crime, "Involvement of Organized Crime," available at http://www.unodc.org/unodc/en/trafficking_victim_consents.html (last visited Oct. 26, 2005) (observing: "The relatively low risks of trafficking and substantial potential profits have, in some cases, induced criminals to become involved as an alternative to other, riskier criminal pursuits.")
38. Joint Report on Human Rights; (where it was observed that "a number of the so-called "victims of trafficking" are actually persons who voluntarily

use traffickers so that they can enter into prostitution for financial reasons. However, some persons who have traveled overseas expecting to be employed as au pair girls or in similar jobs may also end up in prostitution.")

39. For details of how some of these factors may affect women in other continents, see A. Miller and A. Stewart, "Report from the Roundtable on the Meaning of 'Trafficking in Person': A Human Rights Perspective" 20 (1998) *Women's Rts. L. Rep.* 14; hereinafter Report from Roundtable.
40. *Trafficking to Italy*, 26 (noting: "Male children are more highly valued than female children, as the male continue with the family name, while the female children marry out of the family.")
41. Ume-Ezeokeke, Desk Review, 15; Nightingale, Labor Migration, 5; (observing: "In most cases, women migrants are trafficked and the decision to migrate is taken by others (relations, friends, husbands, and/or parents). This is another indication of the patriarchal nature of Nigerian society, which subjugates women and erodes their independence of thought, initiative, action and decision.") (Parenthetical emphasis in original); See also Joint Report on Human Rights, 39; (observing that "they were aware of cases in which husbands have sold their daughters and even wives to trafficking agents well aware that these women may be exploited and forced into prostitution overseas."
42. Joint Report on Human Rights, 40–41, 5.2.1–2; (observing: "A contract is made with the woman . . . in the presence of a priest, the madam and the parents (mostly the mother) . . . Even if the mother and the girl or young woman are not fully aware of the implications of the contract and believe that the woman is going abroad to work as a housemaid, in the cleaning business or even to receive an education. . . ."
43. U.S. Department of State, "Office to Monitor and Combat Trafficking in Persons," available at http://www.state.gov/g/tip/, (last visited June 15, 2005). (confirming the obvious fact that women and children are particularly vulnerable to trafficking due largely to the persistent inequalities they encounter in status and opportunities.)
44. *Trafficking to Italy*, 27; (observing that "customs helped to explain the inferior status accorded to women among the Edos [of Nigeria]. Thus sons are preferred to daughters. This influences access to education as parents prefer to send sons to school while girls were withdrawn from school in times of adversity and married off at young ages." and at 21 the Study observed: "High rates of unemployment among girls due to relatively low levels of female education because of unwillingness of their parents to send them to school, provided a pool of girls to be trafficked abroad." And at 7 "Many families unable to cope with exorbitant costs of education are forced to withdraw their girls from school, hence there is a high rate of illiteracy among women.")
45. Statistics from Nigeria's last census indicates that the number of women in the labor market is very few. Notwithstanding that the male-female population ratio was 50–50, out of the 26.6 million people in employed labor, only 9.8 million (36.8 percent) were females. On the other hand, less valued informal jobs like petty trading, processing and sales, tailoring, and beauty salons are dominated by women. See Nightingale, Labor Migration, 3; In a similar

vein, a trafficking Study conducted in 2003 in Nigeria confirms this trend. See *Trafficking to Italy;* (where it was observed: "In Nigeria, women contribute to the domestic economy as farmers, petty traders, domestic workers and homemakers. Their work is grossly undervalued and poorly rewarded, and to worsen their condition, they have no direct access to credit facilities because of low income and lack of collateral. Their lack of formal training means that they are not able to access other opportunities available in the better paying employment sectors of the economy. Consequently, women have become prime targets for recruiters involved in trafficking for sexual exploitation.")

46. Reuters, Mafia Makes Millions; (reporting that, "[i]n Italy, criminals operate an extensive and elaborate ring that lures Nigerian women into the country on the pretext of getting work. They are then sold to pimps for about $12,000 each. 'The girls are slaves. There is no other way to define it. . . . The pimps want to make a four-fold profit on their investment, meaning the girls have to pay $48,000 before they are free.'") (Emphasis in original).
47. This line of reasoning is contrary to the views expressed elsewhere: "sex trafficking cannot be viewed as a cultural practice but rather as a universal crime linked to slave trade." See Susan W. Tiefenbrun, "Sex Sells but Drugs Don't Talk: Trafficking of Women Sex Workers" 23 (2001) *T. Jefferson L. Rev.* 199, 208. It should be noted that Tiefenbrun did not completely rule out the impacts of cultural practices in trafficking. She qualified the above statement with the following words: "That is not to say that legal scholars should disregard the cultural, social, economic and political causes of the worldwide practice of sex trafficking."
48. For a comprehensive engagement of the factors influencing women to migrate for work, see International Labor Organization, *Preventing Discrimination, Exploitation and Abuse of Women Migrant Workers: An Information Guide—Booklet 2: Decision-Making and Preparing for Employment Abroad* (2003): 9–20. See also "Report of the Special Rapporteur, Ms. Gabriela Rodriguez Pizarro," submitted pursuant to General Assembly Resolution 57/218 (U.N. Doc. A/58–275) (12 August 2003).
49. Convention on the Elimination of All Forms of Discrimination Against Women, Sep. 3, 1981, 1249 U.N.T.S. 13 (adopted and opened for signature, ratification and accession by G.A. res. 34/180 of 18 Dec. 1979), available at http://www.safnet.com/cedaw.html (last visited Oct. 1, 2005); hereinafter cited in text as CEDAW.
50. The Constitution of The Federal Republic of Nigeria, 1999, section 42(2): "No citizen of Nigeria shall be subjected to any disability or deprivation merely by reason of the circumstances of his birth" hereinafter cited in text as Nigerian Constitution.
51. The existence of the status of illegitimacy is recognized and endorsed by the Nigerian culture. Describing the position, Coker observed: "It is generally supposed that there is no status of illegitimacy in native law and custom: this, however, is not correct for there is a status of illegitimacy as opposed to that of legitimacy." See G.B.A. Coker, *Family Property Among*

the Yoruba (London: Sweet & Maxwell, 1966): 226. Moreover, Obi after examining the position in Southern Nigeria concluded that a child born of an unmarried mother is illegitimate at birth; See S.N.C. Obi, *Modern Family Law in Southern Nigeria* (London: Sweet & Maxwell, 1966): 294.

52. Nigerian Constitution, section 1, which embodies the Constitutional supremacy clause: "This Constitution is supreme and its provisions shall have binding force on all authorities and persons throughout the Federal Republic of Nigeria. . . . If any other law is inconsistent with the provisions of this Constitution, this Constitution shall prevail, and that other law shall to the extent of the inconsistency be void."
53. See e.g., The Canadian Charter of Rights and Freedom, Part 1 of the Constitution Act, 1982, being schedule B to the Canadian Act 1982 (U.K.), 1982 C.11, section 15 (the bedrock of Canadian equality jurisprudence); hereinafter cited in text as Canadian Charter. The Charter is enforceable against government or government related/controlled bodies. This equality provision has greatly enhanced the status of Canadian women.
54. See e.g. *International Pen and Others (on behalf of Saro-Wiwa Jr.)* v. *Nigeria* (*Ken Saro-Wiwa* case), Communications 137/94, 139/94, 154/96 & 161/97, Twelfth Annual Activity Report, where the complainants died at the hands of the government of a state party. For this decision and other African Commission decisions, see the University of Minnesota Human Rights Library online resources, available at http://www.umn.edu/humanrts/africa/; African Commission's homepage is at http://www.achpr.org; hereinafter collectively called African Commission site.
55. A good example is open murder carried out by the Nigerian government in November 1999 against the people of Odi Community in Bayelsa State. In addition, on October 28, 1999 the Nigerian government deployed a number of soldiers and mobile police to Choba in Rivers State, who reportedly killed four people, injured several others, amputated the arm of one person, and raped at least sixty-seven women and detained twenty-one youths See Human Rights Watch, "The Destruction of Odi and Rape in Choba," in *Nigeria—Human Rights Watch World Report* (Human Rights Watch 2000), also available at http://www.hrw.org/press/1999/dec/nibg1299.htm, last visited (20 Aug. 2005). It should be noted that Odi and Choba communities are ethnic minorities in Nigeria. In another development, Banyamulenge is an ethnic minority in the Democratic Republic of Congo. This Community was denied their Congolese citizenship. In 1996 the Congolese Tutsi were expelled from the Masisi region, which led to a violent inter-ethnic conflict. See H. Wolpe, "The Great Lakes Crisis: An American View" 7 *South African J. Int'l Affairs* 27, (2000): 31. See also Mbata B Mangu Andr, "The Conflict in the Democratic Republic of Congo and the Protection of Rights under the African Charter" 3 *African Hum. Rights Law J.* 235, (2003): 239. Of recent, Amnesty International has drawn the attention of the international community to the "systematic rape and torture of at least 40,000 women and girls . . . in the Democratic Republic of Congo . . . many

victims, aged six to over 70 are being gang raped by up to twenty-five combatants or taken prisoner and used for months or years as sex slaves" See http://www.righttodecide.org//newsletter/article.html; last visited (1 Nov. 2005).

56. For a review of the insecurity in the Democratic Republic of Congo which has been exacerbated by heightened corruption, authoritarianism, ethnic divide, military administration, and mismanagement of national economy see generally Breytenbach, 1998. See also Extract from the Report on UN Deployment.
57. Elizabeth Isichei, "The Maitatsine Risings in Nigeria 1980–1985" XVII, 3, *Journal of Religion in Africa* (1987).
58. Kazah Toure Toure, *Ethno-Religious Conflicts in Kaduna State* (Kaduna, Nigeria: Human Rights Monitor, 2003).
59. Gwamna Dogara Je'adayibe, "The Urban Factor in Ethno-Religious Crisis in Jos and Bauchi Areas" (a Report commissioned by the African Centre for Democratic Governance (AFRIGOV)) (Abuja, Nigeria: African Centre for Democratic Governance, 2002).
60. *Kaduna State of Nigeria White Paper on the Report of Judicial Commission of Inquiry Into Kaduna State Religious Disturbances of February 2000* (Kaduna, Nigeria: The Government Printer, 2001); hereafter cited in text as Report of Judicial Commission. It should be noted that due to political factors and logistic problems, the reported figures are likely to be below the actual number of deaths.
61. Jan H. Boer, *Nigeria's Decades of Blood* (Jos, Nigeria: Stream Christian Books, 2003) (observing that there had already been more than thirty violent incidents of riots in the northern states of Nigeria). See also Joseph Kenny, "Sharia and Christianity in Nigeria" XXVI, 4, *Journal of Religion in Africa* (1996) (noting that although social tension and confrontation between regions and ethnicities have been part of Nigeria for a long time, religious confrontation is a very recent phenomenon).
62. Joint Report on Human Rights; (where the Chief of Mission for the International Organization for Migration (IOM) explained that "a recent survey conducted by IOM showed that it is mostly victims of internal conflicts that are being trafficked and that internally displaced children also are victims of trafficking. Internal conflicts in Nigeria are conducive to establishing illegal trafficking and also for recruiting children.").
63. Meredeth Tushen et al, eds. *What Women Do in Wartime: Gender and Conflict in Africa* (London: Zed Books, 1998).
64. A. Joshi, "The Face of Human Trafficking" 13 *Hastings Women's L.J.* 18 (2002).
65. See generally "IOM Says 120,000 Trafficked into Western Europe Annually," which is a release by the U.S. Mission to the European Union, 2 January 2002, available at www.useu.be/Categories/Justice%20and%20Home%20Affairs/Jan0802IOMHumanTrafficking.html (last visited 8 Jan. 2006).
66. Dan Isaacs, "Nigerian Woman Fights Stoning" BBC (8 Jul 2002), available at http://news.bbc.co.uk/1/hi/world/africa/2116540.stm (last visited

Mar. 15, 2006); Amnesty International, "Nigeria: Amina Lawal Freed," available at http://www.amnesty.org.uk/action/aminalawal.shtml (last visited Mar. 15, 2006); Amnesty International, "Amnesty International Press Release—Nigeria: Amina Lawal's Death Sentence Quashed at Last but Questions Remain about Discriminatory Legislation" (25 September 2003), available at http://web.amnesty.org/library/index/engafr440322003 (last visited Mar. 15, 2006).

67. U.N. Office on Drugs and Crime, "Trafficking in Human Beings," available at http://www.unodc.org/unodc/en/trafficking_human_beings.html (last visited Oct. 26, 2005) (observing that "women and girls are attracted by the prospect of a well-paid job as a domestic servant, waitress or factory worker. Traffickers recruit victims through fake advertisements, mail-order bride catalogues and casual acquaintances.") See also U.N. Office on Drugs and Crimes, "Trafficking in Persons: the New Protocol," available at http://www.unodc.org/unodc/trafficking_protocol_background.html (last visited Oct. 26, 2005) (observing that "[y]o[u]ng women and teenagers are often lured into prostitution rings by advertisements for domestic positions abroad and find themselves bought and sold via catalogues or by close family members.")
68. Melanie R. Wallace, "Voiceless Victims: Sex Slavery and Trafficking of African Women in Western Europe" 30 (Spring 2002) *Georgia J. Int'l & Comp. L.* 569 (asserting that "[t]here are certain consistent patterns by which most African prostitutes are introduced to prostitution in Western Europe. The first scenario involves African women brought from their home countries for the purpose of exploiting them through prostitution (usually with their prior knowledge. Sponsors with ties on both African and European continents lure African women and girls to Europe, promising them a chance to study at a university or take advantage of job opportunities. These women are often promised jobs as maids or au pairs or given loans (with or without their knowledge) to finance their passage and are then forced to repay the loans through prostitution when they arrive.") (all comments in original). See also U.N. Office on Drugs and Crime, "Trafficking in Human Beings," (noting: "Upon arrival at their destination, victims are placed in conditions controlled by traffickers while they are exploited to earn illicit revenues.")
69. BBC Child Asylum Seekers, where BBC reported: "There are 2,500 African prostitutes working on the streets of Turin alone. Seven have been killed in the past four years." BBC also interviewed Marianne, a Nigerian girl trafficked to Italy for prostitution, who observed: "I don't want to die. I want to stay [sic] in life . . . Many of our girls are dying here because of 'I cannot do it.' They organize our boys and beat you. You have to be on the street as if you are not a normal human being." (emphasis in original). It must be pointed out that the BBC observation that seven African prostitutes were killed in the past four years is an understatement. According to official sources from Nigeria, "the wife of Edo State Governor, Mrs. Eki Igbinedion, announced that about 116 Nigerian prostitutes were killed in Italy between 1994 and 1998." See *Trafficking to Italy*, 39.

See also Joint Report on Human Rights, 43, 5.4.4 (where it was observed that a trafficking syndicate or the pimp could trace a returned trafficking victim "if they suspect that she intends to cooperate with the authorities. In such cases the madam or the agent may hire persons from militant groups . . . and in this way have the woman killed as a deterrent to others.")

70. Tiffany St. Claire King, "The Modern Slave Trade" 8 (2002) *U.C. Davis J. Int'l L. & Pol'y* 293, 308–309. See also Lori Romeyn Sitowski, "Congress Giveth, Congress Taketh Away, Congress Fixeth Its Mistake? Assessing the Potential Impact of the Battered Immigration Women Protection Act" 19 (2001) *Law &Ineq.* 259, 280 (observing that Captors force their victims into submission by unleashing various forms of physical coercion on them and "many are thereby exposed to AIDS and other disease, and some are worked or beaten to death.") See also Agbu, 2003; (observing that "[a] report of the International Organization for Migration noted that in many cases traffickers seize their victims' travel documents and sell the women to brothel owners.")
71. *Trafficking to Italy,* 28–29 (With particular reference to the Edos of Nigeria, the authors observed: "Various deities and ancestral deities are worshipped . . . *Osanobua* or *Osa* is the highest God, creator of all things and beings in the world and heaven . . . *Olokun* is described as equivalent of the Greek god Neptune. *Olokun* is the great god of the sea. He is said to be a senior son of *Osanobua* . . . *Ogun* is the deity of iron or metals. *Osun* is the deity of medicine and employed to ensure the effective use of all forms of medicine. *Obiemwen* is a wife of the earth and described as equivalent of the Greek Uranus . . . *Ogiuwu* is the deity in charge of death. *Oruunmila* is the divining deity. Spirits of the departed or ancestors are also worshipped.")
72. BBC Child Asylum Seekers, where a Social Worker Lynne Chitty, reacting to the disappearance of more than 40 African teenagers seeking asylum in the UK, observed that, "traffickers forced girls to go through a voodoo ceremony before they left their home country. They have to swear not to tell anyone and while they are swearing they are being cut. Some girls have 40 or 50 cuts all over their body. They are forced to drink blood and this all happens in a dark and frightening place. One girl when she told me was just trembling, crying 'my body's going to blow up and I'm going to die now.'") (Emphasis in original).
73. See Nightingale, Labor Migration; (observing that in Nigeria only "few trafficked persons have been courageous enough to reveal the identity of their traffickers, due to the oath of secrecy to which they are sworn and fear of repercussions for breaking it. To date, no traffickers have been prosecuted."). See also Joint Report on Human Rights, 5.2.5–6; (where Carol N. Ndaguba, the Executive Secretary/Chief Executive of the Nigerian National Agency for the Prohibition of Traffic in Persons and Other Related Matters (NAPTIP) referred to a recent incident in which six trafficked women had refused to testify against their traffickers because of the juju oath they have been committed to. However, in order to convince the women that nothing would happen to them if they testified, NAPTIP raided two shrines in Edo State

and recovered a number of items including the pictures and hair of the six victims. Two priests were also arrested and paraded before the victims in order to convince them.) Notwithstanding all the institutional wars against shrines and juju oath, the psychological fears in the minds of trafficked victims remain unabated.

74. Ume-Ezeokeke, Desk Review, 19; (observing that "an officer of the Trafficking Unit in Edo [State of Nigeria] Police Commission said that it is difficult to arrest or even prosecute the Barons because complainants and witnesses are not willing to testify against them in the court for fear of being assassinated.")
75. See Anti-Slavery, "Human Traffic, Human Rights: Redefining Victim Protection" 10. Nigeria 159 at 165, available at http://www.antislavery.org/homepage/resources/humantraffichumanrights.htm (last visited May 2, 2005) (although the girl was eventually persuaded to give evidence to the police, shortly after relaying her experiences, she injured herself unconsciously and blamed the injury on the oaths.)
76. Edo State Criminal Code (Amendment Law) 2000, sections 223a-223d; hereafter cited in text as Edo Criminal Code, (specifically, 223A punishes any person who "sponsors a girl or woman by giving her any financial, physical or material assistance to enable her travel out of Nigeria" for prostitution or any immoral act or administers any oath on any woman or girl or performs any fetish ritual in order to enable her travel out of Nigeria to become a prostitute or engage in sexual dealings with any person; 223B punishes any female person who engages in prostitution or other immoral acts within or outside Nigeria; 233C punishes any man who patronizes prostitutes; 223D punishes any woman who lures or induces any man to engage in sexual intercourse with her for any gratification). Analytically, this amendment is a paradox: it initially set out to punish traffickers and save victims of trafficking, however, its substance reveals that it punishes victims rather than traffickers. What purpose does it serve to punish a woman who engages in prostitution abroad, without making exceptions respecting the reasons for her actions? Most trafficking victims do not know that they would end up as prostitutes. As such punishing a trafficking victim who engages in prostitution does not seem reasonable. Rather than reduce trafficking, this law has the effect of making trafficking go underground because a woman who reveals her trafficker stands the risk of being implicated as well. Hence it appears that women would rather keep quiet than reveal their ordeals. Revelation will lead to double jeopardy. Moreover, the law lays emphasis on prostitution rather than trafficking. This is a misconception. Trafficking and prostitution are two different concepts although they may be inextricably intertwined. The inability of the law to draw this distinction is rather unfortunate. It is note within the scope of this analysis to delineate the contours of the trafficking-prostitution debate that has amassed volumes of feminist literature. For a close-contextual engagement of this issue, see Victor N. Opara, "Legal Aspect of Migration and Human Trafficking" in Hakeem I. Tijani, ed. *Africa and the Wider World* (New

York: McGraw-Hill Higher Education Publisher, 2006) (Part VII, forthcoming).

77. For a compendium of the controversies, see Chigbo, 2005.
78. This back-stabbing attitude is contrary to U.N. Principles and Guidelines. See U.N. Principles, Guideline 5; (asserting that "[a]n adequate law enforcement response to trafficking is dependent on the cooperation of trafficked persons and other witnesses. In many cases, individuals are reluctant or unable to report traffickers or to serve as witnesses because they lack confidence in the police and the judicial system and/or the absence of any effective protection mechanisms. *These problems are compounded when law enforcement officials are involved or complicit in trafficking. Strong measures need to be taken to ensure that such involvement is investigated, prosecuted and punished. Law enforcement officials must also be sensitized to the paramount requirement of ensuring the safety of trafficked persons.*") (Emphasis added).
79. U.N. Office on Drugs and Crime, "Trafficking in Human Beings" available at http://www.unodc.org/unodc/en/trafficking_human_beings.html (last visited Oct. 26, 2005) (where it was observed: "The support and protection of victims who give evidence is key to prosecuting the ringleaders behind the [trafficking] phenomenon" See also U.N. Office on Drugs and Crime, "Involvement of Organized Crime" available at http://www.unodc.org/unodc/en/trafficking_victim_consents.html (last visited Oct. 26, 2005) (cautioning that "[t]rafficked persons should also be seen as victims of crime. Support and protection of victims is a humanitarian objective and an important means of ensuring that victims are willing and able to assist in criminal cases.")
80. Such measure has been effected in Nigeria, although its enforcement remains to be seen. See Nigerian Trafficking Act, at section 45 (Mandating that "[w]here a person volunteers to the Agency or an official of the Agency any information, which may be useful in the investigation of an offence under this Act, the Agency shall take all reasonable measures to protect the identity of that person and the information so volunteered shall be treated as confidential.")
81. Reuters, Mafia Makes Millions; (observing: "In Italy, criminals operate an extensive and elaborate ring that lures Nigerian women into the country on the pretext of getting work. They are then sold to pimps for about $12,000 each . . . The pimps want to make a four-fold profit on their investment, meaning the girls have to pay $48,000 before they are free. They are told that if they flee or talk to the police, their families in Nigeria will be killed.")
82. S. McClelland, "Inside the Sex Trade" *Macleans* (3 December 2001) 22.
83. Edward Lawson, Encyclopedia of Human Rights 144 (Edward Lawson, ed., 1988).
84. International Agreement for the Suppression of the White Slave Traffic, 18 May 1904, 35 Stat. 426, 1 L.N.T.S. (as amended by Protocol, Dec. 3, 1948), available at http://www.un.org/Depts/Treaty/final/ts2/newfiles/part_boo/vii_8.html (last visited October 1, 2005).

85. International Convention for the Suppression of the White Slave Traffic, 4 May 1910, 211 Consol. T.S. 45, 1912 GR. Brit. T.S. No. 20, at 2670 (as amended by Protocol, 20 Oct. 1947).
86. The International Convention for the Suppression of the Traffic in Women of Full Age, 11 Oct. 1933, 150 L.N.T.S. 431.
87. Convention for the Suppression of the Traffic in Persons and of the Exploitation of the Prostitution of Others, July 25, 1951, 96 U.N.T.S. 271, available at http://www.univie.ac.at/RI/KONTERM/intlaw/konterm/vrkon_en/html/doku/prostitu.htm#1.0 (last visited Oct. 1, 2005); hereafter cited in text as Convention for Suppression of Exploitation.
88. It is not within the scope of this analysis to make extensive use of copious feminist literature on trafficking-prostitution debate. I have addressed this issue elsewhere. For a thorough engagement of the issue, see Victor N. Opara, "Legal Issues in Migration and Human Trafficking in Africa" in Hakeem I. Tijani, ed. *Africa and the Wider World* (New York: McGraw-Hill Higher Education Publisher, 2006) (Part VII, forthcoming).
89. United Nations Office on Drugs and Crime, "Trafficking in Persons: the New Protocol," available at http://www.unodc.org/unodc/trafficking_protocol_background.html (last visited Oct. 26, 2005).
90. U.N. Convention against Transnational Organized Crime, 29 Sep. 2003, G.A. Res 55/25, U.N. GAOR 55th Sess., available at http://www.unodc.org/unodc/en/crime_cicp_signatures_convention.html, also at http://www.undoc.org/unodc/en/crime_cicp_convention.html (last visited Oct. 26, 2005).
91. The Protocol to Prevent, Suppress and Punish Trafficking in Persons, Especially Women and Children, Supplementing the UN Convention against Transnational Organized Crime, G.A. Res. 55/25 of 15 Nov. 2000, annex II, U.N. GAOR, 55th Sess., No. 49, at U.N. Doc. A/45/49 (vol.1) 2001), U.N. Doc. A/53/383 (2000), also available at http://www.unodc.org/unodc/en/trafficking_convention.html; http://www.uncjin.org/Documents/Conventions/dcatoc/final_documents_2/convention_%20traff_eng.pdf; and at http://www.uncjin.org/Documents/Conventions/dcatoc/final_documents_2/index.htm (last visited Oct. 26, 2005); hereinafter cited in text as UN Trafficking Protocol.
92. Yaounde Declaration, "Africa: Preparing for the 21st century" OAU Doc. AHG/Decl.3 (XXXII), pmbl. 2 (July 8–10, 1996), available at http://www.africanreview.org/docs/govern/yaounde.pdf (last visited March 10, 2006).
93. For a tip of the iceberg see Nnimmo Bassey, "Nigeria: Debt and Corruption" (18 July 2005) *Committee for the Abolition of the Third World Debt*, available at http://www.cadtm.rog//article.php3?id_article=1547 (last visited Mar. 18, 2006) (Observing that "[t]he [Nigerian] Senate president, the number three man in the government, got kicked out of office for allegedly helping to grease [sic] of palms of some Senators, so that a government ministry's budget could be laced up with bogus figures. The Senate president did not go down alone. He is currently squirming in the dock with the former minister of education and some other senators.

Another minister was sacked for underhand dealings in a proposed sale of government houses in the high-brow section of Ikoyi, Lagos. Many of President Obasanjo's extended family members were scheduled to become owners of these choice quarters built with public funds. . . . Many agree that the fight against corruption is long overdue, and that although there are shortcomings in the warfare, it is still better than nothing.")

94. Francis Stewart, *Adjustment and Poverty: Options and Choices* 213 (1995) (lamenting that "the exogenous developments that necessitated adjustment were not tackled by these institutions [World Bank and IMF]—the major ones being falling commodity prices and exorbitant debt servicing. These events were taken as constraints to be accepted rather than challenged. The policies of the institutions probably made these 'exogenous' developments worse. Encouragement of adjusting countries to promote expanded production of primary commodities contributed to the continued worsening of the commodity price situation.")
95. For a critique of the implementation of the structural adjustment policies in Africa, see Howard Stein, *Globalization, Adjustment and the Structural Transformation of African Economies?: Role of International Financial Institutions* (Working Paper No. 32/99, CSGR, May 1999), available at http://ssrn.com/abstract=165812) (last visited March 17, 2006). See also Robert Biel, *The New Imperialism: Crisis and Conditions in North/South Relations* 231 (2000) (arguing that the structural adjustment policies of the IMF were not designed to assist developing countries but to integrate them into the capitalist system).
96. Economic Commission for Africa, African Alternative Framework to Structural Adjustment Programs for Socio-Economic Recovery and Transformation, available at www.uneca.org/publications/ESPD/old/aaf_sap.pdf) (last visited March 17, 2006).
97. David Dollar & Jacob Svensson, *What Explains the Success or Failure of Structural Adjustment Program?* (Policy Research Working Paper, World Bank, 1998) available at http://www.worldbank.org/html/dec/publications/workpapers/WPS1900series/wps1938/wps1938.pdf) (indicating that the World Bank has acknowledged that for economic reforms to be successful, democratic institutions should be allowed full participation) (last visited Dec. 15, 2005). See also Yvonne Tsikata, *Owning Economic Reforms* (United Nations University, Discussion Paper No. 2001/53, 2001), available at http://www.wider.unu.edu/publications/dps/dp2001.53.pdf (last visited Jan. 10, 2006) (stating that local ownership plays crucial role to the success of economic reforms).
98. Eric Toussaint & Damien Millet, "IMF Threat on G8 Proposal of Debt Cancellation" (17 July 2005) *Committee for the Abolition of the Third World Debt,* available at http://www.cadtm.org//article.php3?id_article=1544 (last visited Feb. 10, 2006).
99. The Nation (Nairobi), "Odious Debts—Why Kenya Deserves Debt Relief" (3 April 2005), available at http://www.odiousdebts.org/odiousdebts/index.cfm?DSP=content& . . . (last visited Mar. 18, 2006) (Observing: "Do you know that we are on the only continent to have grown poorer in the last 25 years?

While in 1970 Africa housed 10 per cent of the world's poor, it was home to about half the world's poor in 2000. Of what good have the loans been?")

100. See Jubilee (UK) *General Facts and Figures: Rich World, Poor World,* available at http://www.jubileeplus.org/databank/sefustatistics/generalstats.htm (last visited Sep 11, 2005); See also Jubilee (USA), *A Silent War: The Devastating Impact of Debt on the Poor,* available at http://www.jubileeusa.org/ubilee.cgi? (last visited Sep 11, 2005).
101. Trafficking Victims Protection Act of 2000, 22 U.S.C. 7101 (2000); hereinafter cited in text as U.S. Trafficking Act.
102. U.S. Dept. of State, Victims of Trafficking and Violence Protection Act of 2000: Trafficking in Persons Report (July 2001), available at http://www.state.gov/documents/organization/4107.pdf (last visited Feb. 10, 2006); hereinafter cited in text as First U.S. Trafficking Report.
103. See e.g., *The Global Competitiveness Report 2005–2006,* (World Economic Forum (2005), available at http://www.weforum.org/site/homepublic.nsf/Content/Global+Competitiveness+Programme%5CGlobal+Competitiveness+Report (last visited Mar. 1, 2006).
104. U.S. Dept. of State, "The Link between Prostitution and Sex Trafficking" (24 Nov. 2004), available at http://www.state.gov/r/pa/ei/rls/38790.htm (last visited June 16, 2005). (The release concluded that "[a]s a result of the prostitution-trafficking link, the U.S. government conclude that no U.S. grant funds should be awarded to foreign non-governmental organizations that support legal state-regulated prostitution. Prostitution is not the oldest profession, but the oldest form of oppression.")
105. As has been indicated earlier, it is not within the scope of this analysis to make extensive use of copious feminist literature on trafficking/prostitution debate. I have addressed this issue elsewhere. For a thorough engagement of this issue, see Victor N. Opara, "Legal Issues in Migration and Human Trafficking in Africa" in Hakeem I. Tijani, ed. *Africa and the Wider World* (New York: McGraw-Hill Higher Education Publisher, 2006) (Part VII, forthcoming).
106. Declaration A/DC12/12/01on the Fight against Trafficking in Persons, Economic Community of West African States (ECOWAS), 25th Ord. Sess. of Heads of States and Government, Dakar 20–21 Dec. 2001, available at http://www.iss.co.za/af/RegOrg/unity_to_union/pdfs/ecowas/6Dechutraf.pdf (last visited Jan. 29, 2005): hereinafter cited in text as ECOWAS Declaration.
107. ECOWAS Initial Plan of Action against Trafficking in Persons (2002–2003), available at http://www.unodc.org/pdf/crime/trafficking/Minimum_Plano_CEDEAO.pdf (last visited Jan. 29, 2005); hereinafter ECOWAS Initial Plan.
108. See e.g., The Constitution of Nigeria, 1999, which contains provisions that prohibit forced labor, slavery, sexual exploitation and deprivation of personal liberty. Specifically, section 35 guarantees personal liberty while section 34 states that "(a) No person shall be subjected to torture or to inhuman or degrading treatment, (b) No person shall be held in slavery, (c) No person shall be required to perform forced or compulsory labor").

See also the Criminal Code, Laws of the Federation 1990 (Nigeria), Cap. 77, sections 222(a), 223, 224, 225(a), 227, 365, 366 and 369 (briefly, these provisions are: 222(a) punishes any person who directly or indirectly causes the seduction, unlawful carnal knowledge, or prostitution, or the commission of indecent assault upon a girl under 13 years; 223 punishes any person who procures a girl or woman to have sex with other persons within or outside Nigeria; 224 punishes any person who by threats, intimidation or false pretence procures a woman or girl or administers stupefying or overpowering drugs on her to facilitate unlawful sexual relations with a man either within or outside Nigeria; 225(a) punishes any person who exploits female prostitutes for a living; 227 punishes any person who conspires with another to induce any woman or girl, by means of false pretence or other fraudulent means to facilitate unlawful sexual intercourse between her and any man; 365 punishes the unlawful deprivation of the liberty of a person by confinement or detention; 366 punishes any person who compels another to do any act which he/she is lawfully entitled to abstain from doing—this includes use of threats, persistent surveillance or other forms of intimidation; 369 punishes the use of a person as a slave—this includes placing or receiving any person in servitude as a pledge or security for a current or future debt; or conveying, sending or inducing any person to go outside Nigeria to enable the person to be possessed, dealt or traded in, purchased, sold or transferred as a slave or be placed in servitude as a pledge or security for debt; or entering into any contract or agreement with or without consideration for doing any of these acts). See also the Penal Code, Laws of Northern Nigeria 1963, Cap. 89, sections 271, 272, 275–281 (which briefly provide: 271 & 272 punish any person who entices a minor, male below 14 years and female below 16 years, or conveys him/her outside Northern Nigeria, or deceives or induces any person to move to any other place; 257 punishes any person who induces a girl under 18 to move to another place with the intention of forcing or seducing her to have illicit sexual intercourse with another person; 227 punishes any person who knowingly conceals or confines kidnapped or abducted persons; 279 punishes any person who directly or indirectly deals in any person as a slave; 280 punishes forced labor; 281 punishes the procurement, enticement or leading away of any woman or girl (with or without her consent) for immoral purpose.

109. Trafficking in Persons (Prohibition) Law Enforcement and Administration (Nigeria) Act 2003, 2003 Act No. 24; hereinafter cited in text as Nigerian Trafficking Act.
110. Nigerian Trafficking Act, section 50. Compare with UN Trafficking Protocol, art. 3; (Trafficking means "[t]he recruitment, transportation, transfer, harboring or receipt of persons by means of threat or use of force, of deception, of abuse of power or of a position of vulnerability or of giving or receiving of payments or benefits to achieve the consent of a person having control over another person for the purpose of exploitation.")
111. U.N. Principles, Guideline 11; (stating that "trafficking is a regional and global phenomenon which cannot always be dealt with effectively at the

national level . . . International, multilateral and bilateral cooperation can play an important role in combating trafficking activities. Such cooperation is particularly critical between countries involved in different stages of the trafficking cycle"). See also ECOWAS Declaration, preamble; (declaring that "effective cooperation, intelligence gathering, information sharing, and training are essential to the prevention and eradication of trafficking in persons; [and also acknowledged] the importance of enhanced regional and international cooperation in the struggle against trafficking in human beings").

112. Government News Network, "UK and Nigeria Sign Agreement to Stamp Out Modern Day Slavery" 17 Nov. 2004, available at http://www.gnn.gov.uk/content/detail.asp?NewsAreaID=2&ReleaseID=135721&print=true (last visited 7 Jan. 2006); Afrol News, "Nigeria to Fight Human Trafficking" 17 Nov. 2004, available at http://www.afrol.com/printable_article/14827 (last visited 7 January 2006). See also Women's Rights Watch—Nigeria, *2004 Report on the State of Women's Rights in Nigeria,* available at http://www.rufarm.kabissa.org/articles/2004report.htm (last visited Oct. 24, 2005).
113. See ibid. where the Attorney General of Nigeria stated that "Nigeria is unrelenting in its commitment to partner with other countries of the world in fighting human trafficking." This proactive move is a welcome development that will fulfill the U.N. requirements which urge states to "consider adopting bilateral agreements aimed at preventing trafficking, protecting the rights and dignity of trafficked persons and promoting their welfare . . . [as well as] establishing mechanisms to facilitate the exchange of information concerning traffickers and their methods of operation." See U.N. Principles, Guideline 11(1), (6).
114. For example, Greece received international criticism from Human Rights Watch in 2000 with regards to its treatment of trafficking victims: "[T]he government of Greece has failed to combat trafficking, continuing instead to treat trafficking victims as criminals, allowing the real criminals—the traffickers and their protectors within government structures—to profit with impunity. Detained and deported, trafficked women do not have access to even the most minimal human rights guarantees—no shelter, no witness protection, no medical care, psychological support, or assistance. Nor do they have access to justice. The government of Greece has failed abysmally to indict and prosecute traffickers and corrupt officials." See King, 2002, 298.
115. Joint Report on Human Rights, 45, 5.7.4; (Noting that "in many cases returned women have been shown on television").
116. U.N. Principles, Guideline 6(6) (urging states to consider "ensuring that trafficked persons are effectively protected from harm, threats or intimidation by traffickers and associated persons. To this end, there should be no public disclosure of the identity of trafficking victims and their privacy should be respected and protected to the extent possible, while taking into account the right of any accused person to a fair trial").

See also UN Trafficking Protocol, Part II—Protection of Trafficked Persons, art. 6–8; which mandates countries to endeavor to provide for the basic safety and security of victims.

117. A good example is the open murder carried out by the Nigerian government in November 1999 against the people of Odi Community in Bayelsa State, a major oil community in the Niger Delta zone. In addition, on October 28, 1999 the Nigerian government deployed a large number of soldiers and mobile police to Choba Community in Rivers State (another major oil community in the Niger Delta zone), who killed four people, injured several others, amputated the arm of one person, raped at least sixty-seven women, and detained twenty-one youths. The pioneering incident of fatal brutality in oil community / oil companies' showdown climaxed in November 1995 when Ken Saro-Wiwa and eight other leaders of Ogoniland (another major oil community in the Niger Delta) were executed for protesting against environmental damages caused to their community by the activities of oil companies, especially the Shell Oil Company (incorporated and carrying on business in Nigeria under the name Shell Petroleum Development Corporation). See Human Rights Watch, "The Destruction of Odi and Rape in Choba," in *Nigeria—Human Rights Watch Word Report* (2000), available at http://www.hrw.org/press/1999/dec/nibg1299.htm,(last visited 20 Nov. 2005). See also Philip Alston, "The 'Not-a-Cat' Syndrome: Can the International Human Rights Regime Accommodate Non-State Actors?" in Philip Alston, ed., *Non-State Actors and Human Rights* 3, (2005): 11, and Chinedu Reginald Ezetah, "International Law of self-determination and the Ogoni Question: Mirroring Africa's Post Colonial Dilemmas" 19 (1996–97) *Loyola of Los Angeles Int'l & Comp. L.J.* 811. Apart from these government violations of human rights and dignity, there are several other documented incidents of ethnic conflicts and religious riots purely caused by individuals and religious fanatics which do not implicate the Nigerian government. All of these incidents illustrate that extra-judicial killings and summary executions are substantially becoming embedded in the Nigerian political and social framework at the detriment of human rights and freedom.

118. Karl Llewellyn, *The Bramble Bush* (New York: Oceana Publications 1960): 17 (observing that "procedural regulations are the door, and the only door, to make real what is laid down by substantive law.").

119. U.N. Principles, Principle 12 (stating: "States shall adopt appropriate legislative and other measured necessary to establish, as criminal offences, trafficking, its component acts and related conduct"), and Guideline 5(4) (urging States to consider "establishing specialist anti-trafficking units in order to promote competence and professionalism"). See also ECOWAS Declaration, Proclamation 11; (urging States to "create specialized anti-trafficking units within law enforcement agencies and within the prosecutorial services, with a special view to fight the involvement of organized criminal groups").

120. UN Trafficking Protocol, at art. 9(1)(b), as well as Part II—Protection of Trafficked Persons (art. 6–8); which recognize that victims of trafficking are often in greater danger and in greater need of assistance and support, particularly

if repatriated to their countries of origin. It calls for further social assistance to victims in areas such as counseling, housing, education and health care needs.

121. Hyland, 2001, 30; (recounting how NGOs lobbied their governments).
122. I am optimistic that they will succeed in this task considering the fact that majority of African NGOs are run by women, coupled with the fact that African women are getting more sensitive to gender issues, of which trafficking is one.
123. Nigerian Trafficking Act, section 51; ("This Act may be cited as Trafficking in Persons (Prohibition) Law Enforcement and Administration Act, 2003.").
124. See e.g. Nigerian Trafficking Act at sections 11, 12, 13, 14, 17, 18, 19, and 21 which address the core prohibitions.
125. United Nations, *Trafficking in Persons: the New Protocol,* available at http://www.unodc.org/unodc/trafficking_protocol_background.html (last visited Oct. 26, 2005) (emphasis added).
126. It is not within the scope of this analysis to delineate the contours of consent in human trafficking. I have addressed that issue elsewhere. For a thorough engagement of the issue, see Victor N. Opara, "Trafficking Contracts: Myth or Reality? Re-Examination of *Consent* in Human Trafficking" (forthcoming).
127. UN Trafficking Protocol, art. 31; which deals with the alleviation of social conditions and the need for public information campaigns. These are particularly important with respect to trafficking, where the willingness and desperation of potential victims to relocate and their ignorance of trafficking and the true conditions in the destinations to which they are trafficked, have been identified as major contributing factors to increase in trafficking. See also ECOWAS Initial Plan, 6; (stressing the need to prevent trafficking through creation of awareness: "States, in partnership with NGOs, other civil society groups, and public and private media, shall develop and disseminate public awareness materials focusing on (a) raising public understanding that trafficking in persons is a crime, and (b) discouraging the demand that leads to trafficking . . .").
128. This process would be in compliance with U.N. Guidelines on Human Trafficking. See U.N. Principles and Guidelines on Human Rights and Human Trafficking, at Guideline 1(3).

Chapter Nine

Trafficking Contracts: Myth or Reality?: Re-Examination of *Consent* in Human Trafficking

Victor Nnamdi Opara

SYNOPSIS

One issue that has continued to engage the international community is whether trafficking can be legalized by the consent of the person being trafficked. The existence of consent appears to bar the intervention of human rights advocacy since the law presumes that a person who consents to be trafficked knows what she wants and what to expect, and as such has waived any remedies she might otherwise have been entitled to. However, the major problem with this presumption is that it prevents the international community from inquiring into what happens after the contract is formed. In view of this societal attitude, this analysis pierces the veil of trafficking contracts by using true-life narratives of trafficked African and Asian women to illustrate the lopsidedness of trafficking contracts. Using theories of liberty and freedom as well as the doctrinal principles of the law of contract, the analysis explores the potential ramifications of *consent* in order to illustrate the absence of liberty and freedom that characterize trafficking contracts. The analysis aims to advance scholarly considerations of human rights by illustrating that a close doctrinal engagement of the law of contract can assist in closing the gap between social attitude towards victims of trafficking and the reality. In achieving this goal, the analysis supplies the normative clarity necessitated by society in order to understand what lies beneath a trafficking contract. Structurally, the chapter comprises two parts. Part I embodies the introduction, defines trafficking concepts, outlines the history of trafficking in Africa and Asia, lays down a compendium of trafficking statistics, and gives an overview of the recruitment strategies of trafficking syndicates. It also delineates the doctrine of the law of contract vis-à-vis the narratives of trafficked women. Part II examines the intersections between trafficking contracts and contracts for slavery.

PART I: SCOPE AND NUANCES OF TRAFFICKING CONTRACTS

Introduction

Recently, the issue of what legal boundaries should be drawn where a woman willfully consents to be trafficked has been the subject of incisive debate in trafficking discourses. It has engaged the international community as well as human rights practitioners and advocates. In response to this development, the international community has recently demonstrated a strong willingness for a new international instrument that holistically addresses trafficking and the crucial issues that come with it. This willingness has led to the U.N. Protocol to Prevent, Suppress and Punish Trafficking in Persons, Especially Women and Children, Supplementing the U.N. Convention against Transnational Organized Crime (U.N. Trafficking Protocol).[1] Notwithstanding this acclaimed universal will, there were still several issues that required negotiations at the international level, among which some remain unresolved. Initially, one of the most contentious issues was what the definition of trafficking should be. Some states took the view that only trafficking that involves forced prostitution should be addressed by the U.N. Trafficking Protocol, so that in such cases when a victim consented to be trafficked, such consent should remove the conduct from the jurisdiction of the Protocol. At the early stages of the negotiation process, the United States was one of the proponents of this view.[2] However, most NGOs, especially the Coalition Against Trafficking in Women and Equality, opposed the consent argument on the grounds that all forms of prostitution should be addressed because the distinction between forced and voluntary prostitution did not make any sense.[3] Finally it was agreed that to completely ignore the consent of victims could exclude valid defenses, and also had the potential of triggering constitutional and other legal issues at the national level. A middle ground was therefore reached: although a trafficker is free to raise the consent of the victim as an initial defense, such consent to initial recruitment is not synonymous with consent to the entire course of trafficking. Trafficking and any alleged consent to exploitation should be deemed irrelevant if any of the prohibited trafficking mechanisms listed in the definition have occurred. Such prohibited mechanisms include threat or use of force, coercion, abduction, fraud, deception, abuse of power or position of vulnerability, the giving or receiving of money or benefits to achieve the consent of any person who has influence over a person.[4] This international consensus that consent should be taken into consideration when analyzing trafficking cases has resulted in some domestic laws on trafficking which limit statutory protections to persons "under the age of eighteen years."[5]

Notwithstanding this partial consensus on the effect of consent, the issue that has continued to engage the international community is whether trafficking can be legalized by the consent of the person being trafficked. By stating that consent to initial recruitment is not synonymous to consent to the entire course of trafficking, the international community left vague the appropriate strictures of consent. In reality, such vagueness poses difficulties to those consenting to be trafficked. The existence of consent appears to bar the intervention of human rights instruments and the invocation of its norms since the law presumes that an adult who consents to be trafficked knows what she wants and what to expect, and as such has waived any remedies to which she might otherwise have been entitled. However, the major problem with this line of reasoning is that the bar of human rights instruments equally prevents the international community from inquiring into what happens after a trafficking contract is formed. The United Nations Office on Drugs and Crime succinctly captured the social attitude towards this contractual consent in the following words:

> Every year hundreds of men, women and children are trafficked illegally all over the world. Most of us assume that these people are willing participants in a criminal transaction. *We believe that they are simply looking for an escape from poverty. Rarely do we pause to think about the specific problems they encounter when they are being smuggled or what happens to them afterwards. The reality reflects a very different picture, namely that these people are often economically, sexually and physically exploited.* They pay large sums of money in order to be transported under harsh conditions to another country, often unknowingly under a false pretext. They end up forced to work in prostitution or engaged in other criminal activities in the country of destination.[6]

This observation locates the social context of the problems that consenting trafficked women face after the fact. In view of this societal attitude towards victims of trafficking, this analysis attempts to pierce the contractual veil by using true-life narratives of trafficked women in order to illustrate the lopsidedness of a trafficking contract.

This chapter contributes to the efforts of human rights practitioners and advocates in using existing protections to enhance the protection of the vulnerable, rather than waiting for more treaties to be negotiated. The chapter is also aimed at advancing scholarly considerations of human rights, by illustrating that close doctrinal engagement of the law of contract can assist in closing the gap between trafficking contracts and reality by supplying the normative clarity which society requires in order to perceive what lies beneath the former. It is hoped that this will make society more responsive to the plight of trafficking victims. The thrust of this analysis is to ascertain the limits, if any, of *consent* in trafficking contracts.

SCOPE AND CLARIFICATIONS

Human trafficking generally involves coerced recruitment and transportation of people for a variety of forced labor and slavery-like practices, including forced domestic labor, manual or industrial labor, commercial marriages,[7] and sex trade or prostitution. That means that human trafficking is still a broad topic. Accordingly, on a narrower dimension this chapter focuses on trafficking in women for prostitution. In an attempt to further narrow the focus, this paper, while examining trafficking contracts globally, will focus on Africa and Asia, using reports of African women, especially Nigerians, trafficked to Europe for prostitution as well as reports of Asian women, especially Burmese (Myanmar) women, trafficked to Thailand for prostitution, as a case study. The analysis attempts to review some doctrinal thresholds of the law of contract in order to determine whether there is "forced prostitution" within a contract of trafficking for prostitution. Without being exhaustive, the analysis attempts to explore the potential ramifications of the issue of *consent* in order to bring to the fore more thought-provoking illustrations of the absence of liberty and freedom that characterize a trafficking contract. Using theories of liberty and freedom, as well as doctrinal principles of the law of contract, this analysis argues that it is a peremptory norm of mainstream international law, the African Charter on Human and Peoples' Rights, as well as domestic laws of most states that one cannot contract out her liberty and freedom.

It is trite that contracts made with minors are void unless they are made for the interest of the minor. It is also trite that a minor cannot give a valid consent to trafficking. In view of these basic principles, except otherwise stated, this analysis proceeds on the assumption that the trafficking contracts mentioned in this paper involve adults only. It is also trite that contract to engage in illegal conduct is invalid, since an action cannot be founded on illegality: *ex turpi causa non oritur actio*. However, this analysis does not proceed on the premise that trafficking contracts are *ex ante* invalid. Adhering to the orthodox view that trafficking contracts are invalid *ex ante* poses a lot of limitations. First, it raises the issue of women's innocence. In other words, it supports the premise that women who consent to trafficking don't know what they are doing, and should be protected from exploitation. This line of reasoning has the effect of placing women in the same class as children. As such, most feminists may view this line of reasoning as paternalistic. Second, it forestalls all inquiry on the ramifications of the consent of the trafficked woman. Third, it exacerbates the plight of consenting women since they go with the notion that they are doing something that is legally abhorred. This prevents them from crying out for help when the trafficking transaction begins to work hardship on them. This raises a paradox. The invalidation of the trafficking contract was meant to protect the woman, but in reality, it has worsened her plight. Fourth, invalidation of trafficking contracts *ex ante* makes trafficking transactions to go underground. This limits the availability of reliable data on trafficking, and also increases information asymmetry. Information asymmetry in turn increases both the "lemons problem" and "moral hazard" issues in trafficking transactions. The secrecy surrounding trafficking transactions makes it difficult for consenting women to have reliable information about the trafficker before giving their consent. Were adequate information available to them prior to the giving of their consent, the women would have been able to do some background assessments on the trafficker, a sort of 'due diligence' test. As such, a trafficker's reputation in the community would have been relevant in determining whether would-be trafficking victims would give their consent to such transactions. In other words, the general atmosphere of information asymmetry appears to empower traffickers to take advantage of consenting women. Unfortunately, the traditional theory of invalidity of trafficking transactions indirectly assists in encouraging this imbalance. This analysis therefore defies the mainstream notion that trafficking contracts are invalid. If the mainstream notion is correct, why do some domestic trafficking laws limit their protections to persons under the age of eighteen? Why doesn't the protection cover both adults and minors, thereby leaving the burden of proof on the trafficker? The time has come for the international community to face the reality that such *ex ante* invalidations of trafficking contracts are not enough. It only addresses the issue at the periphery, without proper diagnoses. It is like treating a patient without going through the patient's medical history and laboratory results. Of course, the physician's prescriptions may not treat the illness after all. There is therefore the need to appraise trafficking contracts in order to gauge their merits. In view of this need, this chapter proceeds on the assumption that trafficking contracts are valid, and that adult women are capable of giving valid consents to trafficking.

Moreover, it must be noted that although this analysis uses "he" to refer to traffickers, that does not mean that women are not involved in trafficking. In fact, 'Madams' are women who actively participate in trafficking. This analysis uses "he" to refer to traffickers because, in reality, a majority of associates involved in the trafficking chains are men, due to the transnational security networking that trafficking entails.

DEFINITION OF CONCEPTS

Trafficking was originally synonymous with illegal cross-border trade, especially the drug trade. Hence trafficking gives an image of illegal conduct. The phrase *trafficking in people* or *trafficking in persons* generally refers to criminal activities that involve the transfer of persons from one state to the other. It could be domestic or international. The phrase was first used in global vocabulary to describe the exportation of women and children, especially for prostitution.[8] Historically, the social problem known as *forced prostitution* made its debut in the international arena in the early 1890s, when European women were exported to brothels in colonies around the globe, to provide sexual services to European men far from home. The terms *traffic in women* and *White Slavery* were used to describe this practice.[9] Since then, trafficking women for prostitution has remained an ongoing universal problem that has continued to engage the international community and international crime detectives, and has also undermined national sovereignty and security.

The U.N. Protocol to Prevent, Suppress and Punish Trafficking in Persons, especially Women and Children defines *trafficking in Persons* thus:

> Trafficking in Persons shall mean the recruitment, transportation, transfer, harboring, or receipt of persons, by means of the threat or use of force or other forms of coercion, of abduction, of fraud, of deception, of the abuse of power or of a position of vulnerability or of the giving or receiving of payments or benefits to achieve the consent of a person having control over another person, for the purpose of exploitation. Exploitation shall include, at a minimum, the exploitation of the prostitution of others or other forms of sexual exploitation, forced labor or services, slavery or practices similar to slavery, servitude or the removal of organs, (U.N. Trafficking Protocol, art. 3, para. a).

On the other hand, respecting the exchange of sexual services for money, the term *to prostitute* often implies the "indiscriminate" sale of sex,[10] a connotation that many prostitutes and feminist scholars claim is at odds with reality and ignores the possibility of prostitutes' autonomy and control in their work. The term *prostitute* depicts a person who provides sexual services for a fee, and *prostitution* refers to the practice/institution of commercial sex.[11] A woman's willingness to participate in this industry has continued to attract the attention of the international community: "Sometimes the women are willing participants, *selling themselves* in the hopes of establishing a better life, or making enough money to help their families back home. More often than not, however, they are duped into a hell of extortion, abuse and intimidation. 'These women find themselves caught in a web of organized crime. They are *bought and sold* and moved around. They are bound into this cycle of fear and abuse.'"[12] The use of sales imagery in this context conjures a mental picture of a contractual transaction in goods and services, which involves the consent of both parties in order to be effective. It equally raises the issue that some women are the authors of the very system that dehumanizes and abuses them. This invariably means that the consent of those women impacts on, and to a large extent deprives them of their liberty and freedom. They are therefore at the mercy of buyers (the syndicates, Madams/pimps), but this is not the end of the story. This issue is fully analyzed below in the section classical doctrine of contract. Yet it must be pointed out that sometimes, women are forced into prostitution against their will. While it is arguable that most trafficked women consent to trafficking for the sake of better economic prospects, some of them are just kidnapped and trafficked for prostitution. In Sussex, England, more than 40 African teenage girls who were seeking asylum in the United Kingdom, some as young as 14, were taken away from children's homes and sold as prostitutes in Italy.[13] Moreover, in some communities, social and cultural practices that view women as inferior beings make it easier for traffickers and complicit family members to treat women as cheap and less treasured commodities that can be shipped away to foreign lands in order to better the prospects of their family, whether or not the woman consents to assume that role.[14]

HISTORICAL OVERVIEW AND STATISTICS OF TRAFFICKING[15]

The most current international statistics on human trafficking appear in the Fifth Annual Trafficking in Persons Report, released in June 2005 by the U.S. State Department. The Report, authored by John Miller, states that about 600,000 to 800,000 people are trafficked across international borders every year, of which about 80 percent are women and children.[16] This is not significantly different from the number of global trafficking reported by the U.S. State Department in 2004, where it was estimated that between 700,000 and 4,000,000 persons were trafficked annually around the globe, with 50,000 women and children trafficked annually to the U.S. for sexual exploitation.[17] Reports confirm that thousands of African women are trafficked every year to Western Europe and North America,[18] with Canada serving as a conduit for trafficking to the United States.[19] According to a Reuters news report in December 2000, between 700,000 and 2,000,000 women and children are victims of trafficking per year.[20] Anti-Slavery, an NGO concerned with the eradication of trafficking and related slavery-like practices, has observed that "it is impossible to know how many people are trafficked, and statistics are difficult to obtain because trafficking is an underground activity."[21] This observation appears to be correct because a great deal of trafficking cases remain undocumented due largely to its underground nature.[22]

The effect of this revelation is that the reported cases are likely to be below the real trafficking figures. According to the United Nations Office on Drugs and Crime, in the past 21 years there has been a rise in human trafficking, caused by a great number of factors, including the end of the Cold War, which led to the opening of several borders and a rise in the movement of people, the debut of organized crime in the international arena, and the increased demand for sex tourism. There are about 200,000 to 500,000 "illegal" sex workers in the European Union, and Eastern Europe accounts for two-thirds.[23] They are illegal because they are not officially registered as sex workers. In fact, the U.N. Office on Drugs and Crime revealed the contagious nature of the global criminal network: "Over the past decade, trafficking in human beings has reached epidemic proportions. No country is immune. The search for work abroad has been fuelled by economic disparity, high unemployment and the disruption of traditional livelihoods."[24] It is estimated that Nigerian and Albanian women constitute the largest proportion of the approximately 20,000 prostitutes in Italy.[25] The Organization for Migration reports that in 1997 alone, 500,000 women of Russian and Ukrainian origin were trafficked into Western Europe.[26]

On the African scene, Nigeria presents the biggest challenge to the African continent and the international community. Although trafficking for prostitution is a more recent phenomenon in Nigeria, it has climaxed in the last decade. The major obstacle in the assessment of human trafficking in Nigeria is a lack of statistical data.[27] This problem is compounded by the clandestine nature of human trafficking. Moreover, most Nigerians find it difficult to disclose their traveling plans to friends and neighbors due to fears that the information recipient may foil the plans or impose herself on the person facilitating the movement. Notwithstanding these statistical shortfalls, figures of deported trafficking victims exist, which could be used as a basis for statistical inquiry.[28] Between March 1999 and December 2000, 1,178 Nigerians were deported from five countries for trafficking related reasons, and the majority were from Rome. Of this number, only 12 were men.[29] This number remained substantially the same in 2001 as revealed in a homegrown Nigerian trafficking study, (*Trafficking to Italy,* 20) which indicated that more than 1,116 Nigerian women were repatriated in 2001. The Nigeria Police Desk Office on Human Trafficking reported that between 1999 and 2001, over 8,633 trafficked persons were deported back to Nigeria, (Juliet Ume-Ezeokeke, 4). In 2001, the Nigerian Ambassador to Italy reported that there were about 10,000 Nigerian prostitutes in Italy, (Juliet Ume-Ezeokeke, 4). This figure doubled in 2002, as the number of Nigerian women involved in Italian sex trade rose to 20,000.[30] To sum up the figures of deportations so far, between 1999 and 2003, 19,774 Nigerians had been deported from Europe for human trafficking offences relating to prostitution.[31] Thereafter, in 2004, many Nigerians were deported from Italy and Saudi Arabia. Between January and March 2004, over 1000 Nigerians were deported from Saudi Arabia, and an additional 386 Nigerians were also deported from Saudi Arabia in April 2004, all for trafficking offences;[32] while between April and May 2004, 371 Nigerian women were deported from Italy.[33]

A combination of these deportation figures, and the dead and maimed trafficking victims, as well as those that have either legalized their stay or are still working illegally or are stranded abroad somewhat will give expression to the huge number of Nigerian women who have been trafficked to Europe for prostitution. Against this backdrop, it appears that the estimation of the U.S. Diplomatic Mission to Nigeria that as of May 2003, "as many as 300,000 [Nigerian women] have been trafficked since 1997"[34] is reasonably accurate. It is also estimated that over 500,000 African women and children have been trafficked, (Ume-Ezeokeke, Desk Review). A synthesis of the above two estimates, reveals that Nigerian women constitute more than 50% of all Africans who have been trafficked anywhere in the world.

On the Asian scene, trafficking is fuelled mostly by sex tourism.[35] For example, Nepali women are trafficked in large numbers to brothels in India;[36] Burmese women are trafficked to Thailand; Bangladesh women are trafficked to Brothels in Pakistan and India, (Human Rights Watch, 205, 197). For newly developed and developing countries in Asia, sex tourism has been extremely lucrative. For example, in 1986 Thailand earned $1.5 billion from tourism, which amounted to more foreign currency than it earned from a combination of other industries, including rice export, (Enloe, 1989, 37). Sex tourism remains Thailand's primary draw for foreign currency. The connection between Thailand and sex tourism is so strong that Thailand has been described as a "sex industry country" rather than a "newly industrializing country."[37] It is estimated that 70 to 80 percent of Japanese, American, Australian, and Western European male tourists travel to Asia for purposes of sexual recreation.[38] This illustration lends credence to the claim that "tourism-oriented prostitution has become an integral part of the economic base of countries in the South-east Asia," (Hall, 1992, 74). The existence of sex tourism increases the incentive for traffickers to force women and girls into prostitution.[39] Tourism increases the demand for and the profits to be gained from prostitution, (Lucas, 1999, 690).

This statistical inquiry will not be complete without mentioning the ill profits that traffickers make from this transnational trade in women. In 2000, human traffickers realized estimated profits of $7 billion from prostitution alone, (Reuters, Mafia Makes Billions). The profit margin in human trafficking increased in 2004 as the industry earned more than $10 billion.[40] The realizable profit has further risen to $11.8 billion in 2005.[41] This trend of constant increase in profit margin reveals that the penalties for the crime are meager; as such, traffickers seem better off defaulting rather than stopping their nefarious trade.[42] It further illustrates that there are monetary incentives in the industry despite attempts by the international community to stem its tide. That means that the international community needs to increase the punishment for trafficking, including increases in fines and prison terms. Accordingly, one scholar has warned that unless the problem of sex trafficking is addressed from an economic perspective by increasing the cost of running a sex trafficking business and by decreasing the economic benefits of the lucrative sex industry, achieving a lasting solution to this problem might be a mirage.[43] This adjustment to the cost/benefit analysis might well produce a deterrent effect.

RECRUITMENT STRATEGIES OF SYNDICATES VIS-À-VIS VICTIMS' CONSENT

Trafficking syndicates use several opportunistic strategies to achieve their nefarious objectives. They woo their victims with elaborate stories of better lives abroad, and when victims succumb, syndicates compel them to work as prostitutes. The first step in this recruitment process is for syndicates to put up employment advertisements in the media, and then target their victims.[44] Some naïve women and girls respond to such advertisements with the hope of securing a better living abroad only to end up as prostitutes.[45] Upon arrival in the destination country, their job descriptions change drastically.[46] In addition, once trafficked women arrive in a destination country, traffickers utilize a variety of strategies to make them subservient and dependent. Instilment of fear is the most potent psychological weapon that traffickers have used in gaining control over most of their victims. Other coercive strategies include threatened harm to the victim or her family at home, humiliation, threats of deportation, and at times openly killing the most uncooperative as a deterrent to others.[47] Physical coercion is another strategy that has proved potent for traffickers. This mechanism is aimed at getting the unalloyed loyalty of trafficked women, and includes rape, torture, beatings, starving, forced abortions and imprisonment, as well as confiscation of victims' passports, visas, work permits, and other traveling documents.[48]

Psychological coercion has proved most productive for traffickers of African women due largely to the belief in the supernatural or ancestral spirits, which some African communities and families still hold.[49] Traffickers often subject the women to juju rituals before leaving the source country. At the ritual, the woman is made to take oaths of allegiance, secrecy, confidentiality, and repayment of the costs of her journey and other incidental expenses, as solely determined by the trafficker. Traditional priests in the community frequently administer these oaths at a shrine. The entire scenario generates its own aura of fear, coupled with the ritual rites and the presence of the priest in his ceremonial robe. Thereafter, the woman feels obligated to the trafficker, and is sworn not to disclose her sufferings to any other person.[50] A vivid description of the procedure appears below:

> A contract is made with the woman and she has to swear an oath to a shrine. The woman swears the oath in the presence of a priest, the madam and the parents (mostly the mother) usually a number of rituals are a part of the oath swearing—a goat or chicken is slaughtered, "nonsense words" are said and wine spilled on the ground. The woman subjects herself to the bidding of the madam and is obliged to pay back money to her. The oath to the shrine is not an unusual phenomenon but a part of ordinary life and the social system in parts of Nigeria . . . Even if the mother and the girl or young woman are not fully aware of the implications of the contract and believe that the woman is going abroad to work as a housemaid, in the cleaning business or even to receive an education the woman is obliged to the oath and to the bidding of the madam . . . the sworn oath given by the victims and their sense of obligations towards the shrine make them fear of reprisals even before they are sent off to a foreign country, (Joint Human Rights Report, 40–41, 5.2.1–2).

The thought of a juju ritual itself instills fear of reprisal on trafficked African women, compelling them to endure their sufferings in silence. They automatically become afraid of leaving the trafficker or testifying against the trafficker.[51] This has had the adverse consequence of complicating the task of law enforcement agencies and criminal investigators who obviously require both the evidence and tips of trafficked women for thorough investigation and successful prosecution of traffickers.[52] In one reported incident, a Nigerian woman who was trafficked to the U.K. refused to give evidence to the U.K. police because of the fear of the oath she had sworn.[53] To illustrate the immense impact of juju rituals on trafficking in Africa, in 2000 the Edo State of Nigeria (the State most notorious for having the highest number of African women trafficked to Europe for prostitution) enacted the Edo State Criminal Code (Amendment Law).[54] Section 233A of the law categorically criminalizes the administration of any form of oath on a woman or girl or the performance of any fetish ritual aimed at facilitating or enabling a woman or girl to travel out of Nigeria for the purpose of prostitution. In addition, the law also prohibits any person from sponsoring a woman or girl by giving her financial, physical, or material assistance to facilitate her traveling out of Nigeria for the purpose of prostitution or any immoral act, (Edo Criminal Code). The law was strongly opposed by organized crime syndicates who resorted to several vilifying strategies against the Edo State government and legislature, thus throwing the state into a pandemonium.[55]

Despite the good intentions of the Edo State legislature in tackling the juju ritual practice, most trafficked African women are still not willing to volunteer information to their state police because of the implications it would have on their safety and on the safety of their families at home. The Nigerian police, for example, are known to collaborate with criminals, and in some cases high profile confidential tips given to the police with the aim of facilitating criminal investigations have leaked to the criminals, who then retaliate against the whistle-blower.[56] Hence the continued reluctance of deported trafficking victims to give evidence against their traffickers appears justifiable. States should map out adequate protective mechanisms for those who testify.[57] Until such state-oriented institutional measures are executed, trafficking victims may remain lukewarm in assisting trafficking crime investigators.[58] Realistically, it must be admitted that mapping out adequate protective mechanisms in order to obtain the testimony of trafficking victims involves extensive and comprehensive reform of the police force and other law enforcement agencies. If this remains the case, such a police reform in the context of Africa is at best unachievable at present.

Another method of psychological coercion which traffickers utilize in controlling their victims is to place them in debt bondage. This appearance of indebtedness makes a trafficked woman feel bound to her trafficker.

Through this mechanism, traffickers are able to control all the earnings of their victims. Since only the trafficker knows the costs incurred in effecting a woman's trafficking, the general assessment is unduly lopsided. A trafficked woman takes whatever figure the trafficker quotes as the amount to be repaid. In addition, upon arriving at the destination country, there is a simulated change of control all in an attempt to further exploit trafficked women: the trafficker sells the woman to a Madam or pimp. The Madam owns the apartment that accommodates the trafficked woman, and also sets the conditions of sexual services and remittance of proceeds. The Madam is also in charge of receiving payments from clients. The amount that a trafficked African woman is expected to repay to the Madam usually ranges from $20,000 to $45,000; (Ume-Ezeokeke, Desk Review, 16) sometimes extending to as much as $48,000.[59] Unfortunately, because the Madam is in control of the proceeds, coupled with the fact that a trafficked woman does not keep a record of her income, there is no accountability. Suffice it to say that notwithstanding the huge profits that a trafficked woman generates, she still remains indebted to the Madam because payments made by clients disappear into the Madam's coffers. As such, a trafficked woman is thrown into a vicious cycle of debt repayment. This strategy assists the Madam in ensuring that trafficked women do not leave the brothel, (McClelland, 2001). This strategy has been most effective for syndicates who traffic African women, as they have been able to use it as a mechanism of controlling their victim's conscience. The juju ritual mentioned earlier correlates with this model to compel the woman to remain in the brothel, as she believes that she is indebted to the Madam until the debts are repaid. In order to facilitate the efficiency of this strategy, the Madam and trafficker confiscate the traveling documents of trafficked women, (Ume-Ezeokeke, Desk review). The above analysis provides some insight into the lives and predicaments of trafficked African women.

All the strategies mentioned above constitute offences under Nigerian law and related international instruments. The Constitution of Nigeria in sections 34 and 35 prohibits sexual exploitation and deprivation of personal liberty.[60] In a similar vein, the Nigerian Criminal Code in section 227 punishes any person who conspires with another to induce any woman or girl, by means of false pretence or other fraudulent means to facilitate unlawful sexual intercourse between her and any man.[61] The key element of this crime is the use of false pretense or fraudulent means to accomplish sexual intercourse between a woman and a third party. Section 369 of the Criminal Code punishes the placement or receiving of any person in servitude as a pledge or security for a current or future debt; or conveying, sending or inducing any person to go outside Nigeria to enable the person to be possessed, dealt with or traded in, purchased, sold or transferred as a slave or be placed in servitude as a pledge or security for debt; or entering into any contract or agreement with or without consideration for doing any of these acts, (Criminal Code, 369). By this provision, the trafficker, Madam, juju priest, and any of the woman's family members who participate in the contract are all accomplices, and as such are liable under the law. Applying international standards to the trafficking strategies will also reveal that they are prohibited. The U.N. Trafficking Protocol in article 3 prohibits "[t]he recruitment, transportation, transfer, harboring or receipt of persons by means . . . of deception, . . . of giving or receiving of payments or benefits to achieve the consent of a person having control over another person for the purpose of exploitation," (U.N. Trafficking Protocol, art. 3).

On the other hand, with respect to trafficked Burmese women, Human Rights Watch offers the following indications of their condition: "[Human Rights Watch] interviewed thirty Burmese women and girls in depth, most from remote rural villages in Shan state, most from peasant or agricultural laborer background. . . . All but one had been lured to Thailand by the prospect of improving their economic situation. Only four knew they would be working as prostitutes, and even those four had no idea of what the actual work would be like," (Human Rights Watch, 2). The fact above gives rise to two presumptions: that although some trafficking victims do not give informed consent (since the job description changes automatically on their arrival to the destination country), some nevertheless are aware that they will be working as prostitutes in the destination country, hence they gave informed and full consent. That they "had no idea of what the actual work would be like," does not rule out the fact that they consented. In fact, at first blush, it appears that the principle of *volenti non fit injuria* might be invoked to stop them from complaining, since in tort law, they may be presumed to have waived whatever legal remedies they otherwise would have had. However, on closer examination, it is worthy of note that notwithstanding the women consented, the law of contract does not permit them to contract out their liberty. In other words, the consent does not in any way abrogate their right to choose clients that they want to service. In that case, compelling a woman to service clients against her wish would not only amount to psychological violence but also wrongfully causing harm to another since she is exposed to a lot of deadly diseases, including HIV/AIDS. Some may argue that prostitutes are generally exposed to diseases even when they make the choice of clients, but it is more tolerable for one to injure oneself than for one to be forced into injury. A prostitute might see some physiological or epidemiological features in a client that she resents. Compelling her to have sex with that particular client against her wish is detrimental to her health, dignity, and well being.

CLASSICAL DOCTRINE OF CONTRACT

Contract is "an agreement which the law will enforce or recognize as affecting the legal rights and duties of the parties . . . [or] a promise or set of promises the law will enforce."[62] A contract could be unilateral, bilateral, or multilateral. This chapter however focuses on bilateral contracts between a trafficked woman and her trafficker. Although legal scholars have defined bilateral contracts in different ways, its underlying features remain the same: "A bilateral contract consists of an exchange of promises; the offeror promising to do something in exchange for the offeree promising to do something else in return," (Sagay, 1985, 5). "A bilateral contract consists of mutual promises, made in exchange for each other by each of the two contracting parties. . . . In a bilateral contract both parties are promisors and both parties are promisees; and *the legal effect of such a contract is that there are mutual rights and mutual duties*."[63] These observations reveal the important features of a valid bilateral contract, which every trafficking contract is supposed to have: the recognition of the rights and duties of both the trafficked woman and the trafficking syndicate. In other words, each of the two contracting parties has rights which cannot be trumped by the other, as well as obligations which cannot be abandoned, but rather must be fulfilled. If one party evades his or her obligations under this classical contract doctrine, the agreement ceases to be mutual. Where these requirements are lacking, the contract is likely to collapse. The requirement of mutual rights and duties will be exhaustively analyzed below.

Every contract consists of two acts that establish a right: "a promise and its acceptance."[64] One of the parties must make an offer or promise, which the other may act upon. If the other accepts the offer or promise as made, that is, without any conditions or amendments, then a contractual relationship arises. This principle is given more content and expression by Corbin: "An offer is an expression by one party of his *assent to certain definite terms, provided that the other party involved in the bargaining transaction will likewise express his assent to the identically same terms*. An offer looks forward to an agreement—*to mutual expression of assent*. . . . It will not be disputed by any one that, after an offer is made, a *voluntary expression of assent* [acceptance] by the offeree is all that is necessary to create what we call contract."[65]

Some distinct principles may be distilled from this definition: (a) the contract must be specific as to what the offeree is consenting to or accepting;

(b) both parties have to consent to the same terms; and (c) the consent must be voluntary. Hence every valid contract is expected to have specific terms, be mutual, and be voluntary. The constant repetition of mutual in the definitions of "bilateral contract" and "offer" above appears to suggest that the law of contract may not recognize a contract that is lopsided. The "mutual" requirement of contract means that there are shared rights and obligations which each party is expected to fulfill. Hence it is necessary to note that contract is founded on two mutual principles: "voluntariness" and "consideration." Where one is lacking, the contract is likely to collapse. Before undertaking inquiries into these underpinning features, it will be necessary to say a word about "acceptance" which complements an "offer." Without the acceptance of an offer, there cannot be a contract. Acceptance is a final expression of assent to the terms of an offer, (Sagay, 1985, 13).

CONSIDERATION

Consideration is the price paid by a party in a contract. In a typical trafficking contract, consideration would be the price paid by a trafficked woman and the trafficker in the trafficking contract. Consideration is not limited to money. It could be either in monetary terms or in material value. The most essential requirement of consideration is that there must be a sacrifice from each party. One of the leading authorities of contract law in Africa has observed:

> There must be an exchange, either of promises, or a promise for an act. The basic feature of the doctrine is reciprocity. Something of value in the eyes of the law must be given for a promise in order to make it enforceable as a contract. Thus for a party to be entitled to bring an action on an agreement he must demonstrate that he contributed to the agreement. It is this contribution that is called consideration . . . *The problem however, has always been how to determine what type of contribution is of sufficient value 'in the eye of the law' to qualify as consideration*, (Sagay, 1985, 42).

The last sentence of this observation echoes the problem of most trafficking contracts—sufficiency of consideration. Although in contract law, consideration is not necessarily required to be sufficient, in practice, where the consideration paid by a party is very insufficient compared to the consideration of the other party, courts of equity have intervened to provide equitable remedies.[66] The most comprehensive and oft cited definition of consideration is that laid down by Lush J. in *Currie* v. *Misa:* "A valuable consideration in the eye of the law may consist either in some right, interest, profit or benefit accruing to the one party, or some forbearance, detriment, loss or responsibility, given, suffered or undertaken by the other. Thus consideration does not only consist of profit by one party but also exists where the other party abandons some legal right in the present, or limits his legal freedom of action in the future as an inducement for the promise of the first," (Grotius , BK II, c. 12). In *Mills* v. *Wyman*[67] the Court opined: "The rule that a mere verbal promise, without any consideration, cannot be enforced by action, is universal in its application, and cannot be departed from to suit a particular case. . . . It is only when the party making the promise gains something, or he to whom it was made loses something, that the law given [sic] the promise validity."[68]

VOLUNTARINESS

The second requirement of a valid contract is "voluntariness." This means that both parties must desire the contract out of their own free will. Hence there is the need to examine whether undue influence plays any role in a trafficking contract. In a typical trafficking contract, it is evident that most of the women who enter into it are lured by promises of greener pastures abroad.[69] However, as soon as they arrive in the destination country they realize that all the sugarcoated words of the trafficker are mere hoax gimmicks or mere rhetoric. This scenario places trafficked women in a precarious and vulnerable state. The law has always revoked contracts where there are no fair exchanges as a result of the overriding influence of one of the parties. This gesture aims at protecting a party who was unusually vulnerable to persuasion against "any possible use of the relevant influence, irrespective of the intentions of the person possessing it . . . unless and until . . . the transaction has been shown to be truly for the benefit of the person influenced."[70] The question is whether a trafficking contract entered into by a woman is in her best interest. This issue will be revisited below under the section "Narratives of African and Asian Women," where the analysis applies contract theories to true-life narratives of trafficked women.

Voluntariness implies freedom of contract and can only flourish in an atmosphere of free will. The will of the trafficked woman must be conjoined with the will of the trafficking syndicate for there to be freedom. In most trafficking contracts, there is no conjunction of wills, and there is no adherence to the universal law of freedom. A party cannot contract out her liberty and freedom. A lopsided contract cannot be supported on any rational principle. It is trite that traditional doctrines of contract give relief where a party is in a weak position because of ignorance, inexperience, need, or a relationship of trust, and the other party has taken advantage of this to make a contract under which the weaker party is exploited in value for money terms.[71] The involuntariness in trafficking contracts, coupled with the obvious fact of information asymmetry and the critical financial dilemma of trafficked women, intensifies the vulnerability of trafficked women. This inference is fleshed out below.

NARRATIVES OF TRAFFICKED AFRICAN AND ASIAN WOMEN

Human Rights Watch begins its report on the rising incidence of trafficking of Burmese women into Thailand with a pathetic non-fictional story of a Burmese woman, Lin Lin, who was recruited and trafficked into Thailand for prostitution after her father took US$480 from a trafficking syndicate (albeit on the belief that his daughter would pay the loan through her "legitimate" earnings).[72] Lin Lin having worked in four different brothels in Thailand as a prostitute in an attempt to pay off her father's debt, tested positive for HIV, (Human Rights Watch, 1). The four different brothels that Lin Lin worked for were owned by one family. Lin Lin worked for two years as a prostitute in those brothels. The syndicate's clients paid $4 per hour for sexual services they received from Lin Lin. The clients could take her out all night for $30 by leaving an identity card or passport. During the weekdays Lin Lin had six to seven clients a day. She worked every day except for the two days off each month for her menstrual period. On one occasion, Lin Lin had to borrow money to pay for medicine to treat a painful vaginal infection, (Human Rights Watch, 1, 38–39). From an analytical perspective, to pay the loan of $480, simple arithmetic reveals that Lin Lin needs to service 120 men for 120 hours, on the assumption that each client receives one-hour service on each occasion, and each client pays the regular service fee of $4 per hour. As revealed by the facts of the case, Lin Lin services six to seven clients a day on weekdays. Assuming she services just 6 men a day, she would need to work for 20 days to pay off her father's debt of $480.[73] This estimation is based on the assumption that each client receives just one hour of service. But in reality, it is rare for a trafficked woman to work for just 6 hours a day. Reports from other trafficking sources reveal that trafficked women work for up to 18 hours per day (which could translate to each client receiving three hours service per day).[74]

Unfortunately, Human Rights Watch only documents that Lin Lin services six to seven clients per day, without telling us how many hours she actually worked. However, this extra 12 hours per day are not included in the estimations made in this analysis. In other words, rendering sexual services to 6 men (where each man receives one hour service) every day for 20 days at the rate of $4 each would pay off the debt of $480 which Lin Lin allegedly owes to the trafficker (6 x 20 x 4 = 480). However, Lin Lin worked for two years for a debt which would have been repaid in less than one month and sadly ended up with HIV/AIDS. The alleged contract, therefore, is unfair in all ramifications. Hugo Grotius, while emphasizing that there should be equality in the subject of every contract explains: "There remains equality in the subject of the contract, consisting in this, that *although nothing has been concealed which ought to have been said*, and no more has been exacted than was considered due, nevertheless *if an inequality has been detected in the transaction,* although without the fault of either party—*because, for example, the fault was hidden or because there was a mistake in the price—this inequality should be made good, and something should be taken from the one who has more and given to the one who has less,*" (Grotius, 344, emphasis added). This translates to the point that, notwithstanding that Lin Lin had allegedly consented to prostitute herself across the border (that is, in Thailand, outside her Burmese home), since it is obvious that there is pronounced inequality, the inequality matrix should be remedied. The inequality is even more compounded when we consider the fact that the syndicate is the author of the existing inequality. The general scenario conveys a picture of Lin Lin's vulnerability in the alleged contract. This in turn raises the issue of Lin Lin's bargaining power in the alleged contract. It is worth noting that equity has always been invoked to protect a person who, without independent advice, enters into a contract on terms which are very unfair, or for a consideration which is grossly inadequate. Of course, this equitable intervention is made notwithstanding the traditional doctrine of contract law that consideration need not be sufficient. A cursory look at some cases reveals that the law of equity has usually intervened to protect a vulnerable party in any contract where the bargaining powers of the parties are visibly unequal. In an appeal from New Zealand, *Hart v. O'Connor,*[75] the Privy Council recognized the existence of the doctrine of inequality of bargaining power, although relief was refused on the ground that even if there were inadequacy of consideration, the transaction was not the product of any unconscionable conduct on the part of the appellant. According to the Court: "There was no equitable fraud, no victimization, no taking advantage, no overreaching or other description of unconscionable doings which might have justified the intervention of equity. . . ." (*Hart v. O'Connor*, 894). The Privy Council's opinion in *Hart* is an acknowledgment that equity would intervene in situations of insufficient consideration, so long as the prerequisite conditions of victimization, taking of advantage, or overreaching are present in the transaction. As such, it is no longer the case that insufficiency of consideration is immaterial in the assessment of contracts. Victimization was highlighted above under the contractual doctrine of *voluntariness*. It is obvious that the facts of Lin Lin's case reveal that she has been taken advantage of, and that the trafficking syndicate has overreached himself at her expense and detriment. This appears to open the door for equity to step into this alleged contract.

Beale, while commenting on *Hart* said that the decision of the Court appears to require no more than that one party should have consciously taken advantage of the other's ignorance and lack of advice: "[I]n the case the appellant was unaware that the seller was of unsound mind and the seller appeared to be represented by his own solicitor. *If the three conditions—sale at undervalue, the taking of advantage of poverty or ignorance and lack of independent advice—are satisfied, there seems no reason why this jurisdiction cannot be used in this country today . . . the inexperienced person who signs a guarantee of another's debts without realizing the implications of the document, might well qualify for relief.*" [76] Indeed, Lin Lin appears to qualify for Beale's hypothetical "inexperienced person who signs a guarantee of another's debts without realizing the implications of the document." After all, she consented to be trafficked to Thailand for the sole reason of repaying her Father's debt. It remains to add that what counts as "poverty" and "ignorance" is not clearly defined by the courts. In *Cresswell* v. *Potter*,[77] Megarry, J. translated them to mean "a member of the lower income group" and "less highly educated."

It follows that the status of the persons the courts have in mind are even far better than those of Burmese women who are mainly illiterate and hail from the poorest villages of Burma that can hardly feed themselves. According to Human Rights Watch, "All but one of the women we interviewed for this report *were lured from their homes on a promise of economic benefits*. . . . We interviewed thirty Burmese women and girls in depth, twenty-six of whom had been trafficked into Thailand. . . . Of the thirty, *nineteen had parents who were peasant farmers or farm laborers*. . . . They ranged in age from twelve to twenty-two . . . *only four had ever been to school and could read or write in their own language*," (Human Rights Watch, 45–46; emphasis added). This shows the penurious circumstances and illiterate background of the Burmese women who entered into the alleged trafficking contract. Beale has observed that, "the "weaknesses" which seem more relevant in the old cases are ignorance of the value of the property or the nature of the obligation in question, coupled with urgent need or simply surprise, precluding reflection or "shopping around,'" (Beale, 1986, 126–127). This observation fits into the context under review.

In the first place, the Burmese women are ignorant of the value of their bodies (which constitute the subject or 'property' of the transaction); they are equally ignorant of the nature of the obligation required in view of the information asymmetry that is generated by trafficking generally. Arguably, a woman may have consented to be trafficked to prostitute with the belief that she would have the capacity and liberty to choose her clients, but the contrary, which eliminates those options and compels her to service all clients without objections, occurs. The few courageous women who venture to resist some clients are tortured, bruised, battered, and gang-raped.[78] Moreover, the women did not have access to any independent legal advice, which equally highlights the inequality of the contract. Hence trafficking contracts, as seen through the above lenses, are extremely weak and largely unfair. It does not qualify as a contract strictly speaking. It therefore must collapse.

At this juncture, this analysis will consider some narratives of African women in order to balance the regional equation. Like the Burmese women, most Nigerian women are also deceived by traffickers with respect to the kind of work they will perform abroad. Among eighty-seven prostitutes rescued few years ago from a ring in Italy was a Nigerian woman named Joy Eghosa, who came to Italy on the belief that she would work as a fashion designer. However, on arriving to Italy, she was forced into prostitution by her traffickers, (Wallace, 2002). This shows absence of informed consent. Trafficked women like Joy Eghosa cannot be taken to have consented in the first place. As such there is no need to engage in any further inquiry as to whether there is a trafficking contract. On the other hand, even where there appears to be informed consent of African women, the terms of the trafficking contract reveals the same lopsided bargaining power and outcome that were illustrated in Lin Lin's case.

Trafficked African women in the sex industry work for up to 18 hours a day. A trafficker in Belgium reportedly imported African women into Europe and sold them for $8,000 each.[79] The women earn up to $3,492 a month. They are usually required to pay off debts to the Madams for accommodation and travel expenses in the range of $58,200—$69,840 in order to be free.[80] Unlike Lin Lin's case, there is no data for the amount that each client pays per hour. Accordingly, the simple arithmetic employed here is to divide the "cost" price of the woman by the proceeds from "sales" which she is required to generate. The cost price is the $8,000 that the trafficker received from the Madam, and the proceeds from sales are the $58,200—$69,840 that the woman is obligated to pay in order to be free. The average of $58,200 and $69,840 is $64,020. When this amount is divided by $8,000 the result is roughly eight. This means that trafficked

African women are required to pay debts as much as eight times over the alleged contractual amount. It must be noted that the trafficker has already taken his cut. The $64,020 that the women are required to pay are payable to the Madam. This reveals the vicious cycle of exploitation that surrounds trafficking contracts. At each stage of the transaction, trafficked women are exploited by the transactional intermediary. Like Lin Lin's case, this illustrates that the contract is lopsided. It is anything but mutual.

In *Cooke* v. *Oxley*,[81] the court was of the opinion that, "[i]n order to sustain a promise, there must be either damage to the plaintiff or an advantage to the defendant," (Judge J. Buller in *Cooke* v. *Oxley*). In the case of African women under review, the promise or trafficking contract cannot be sustained because there is no damage to the trafficker and the Madam. Instead there is advantage to them. On the other hand, the trafficked women have suffered damages as a result of the opportunistic behaviors of the trafficker and the Madam. They can thus bring actions as plaintiffs. Of course, the trafficked women cannot be defendants since they have not enjoyed any advantage in the deal. On the whole, trafficked women should be free to renege on any contract they have made with traffickers, irrespective of their initial commitments. Traffickers cannot sustain a claim under such contracts. This conclusion is reached without regard to arguments of morality and public policy.[82] The above analysis has been made on the assumption that trafficking contracts are valid contracts that independent parties can freely enter into. Applying Grotius' theory of equality in every contract,[83] it means that notwithstanding that most African women allegedly consented to be trafficked for prostitution like their Asian counterparts, since it is obvious that there is pronounced inequality, the matrix of inequality should be remedied through the intervention of equity, and the provision of equitable remedies.

PART II: INTERSECTIONS BETWEEN TRAFFICKING CONTRACT AND CONTRACT OF SLAVERY

From the analysis in Part I, it could be inferred that a trafficking contract is a sham. The analysis captured the covert matrix of inequality, domination, threat, exploitation, dehumanization, and lack of liberty and freedom that characterize the sham contract. This discovery would prevent any of the parties from relying on the contract as a shield to prevent the intervention of international instruments, human rights law, equity, and tort. Continuation of the relationship is nothing short of forced labor. Bassiouni, while equating forced labor with slavery observed: "With regard to forced labor, the phenomenon is the same. . . . The key legal element in all of these [forced labor] practices is that the "employer" claims that the "worker" has agreed, of his/her own free will, to terms or conditions of "employment," and that the "worker" is "free" to leave the "employment" at any time. *These supposed elements of free choice, consent, and freedom to leave technically negate the applicability of international instruments on the subject.*"[84] However, the piercing of the alleged trafficking contract has revealed that what actually exists in trafficking contexts is not a contract but merely a sham disguised as contract. Accordingly, this discovery opens the door for both domestic laws and international instruments to intervene in order to save trafficked women from further exploitation. The discovery should also serve as an enlightenment tool to society generally, so that the preconceived notion that trafficking victims are the architects of their sufferings, who deserve no public support, ought to be abandoned.

Gorden, while commenting on the violation of the contractual rights of thousands of Haitian workers who were illegally imported into the Dominican Republic to work on the sugarcane estates for the duration of the harvest season, observed that "[the] workers are forced to live in dwellings that are little more than shanks, denied enforcement of their contractual rights, cheated out of their wages, and most shocking of all, prevented from terminating their at-will employment."[85] Gorden's observation is not different from the experiences of trafficked women. As has been illustrated in this analysis, trafficked women are incapable of ending their contracts. Such decisions are often accompanied by threats to the woman or her family back home, which in some cases leads to death of the woman or a family member. In a true contract, each of the parties should be at liberty to end the deal whenever it begins to work hardship on them. Anything short of that is compulsion and slavery. It is trite that prohibition against slavery and slave-related practices has attained the status of *jus cogens* (Bassiouni, 1991, 207) or peremptory international norm, as provided in Articles 53 and 64 of the Vienna Convention on the Law of Treaties.[86] There are many conventions and treaties that prohibit such practices. Article 38 of the Permanent Court of International Justice ("PCIJ") and International Court of Justice ("ICJ") statutes[87] reflect the prohibitions of these practices.

Under these sources of international law, the prohibited practices of slavery, slave-related practices, and forced labor constitute "a common international crime when committed by a public official or private persons against any person," (Statute of the Permanent Court, article 38 of Statutes of PCIJ & ICJ). Slavery and servitude are also banned by Article 4 of the Universal Declaration of Human Rights: "No one shall be held in slavery or servitude; slavery and the slave trade shall be prohibited in all their forms."[88] In addition, in October 2000, the U.S. Congress enacted the

Trafficking Victims Protection Act of 2000,[89] which expressly recognizes human trafficking as a form of slavery outlawed by the U.S. Constitution.[90] In a similar vein, in July 2003, the Nigerian National Assembly enacted the Trafficking in Persons (Prohibition) Law Enforcement and Administration Act of 2003, (Nigerian Trafficking Act) which expressly defines "slave" to mean "a person who is held in bondage whose life, liberty, freedom and property are under absolute control of someone [else]," (Nigerian Trafficking Act, section 50).

One's liberty cannot be contracted out. Article 3 of the Universal Declaration of Human Rights mandates: "Everyone has the right to life, liberty, and security of the person," (Universal Declaration of Human Rights). Consent is not a probative issue in the definition of sex trafficking because one cannot legally consent to slavery, and sex trafficking is clearly a variant of slavery, (Tiefenbrun, 205). The Thirteenth Amendment to the United States Constitution outlaws slavery and prohibits an individual from selling herself into bondage.[91] Multilateral treaties and customary international law condemn slavery.[92] Since its inception, the United Nations has always been committed to the abolition or elimination of slavery, (Rassam, 1999, 304).

From the 19th to 20th century, a number of international instruments were developed to address the abolition of slavery and slave-related practices. Between 1815 and 1957, twenty-four relevant documents impacting slavery and slave-related crimes were developed, in addition to fifty-five other documents, which are applicable to this category of crime, (Bassiouni, 1991, 453). These instruments reveal the intimate connection between the interests of the individual and international law.[93] Forced labor, either in sex work or any other form of work, is synonymous with slavery, (Bassiouni, 1991, 458). The mistake of equating trafficking contracts with contract *simpliciter* is that overtly, trafficking contract seems to have the contractual pillars of "compensation or consideration" and "voluntariness," but, covertly, these essential requirements are absent. The problem is that nobody seems to ask what happens after the formation of trafficking contracts. If the above narratives of trafficked African and Asian women are what the contract is all about, then the contract is on shaky legal grounds. The total restriction of liberty and freedom, coupled with the grossly insufficient consideration, makes trafficking contracts analogous to contracts for slavery. The law of contract, therefore, would not recognize a trafficking contract, not because it is immoral or because it is invalid *ex ante,* but because it falls apart in the same way that contract for slavery collapses. It is simply a simulated contract, which institutes no obligation at all.

Kant, while examining the relationship between the head of a household and his servant, observed that, "[t]his would be a society of unequals (one party being in command or being its head, the other obeying, i.e., serving)," (Kant, 1996, 66). He further observed that servants are included in what belongs to the head of a household, and as far as the form or manner of possession is concerned, they (the servants) are his by a right that is like a right to a thing; "for if they run away from him he can bring them back in his control by his unilateral choice," (Kant, 1996, 66).

Hence there is a right to persons akin to a right to things. This is basically in conformity with most trafficking contracts. Trafficked women are treated as properties of traffickers and pimps, who determine what they should do, how many clients they have to service each day, what amount they should have as allowance, and whether they should be killed, when necessary.[94] This lack of freedom and liberty is what distinguishes a contract for slavery or trafficking from a normal contract:

> [F]or it is by a contract that he has brought them under his control, and *a contract by which one party would completely renounce its freedom for the other's advantage would be self-contradictory, that is, null and void*, since by it one party would cease to be a person and so would have no duty to keep the contract but would recognize only force. (The right of ownership with regard to someone who has forfeited his personality by a crime is not under consideration here.) . . . So we see here . . . that there is a right to persons akin to a right to things (of the head of the house over servants); for he can fetch servants back and demand them from anyone in possession of them, as what is externally his, even before the reasons that may have led them to run away and their rights have been investigated.[95]

Kant's observation is analogous to trafficking contracts. It illustrates that one cannot renounce her freedom and liberty for the benefit of another party in a contract. The contract collapses because it renders the person giving up the right a non-person. Moreover, the fact that one party has absolute control over the other, even to the extent of bringing her back into his control when she runs away, illustrates that there is complete absence of liberty and freedom. There cannot be a contract where one party is all powerful and the other totally powerless. In the same vein, Blackstone in his commentary posited: "Every sale implies a price . . . an equivalent given to the seller in lieu of what he transfers to the buyer: but what equivalent can be given for life, and liberty, both of which (in absolute slavery) are held to be in the master's disposal? His property also, the very price he seems to receive, devolves ipso facto to his master, the instant he becomes his slave. In this case therefore, the buyer gives nothing, and the seller receives nothing: of what validity then can a sale be, which destroys the very principle upon which all sales are founded?" [96] Blackstone's observation is very much applicable to trafficking contracts. It reveals the implications of a "contract" that lacks the pillars of liberty and freedom. It also reveals the implications of a 'sale' that lacks the principles of bargain: a complete rip-off. Accordingly, trafficking contracts are simulated contracts because the essential pillars of freedom and liberty, which impact on the voluntariness of action, are lacking; and also because they defy basic sales doctrines. Trafficking contracts, therefore, collapse in the same way that a contract for slavery will fall apart.

Human trafficking is detrimental to both humanity and society, and should not be allowed to flourish in a free market economy. Some might query whether all other professions and vocations are sacrosanct. Of course, morality might move some people to see some professions like boxing as being a degradation to humanity. The difference between consenting to a boxing contract and consenting to trafficking is very glaring. Boxing serves as sports to the participants. Like every other type of sport, it has got its own side effects, which do not necessarily lead to death. Moreover, because most members of society do not see anything wrong with it, the context is always transparent. On the other hand, trafficking leads to exploitation and harm to trafficked women. Besides, there is the possibility that there might be many naïve victims. Fear of AIDS has led patrons of brothels and pimps to go in search of younger females in the belief that young women are less likely to transmit the AIDS virus.[97] Unfortunately, most of these naïve young women end up being infected with the dreaded killer disease, HIV/AIDS.[98]

CONCLUSION

This chapter has explored the limits of a woman's consent to trafficking. In the course of the analysis, the study applied theories of liberty and freedom to true-life narratives of trafficked women and uncovered the hidden matrix of inequality, domination, exploitation, oppression, dehumanization, threat, and lack of liberty and freedom that essentially characterize trafficking contracts. The chapter also applied doctrinal concepts of the classical law of contract to trafficking transactions. The outcome of the finding was that trafficking transactions do not qualify as contracts strictly speaking because they lack the two pillars of a valid contract: voluntariness and consideration. Accordingly, trafficking transactions are mere simulated deals masquerading as contracts. As such, they institute no legal obligations at all. The study therefore argued that trafficking contracts are analogous to contracts of slavery since the information asymmetries and inequality of bargaining power that characterize trafficking transactions essentially compel trafficked women to contract out their liberty and freedom. The study also calls on society to change its perceptions of trafficking victims and to assist in preventing traffickers from further exploiting their victims.[99]

NOTES

1. U.N. Protocol to Prevent, Suppress and Punish Trafficking in Persons, Especially Women and Children, Supplementing the United Nations Convention Against Transnational Organized Crime, U.N. Doc. A/53/383 (2000), G.A. Res. 55/25 of 15 Nov. 2000, annex II, U.N. GAOR, 55th Sess., No. 49, at U.N. Doc. A/45/49 (vol.1) 2001), available at http://www.unodc.org/unodc/en/trafficking_convention.html, also at http://www.uncjin.org/Documents/Conventions/dcatoc/final_documents_2/convention_%20traff_eng.pdf, and at http://www.uncjin.org/Documents/Conventions/dcatoc/final_documents_2/index.htm (last visited Sep. 20, 2005); hereinafter cited in text as U.N. Trafficking Protocol.
2. William J. Bennett & Charles W. Colson, *The Clintons Shrug at Sex Trafficking, Wall Street Journal*, (Jan 10, 2000): A26.
3. *Equality NOW Prostitution Statement,* available at http://www.equalitynow.org/english/actions/action_2301_en.html (last visited Sep. 5, 2005).
4. U.N. Office on Drugs and Crime, *Protocol to Prevent, Suppress and Punish Trafficking in Persons, Especially Women and Children* (Summary), available at http://www.unodc.org/unodc/en/trafficking_convention.html (last visited Sep. 5, 2005).
5. See e.g. Trafficking in Persons (Prohibition) Law Enforcement and Administration (Nigeria) Act 2003, 2003 Act No. 24, especially sections 11, 12, 13, 14, 17, 18, 19, and 21 which address the core prohibitions, but unfortunately limit their protections only to minors; hereinafter cited in text as Nigerian Trafficking Act. This limitation of protection to persons under eighteen years appears to give the impression that the legislative intent is to protect minors. As such, it could be argued that the policy behind the Act envisions that adults can protect themselves. This raises the issue of consent. In other words, the drafters of the Act seem to conclude that an adult who consents to be trafficked doesn't require the protection of the law. But in reality, this line of policy is myopic. Empirical data on trafficking reveals that there are lots of information asymmetries, and that majority of those who consent to trafficking (both adults and minors) encounter obstacles that were never anticipated when their consent was given. In other words, women who consent to trafficking face both 'lemons' problem (as a result of information asymmetry), and 'moral hazard' problem (as a result of the opportunistic behavior of the trafficker after the consent is given).
6. United Nations, *Trafficking in Persons: the New Protocol,* available at http://www.unodc.org/unodc/trafficking_protocol_background.html (last visited Oct. 26, 2005) (emphasis added).

7. Report of the Special Rapporteur on Violence Against Women, its Causes and Consequences, U.N. ESCOR, Commission on Human Rights 53rd Sess., Provisional Agenda Item 9(a), at 19, U.N. Doc. E/CN.4/1997/47 (1997).
8. Kelly E. Hyland, "The Impact of the Protocol to Prevent, Suppress and Punish Trafficking in Persons, Especially Women and Children" 8 *Hum. Rights Br.* 30 (2001): 30.
9. Laura Reanda, "Prostitution as a Human Rights Question: Problems and Prospects of U.N. Action" 13 Hum. Rts. Q. 202 (1991): 207.
10. Webster's Ninth New Collegiate Dictionary (1985), 946.
11. A. Lucas, "Women and Prostitution" in K.D. Askin & D.M. Koenig, eds. *Women and International Human Rights Law Volume 1*, (New York: Transnational Publishers Inc., 1999) 683 at 684.
12. S. McClelland, "Inside the Sex Trade" Maclean's (3 December 2001) 22, quoting Hedy Fry, Canadian Secretary of State for multiculturalism and the status of women; hereinafter cited in text as Inside the Sex Trade. (emphasis added).
13. BBC News Online, "Child Asylum Seekers Sold for Sex" (Thursday, March 8, 2001), available at http://news.bbc.co.uk/1/hi/uk/1208611.stm (last visited May 26, 2005); hereafter cited in text as Child Asylum Seekers.
14. Juliet Ume-Ezeokeke, "Desk Review for the Program of Action against Trafficking in Minors and Young Women from Nigeria into Italy for the Purpose of Sexual Exploitation," 15 (A joint trafficking project by the UN Interregional Crime and Justice Research Institute and the UN Office on Drugs and Crime), available at http://www.unicri.it/wwd/trafficking/nigeria/docs/dr_nigeria_eng.pd (last visited Oct. 26, 2005); hereafter cited in text as Desk Review. See also Florence Nightingale, "Nigeria: An Assessment of the International Labor Migration Situation." *GENPROM Working Paper No. 7*, at 5 (Gender Promotion Program of International Labor Office, Geneva), available at http://www.ilo.org/public/english/employment/gems/download/swmnig.pdf (last visited June 5, 2005) (observing: "In most cases, women migrants are trafficked and the decision to migrate is taken by others (relations, friends, husbands, and/or parents). This is another indication of the patriarchal nature of Nigerian society, which subjugates women and erodes their independence of thought, initiative, action and decision.") (parenthetical emphasis in original). See also The Joint British-Danish Fact-Finding Mission, *Report on Human Rights Issues in Nigeria,* (Jan. 2005), 39, available at The Danish Immigration Service website: www.udlst.dk (last visited June 5, 2005); hereafter cited in text as Joint Report on Human Rights. Copies could also be obtained by e-mail: dok@ udlst.dk." (observing that "they were aware of cases in which husbands have sold their daughters and even wives to trafficking agents well aware that these women may be exploited and forced into prostitution overseas."
15. It should be noted that part of the statistical data in this subsection C was used in my earlier work. See chapter 8, pages 170–172. The reason for the substantial repetition is because this section deals partly with statistics of trafficking in Africa. Since statistics do not change easily, coupled with the fact that trafficking statistics in Africa are rare to gather and synthesize, it

becomes pertinent to substantially reproduce the statistics on trafficking in Africa. The reproduced statistics on Africa are mostly field surveys by the UN, African governments and NGOs. In essence, it will take a while for further field works to be done in Africa due to the cost associated with such projects. Hence the statistics will remain the same for some time. In any event, any major work on trafficking in Africa, will almost always cite these statistics.

16. U.S. Department of State, "The 2005 Trafficking in Persons Report" available at http://www.state.gov/g/tip/rls/tiprpt/2005/46903.htm (last visited Nov. 20, 2005); hereinafter U.S. Trafficking Report. See also Marina Jiméenez, "B.C. is a Hub for Human Trafficking, Report Says," *The Globe and Mail,* (Thursday, June 9, 2005) which carried the highlights of the Report.
17. U.S. Department of State, "Office to Monitor and Combat Trafficking in Persons," available at http://www.state.gov/g/tip/, (last visited June 15, 2004). For a confirmation of this figure *see* the United Nations Office on Drugs and Crime, *Fact Sheet on Human Trafficking,* available at http://www.unodc.org/unodc/en/trafficking_victims_consents.html (last visited Oct. 26, 2005) (observing that, "a recent CIA report estimated that between 45,000 to 50,000 women and children are brought to the United States every year under false pretences and are forced to work as prostitutes, abused laborers or servants.")
18. See http://europe.cnn.com/2001/WORLD/europe/02/04/immigration/index.html (last visited 10 Dec. 2005). See also J. Chuang "Redirecting the Debate over Trafficking in Women: Definitions, Paradigms, and Contexts" 11 *Harvard Human Rights Journal* 65 (1998).
19. Jiméenez, 2005; which carried the highlights of a U.S. State Department's Fifth Annual Trafficking in Persons Report. The Report noted that "[t]he RCMP [Royal Canadian Mountain Police] estimates that about 800 people are trafficked into Canada annually and an additional 1,500–2000 are trafficked through Canada to the United States." See also "Trade in Humans Targeted" *Metro News,* Toronto, (Tuesday, March 9, 2004) where Canadian Minister of Justice Irwin Cotler, observed that "Canada serves not only as a country of destination but also a country of transit for criminals flooding men, women and children into the United States."
20. Reuters Ltd, "Mafia Makes Billions from Trafficking People—UN" (Dec. 15, 2000), available at http://www.vachss.com/help_text/styles/archive-print.php, (last visited June 15, 2005); hereafter cited in text as Mafia Makes Billions.
21. Anti-Slavery "Human Trafficking Q&A" available at http:www.antislavery.org/homepage/antislavery/trafficking.htm (last visited June 10, 2005); hereafter cited in text as Anti-Slavery.
22. E.E. Okojie, Obehi Okojie, Kokure Eghafona, Gloria Vincent-Osaghae & Victoria Kalu, *Trafficking of Nigerian Girls to Italy,* (July 2003): 17 (A study commissioned by U.N. Interregional Crime and Justice Research Institute), available at http://www.unicri.it/wwd/trafficking/nigeria/docs/rr_okojie_eng.pdf;hereinafter cited in text as *Trafficking to Italy*] (last visited Oct. 26, 2005) (observing: "There is generally a paucity of data on the

scale and trends in human trafficking around the world largely because of the criminal and underground nature of trafficking. Thus most available data are estimates by various researchers and NGOs working on the subject.")

23. United Nations Office on Drug and Crime, "Analysis and Statistics," available at http://www.unodc.org/unodc/en/analysis_and_statistics.html, also at http://www.unodc.org/unodc/trafficking_protocol_background.html (last visited June 15, 2005).
24. U.N. Office on Drugs and Crime, "Fact Sheet on Human Trafficking," available at http://www.unodc.org/unodc/en/trafficking_victim_consents.html (last visited Oct. 26, 2005).
25. *Trafficking to Italy,* 5; (the Study further reveals the history of human trafficking in Italy: "Trafficking of women to Italy dates back to the end of the 1980s when the fear of AIDS rendered drug-addicted Italian girls unattractive on the prostitution market, and the first Nigerian girls began to appear on the streets, especially in the central and northern Italy. Nigerians thus constituted Italy's first cohort of 'forced prostitutes.' . . .")
26. Michael Specter, "Traffickers' New Cargo: Naïve Slavic Women," *N.Y. Times* (Jan. 15, 1998), 6.
27. *Trafficking to Italy,* 14; (noting that "[g]iven the poor state of record keeping in Nigeria, most of them [respondents in a trafficking sudy] had no data to fall back on. As a result, many of the answers were left blank as the respondents said they don't know much about the details of human trafficking although they are aware the problem exists . . . Most of the answers were the impressions or guesses of the respondents based on hearsay . . . In general, obtaining hard data was very difficult, and most of what was obtained represents personal estimates by respondents to the questionnaires. Some of the agencies which had data were very secretive, and reluctant to divulge them. Very little published data by these agencies are available, mainly because there have been no coordinated efforts to keep good records of human trafficking. Most of the available data are records of those repatriated, not of those who had been trafficked.")
28. At the outset, it should be noted that on a general level it is not all deportations that are trafficking related. However, in this analysis, unless otherwise indicated, all the references to deportations are trafficking related. This brief explanatory note is meant to serve as a backgrounder to the reader in assessing the figures.
29. Florence Nightingale, "Nigeria: An Assessment of the International Labor Migration Situation." *GENPROM Working Paper No. 7*, at 3–4 (Gender Promotion Program of International Labor Office, Geneva), available at http://www.ilo.org/public/english/employment/gems/download/swmnig.pdf (last visited June 5, 2005); hereafter cited in text as Labor Migration.
30. Osita Agbu, "Corruption and Human Trafficking: The Nigerian Case" *West Africa Review* (2003), available at http://www.westafricareview.com/vol4.1/agbu.html (last visited June 15, 2005) (Observing that "[a]t a March 2002 seminar organized in Lagos by the International Federation of Women Lawyers (FIDA), WOTCLEF [Women Trafficking and Child Labor

Eradication Foundation] reported that there are about 20,000 Nigerian women involved in the sex industry in Italy. The *Daily Champion* of 12 July 2002 reported that 80% of foreign prostitutes in Italy were Nigerian women.") (Emphasis in original).

31. Warm Africa, "Traffickers hold thousands of children, women in bondage" (12 Nov. 2003), available at http://www.warmafrica.com/index/geo/4/cat/3/a/a/artid/382 (last visited May 2, 2005).
32. Women's Rights Watch—Nigeria, "2004 Report on the State of Women's Rights in Nigeria" available at http://www.rufarm.kabissa.org/articles/2004report.htm_(last visited May 24, 2005)
33. Joint British-Danish Fact-Finding Mission, *Report on Human Rights Issues in Nigeria,* (Jan. 2005), 45, 5.7.2; available at The Danish Immigration Service website: www.udlst.dk (last visited June 5, 2005). Copies could also be obtained my e-mail: dok@udlst.dk; hereinafter cited in text as Joint Report on Human Rights.
34. Sani Mohammed, "Gaudy Promises Lure Children, Women into Slavery" *Crossroads* Vol. 10, No. 4 (May 2003), available at http://nigeria.usembassy.gov/wwwhxmay)3.html (last visited May 2, 2005).
35. Historically, military forces and policies were directly involved in the development of both sex tourism and forced prostitution. See K. Howard, ed. (Y. J. Lee trans.), *True Stories of the Korean Comfort Women* (Cassell, 1995) (1993); S.P. Sturdevant & B. Stoltzfus, *Let the Good Times Roll: Prostitution and the U.S. Military in Asia* (1993); C. Enloe, *Bananas, Beaches and Bases: Making Feminist Sense of International Politics* (1989); N. V. Demleitner, "Forced Prostitution: Naming an International Offence" 18 *Fordham Int'l L.J.* 163 (1994): 180—185; I. L. Sajor, ed. *Common Grounds: Violence against Women in War and Armed Conflict Situations* (Philippines : Asian Center for Women's Human Rights (ASCENT), 1998).
36. Human Rights Watch, "The Human Rights Watch Global Report on Women's Human Rights" (1995) 230.
37. A. Usher, "The Dangerous Truth of 'Foreign Bodies'" (1998) The Nation (Bangkok, Aug. 19), 31 cited in Lucas, 690.
38. C. M. Hall, "Sex Tourism in South-east Asia" in D. Harrison, ed. *Tourism and the Less Developed Countries* (1992) 64; B. Sullivan, "Global Prostitution: Sex Tourism and Trafficking in Women" (July 1996) [Unpublished, archived at University of Strathclyde Law School Library] Paper presented at the Annual Meeting of the Law and Society Association, University of Strathclyde, Glasgow, Scotland, July 11–13, 1996).
39. S. Schlosstein, *Asia's New Little Dragon* (Chicago: Contemporary Books, 1991) 196–197; (observing that tourism generates some US$3 billion annually and sex is one of its most valuable sub sectors).
40. "Trade in Humans Targeted" Toronto *Metro News* (Tuesday, March 9, 2004) (Quoting Canadian Justice Minister Irwin Cotler).
41. For highlights of this report see Jiméenez, 2005. See also the U.S. Trafficking in Persons Report.
42. United Nations Office on Drugs and Crime, "Involvement of Organized Crime," available at http://www.unodc.org/unodc/en/trafficking_victim_

consents.html (last visited Oct. 26, 2005) (observing: "The relatively low risks of trafficking and substantial potential profits have, in some cases, induced criminals to become involved as an alternative to other, riskier criminal pursuits.").

43. See generally S. Tiefenbrun, "Sex Sells but drugs don't Talk: Trafficking of Women Sex Workers" 23 *Thomas Jefferson L. Rev.* (2001): 199.
44. U.N. Office on Drugs and Crime, "Trafficking in Human Beings," available at http://www.unodc.org/unodc/en/trafficking_human_beings.html (last visited Oct. 26, 2005) (observing that "women and girls are attracted by the prospect of a well-paid job as a domestic servant, waitress or factory worker. Traffickers recruit victims through fake advertisements, mail-order bride catalogues and casual acquaintances.") See also U.N. Office on Drugs and Crimes, "Trafficking in Persons: the New Protocol," available at http://www.unodc.org/unodc/trafficking_protocol_background.html (last visited Oct. 26, 2005) (observing that "young women and teenagers are often lured into prostitution rings by advertisements for domestic positions abroad and find themselves bought and sold via catalogues or by close family members.")
45. Reuters, Mafia Makes Billions; (reporting that, "[i]n Italy, criminals operate an extensive and elaborate ring that lures Nigerian women into the country on the pretext of getting work. They are then sold to pimps for about $12,000 each. 'The girls are slaves. There is no other way to define it . . . The pimps want to make a four-fold profit on their investment, meaning the girls have to pay $48,000 before they are free.'") (Emphasis in original).
46. Melanie R. Wallace, "Voiceless Victims: Sex Slavery and Trafficking of African Women in Western Europe" 30 (Spring 2002) *Georgia J. Int'l & Comp. L. 569* (asserting that "[t]here are certain consistent patterns by which most African prostitutes are introduced to prostitution in Western Europe. The first scenario involves African women brought from their home countries for the purpose of exploiting them through prostitution (usually with [without?] their prior knowledge. Sponsors with ties on both African and European continents lure African women and girls to Europe, promising them a chance to study at a university or take advantage of job opportunities. These women are often promised jobs as maids or au pairs or given loans (with or without their knowledge) to finance their passage and are then forced to repay the loans through prostitution when they arrive.") (all comments in original). See also U.N. Office on Drugs and Crime, "Trafficking in Human Beings," (noting: "Upon arrival at their destination, victims are placed in conditions controlled by traffickers while they are exploited to earn illicit revenues.")
47. BBC, Child Asylum Seekers; where BBC reported: "There are 2,500 African prostitutes working on the streets of Turin alone. Seven have been killed in the past four years." BBC also interviewed Marianne, a Nigerian girl trafficked to Italy for prostitution, who observed: "I don't want to die. I want to stay [sic] in life . . . Many of our girls are dying here because of 'I cannot do it.' They organize our boys and beat you. You have

to be on the street as if you are not a normal human being" (emphasis in original). It must be pointed out that the BBC observation that seven African prostitutes were killed in the past four years is an understatement. According to official sources from Nigeria, "the wife of Edo State Governor, Mrs. Eki Igbinedion, announced that about 116 Nigerian prostitutes were killed in Italy between 1994 and 1998." See *Trafficking to Italy*, 39. See also Joint British-Danish Fact-Finding Mission, 43, 5.4.4 (where it was observed that a trafficking syndicate or the pimp could trace a returned trafficking victim "if they suspect that she intends to cooperate with the authorities. In such cases the madam or the agent may hire persons from militant groups . . . and in this way have the woman killed as a deterrent to others.")

48. Tiffany St. Claire King, "The Modern Slave Trade" 8 (2002) *U.C. Davis J. Int'l L. & Pol'y* 293, 308–309. See also Lori Romeyn Sitowski, "Congress Giveth, Congress Taketh Away, Congress Fixeth Its Mistake? Assessing the Potential Impact of the Battered Immigration Women Protection Act" 19 (2001) *Law &Ineq.* 259, 280 (observing that Captors force their victims into submission by unleashing various forms of physical coercion on them and "many are thereby exposed to AIDS and other disease, and some are worked or beaten to death."); Osita Agbu, *supra* note 33 (observing that "[a] report of the International Organization for Migration noted that in many cases traffickers seize their victims' travel documents and sell the women to brothel owners."); Human Rights Watch, *A Modern Form of Slavery: Trafficking of Burmese Women and Girls into Brothels in Thailand* (New York: Human Rights Watch, 1993): 1; hereinafter Human Rights Watch; McClelland, 2001, 22.
49. *Trafficking to Italy*, 28–29; (With particular reference to the Edos of Nigeria, the authors observed: "Various deities and ancestral deities are worshipped . . . *Osanobua* or *Osa* is the highest God, creator of all things and beings in the world and heaven . . . *Olokun* is described as equivalent of the Greek god Neptune. *Olokun* is the great god of the sea. He is said to be a senior son of *Osanobua* . . . *Ogun* is the deity of iron or metals. *Osanyin* is the deity of medicine and employed to ensure the effective use of all forms of medicine. *Obiemwen* is a wife of the earth and described as equivalent of the Greek Uranus . . . *Ogiuwu* is the deity in charge of death. *Orunmila* is the divining deity. Spirits of the departed or ancestors are also worshipped.")
50. BBC, Child Asylum Seekers; where a Social Worker Lynne Chitty, reacting to the disappearance of more than 40 African teenagers seeking asylum in the UK, observed that, "traffickers forced girls to go through a voodoo ceremony before they left their home country. They have to swear not to tell anyone and while they are swearing they are being cut. Some girls have 40 or 50 cuts all over their body. They are forced to drink blood and this all happens in a dark and frightening place. One girl when she told me was just trembling, crying 'my body's going to blow up and I'm going to die now.'") (Emphasis in original).
51. Nightingale, Labor Migration; (observing that in Nigeria only "few trafficked persons have been courageous enough to reveal the identity of their

traffickers, due to the oath of secrecy to which they are sworn and fear of repercussions for breaking it. To date, no traffickers have been prosecuted."). See also Joint Human Rights Report, 5.2.5–6; (where Carol N. Ndaguba, the Executive Secretary/Chief Executive of the Nigerian National Agency for the Prohibition of Traffic in Persons and Other Related Matters (NAPTIP) referred to a recent incident in which six trafficked women had refused to testify against their traffickers because of the juju oath they have been committed to. However, in order to convince the women that nothing would happen to them if they testified, NAPTIP raided two shrines in Edo State and recovered a number of items including the pictures and hair of the six victims. Two priests were also arrested and paraded before the victims in order to convince them.) Notwithstanding all the institutional wars against shrines and juju oath, the psychological fears in the minds of trafficked victims remain unabated.

52. Ume-Ezeokeke, Desk Review, 19 (observing that "an officer of the Trafficking Unit in Edo [State of Nigeria] Police Commission said that it is difficult to arrest or even prosecute the Barons because complainants and witnesses are not willing to testify against them in the court for fear of being assassinated.")
53. See Anti-Slavery, "Human Traffic, Human Rights: Redefining Victim Protection" 10. Nigeria 159 at 165, available at http://www.antislavery.org/homepage/resources/humantraffichumanrights.htm (last visited May 2, 2005), (although the girl was eventually persuaded to give evidence to the police, shortly after relaying her experiences, she injured herself unconsciously and blamed the injury on the oaths).
54. Edo State Criminal Code (Amendment Law) 2000, sections 223a-223d; hereafter cited in text as Edo Criminal Code, (specifically, 223A punishes any person who "sponsors a girl or woman by giving her any financial, physical or material assistance to enable her travel out of Nigeria" for prostitution or any immoral act or administers any oath on any woman or girl or performs any fetish ritual in order to enable her travel out of Nigeria to become a prostitute or engage in sexual dealings with any person; 223B punishes any female person who engages in prostitution or other immoral acts within or outside Nigeria; 233C punishes any man who patronizes prostitutes; 223D punishes any woman who lures or induces any man to engage in sexual intercourse with her for any gratification). Analytically, this amendment is a paradox: it initially set out to punish traffickers and save victims of trafficking, however, its substance reveals that it punishes victims rather than traffickers. What purpose does it serve to punish a woman who engages in prostitution abroad, without making exceptions respecting the reasons for her actions? Most trafficking victims do not know that they would end up as prostitutes. As such punishing a trafficking victim who engages in prostitution does not seem reasonable. Rather than reduce trafficking, this law has the effect of making trafficking go underground because a woman who reveals her trafficker stands the risk of being implicated as well. Hence it appears that women would rather keep quiet than reveal their ordeals. Revelation

will lead to double jeopardy. Moreover, the law lays emphasis on prostitution rather than trafficking. This is a misconception. Trafficking and prostitution are two different concepts although they may be inextricably intertwined. The inability of the law to draw this distinction is unfortunate.

55. For a compendium of the controversies, see Maureen Chigbo, "Igbinedion Versus Prostitutes" *Online Nigeria Portal,* available at http://www.onlinenigeria.com/aids/edo_prosti.asp (last visited June 3, 2005).
56. This back-stab attitude is contrary to U.N. Principles and Guidelines. See U.N. High Commissioner For Human Rights Principles and Guidelines on Human Rights and Trafficking, E/2002/68/Add.1 (2002), at Guideline 5, available at http://www1.umn.edu/humanrts/instree/traffickingGuidelinesHCHR.html (last visited Sep 28, 2005); hereinafter cited in text as U.N. Principles; (asserting that "an adequate law enforcement response to trafficking is dependent on the cooperation of trafficked persons and other witnesses. In many cases, individuals are reluctant or unable to report traffickers or to serve as witnesses because they lack confidence in the police and the judicial system and/or the absence of any effective protection mechanisms. *These problems are compounded when law enforcement officials are involved or complicit in trafficking. Strong measures need to be taken to ensure that such involvement is investigated, prosecuted and punished. Law enforcement officials must also be sensitized to the paramount requirement of ensuring the safety of trafficked persons.*") (Emphasis added).
57. U.N. Office on Drugs and Crime, "Trafficking in Human Beings" available at http://www.unodc.org/unodc/en/trafficking_human_beings.html (last visited Oct. 26, 2005) (where it was observed: "The support and protection of victims who give evidence is key to prosecuting the ringleaders behind the [trafficking] phenomenon" See also U.N. Office on Drugs and Crime, "Involvement of Organized Crime" available at http://www.unodc.org/unodc/en/trafficking_victim_consents.html (last visited Oct. 26, 2005) (cautioning that "trafficked persons should also be seen as victims of crime. Support and protection of victims is a humanitarian objective and an important means of ensuring that victims are willing and able to assist in criminal cases.")
58. For e.g., such measure has been effected in Nigeria, although its enforcement remains to be seen. See Nigerian Trafficking Act, section 45; (Mandating that "[w]here a person volunteers to the Agency or an official of the Agency any information, which may be useful in the investigation of an offence under this Act, the Agency shall take all reasonable measures to protect the identity of that person and the information so volunteered shall be treated as confidential.")
59. Reuters, Mafia Makes Billions; (observing: "In Italy, criminals operate an extensive and elaborate ring that lures Nigerian women into the country on the pretext of getting work. They are then sold to pimps for about $12,000 each . . . The pimps want to make a four-fold profit on their investment, meaning the girls have to pay $48,000 before they are free.

They are told that if they flee or talk to the police, their families in Nigeria will be killed.")

60. The Constitution of Nigeria, 1999, section 35 guarantees personal liberty while section 34 states that "(a) No person shall be subjected to torture or to inhuman or degrading treatment, (b) No person shall be held in slavery, (c) No person shall be required to perform forced or compulsory labor."
61. Criminal Code, Laws of the Federation 1990 (Nigeria), Cap. 77, section 227; hereafter cited in text as Criminal Code.
62. I.E. Sagay, *Nigerian Law of Contract*, (London: Sweet and Maxwell, 1985): 1.
63. *Corbin on Contracts,* (1952) no. 21, 21 (emphasis added).
64. I. Kant, *The Metaphysics of Morals*, Trans. and ed. M. Gregor, (Cambridge: Cambridge University Press, 1996): 67.
65. *Corbin on Contracts*, no. 11; (emphasis mine).
66. Hugo Grotius, *The Law of War and Peace,* BK II, c. 12.
67. (1825), 3 Pick. (Mass.) 207. (Supreme Judicial Court of Massachusetts).
68. Ibid. per Parker, C.J., 47–48.
69. Part I Section 'Recruitment Strategies of Syndicates vis-à-vis Victims' Consent.'
70. Cotton, L.J. in *Allcard* v. *Skinner* (1887) 36 Ch. D. 145, 171.
71. H. Beale, "Inequality of Bargaining Power" 6 *Oxford J. Legal Stud.* 123 (1986): 128.
72. In Nigeria, Lin Lin's Father and the syndicate will both be committing an offence by this act. See s. 369 of the Nigerian Criminal Code, which punishes the placement or receiving of any person in servitude as a pledge or security for a current or future debt. However, notwithstanding this provision, as a practical matter, this kind of practice goes on in Nigeria, and no prosecutions are brought. Suffice it to say that prohibiting a conduct through a statute is not synonymous with enforcing that statute.
73. Notwithstanding that at times some men pay $30 to have her all-night sexual services which calculations are not included in the above summations since they were night jobs. In other words, this all-night sexual services are synergies that increase the profit margin that Lin Lin generates for the syndicate.
74. United Nations Office on Drugs and Crime, *Trafficking in Persons: the New Protocol,* available at http://www.unodc.org/unodc/trafficking_protocolbackground.html (last visited Oct. 26, 2005) (observing that trafficked women in the sex industry work for up to 18 hours a day).
75. *Hart v. O'Connor* (1985) 2 All E.R. 880.
76. Beale, 1986, 126; (emphasis added).
77. (1968) [1978] 1 WLR 255 n.
78. Human Rights Watch, 1. See also BBC, Child Asylum Seekers; where BBC interviewed Marianne, a Nigerian girl trafficked to Italy for prostitution, who observ"I cannot do it. They organize our boys and beat you. You have to be on the street as if you are not a normal human being."
79. United Nations Office on Drugs and Crime, Trafficking in Persons: the New Protocol, available at http://www.unodc.org/unodc/trafficking_protocolbackground.html (last visited Oct. 26, 2005).

80. Joint Human Rights Report, 47, 5.7.12; See also Reuters, Mafia Makes Billions; which reports that Nigerian women trafficked into Italy are "sold to pimps for about $12,000 each.," and the pimps "make a four-fold profit on their investment, meaning the girls have to pay $48,000 before they are free.")
81. *Cooke* v. *Oxley,* (1790) 100 E.R. 785 (K.B.), A. having promised to sell goods to B., gave him certain time at his request to determine whether he would buy them or not; B. within the time determined to buy them, and gave notice thereof to A.; yet A. was not bound in an action for not delivering them, for B. not being bound by the original contract, there was no consideration to bind A.
82. For a review of morality and public policy debate vis-à-vis trafficking of women for prostitution, see generally Victor N. Opara "Legal Issues in Migration and Human Trafficking in Africa" in Hakeem I. Tijani, ed. *Africa and the Wider World* (New York: McGraw-Hill Higher Education Publisher, 2006) (Part VII, forthcoming).
83. See Grotius, supra note 99.
84. M.C. Bassiouni, "Enslavement as an International Crime" 23 *N.Y.U. J. Int'l L. & Pol.* 445 (1991); see also Tiefenbrun, 2001, 458; (emphasis added).
85. M.E. Gorden, "Haitian Forced Labor in the Dominican Republic" 15 *Comp. Labor L.J.* 206 (1994).
86. Vienna Convention on the Law of Treaties (with annex). Arts.53 and 64. Concluded at Vienna, 23 May 1969. Entered into force, 27 January 1988. 1155 U.N.T.S. 331; 1969 U.N.J.Y.B. 140; 1980 U.K.T.S. 58, Cmnd. 7964; reprinted in 8 I.L.M. 679 (1969) & 1 Weston I.E.l.
87. Statute of the Permanent Court of International Justice, art. 38 reprinted in *Statute et Reglement de la Cour 22 (1940)*; The *Statute of the International Court of Justice,* art. 38, reprinted in 1970 U.N.Y.B. 1013, 1017, U.N. Sales no. E.72.I.1; hereafter cited in text as Statute of the Permanent Court.
88. Universal Declaration of Human Rights, G.A. res. 217 A (III), 10 Dec. 1948; available at http://www.un.org/overview/rights.html (last visited 14 April 2002).
89. Trafficking Victims Protection Act of 2000, 22 U.S.C. 7101 (2000); hereinafter U.S. Trafficking Act.
90. U.S. Const. amend. XIII.
91. Amy O'Neill Richard, International Trafficking in Women to the United States: A Contemporary Manifestation of Slavery and Organized Crime, DCI Exceptional Intelligence Analyst Program: An Intelligence Monograph, November 1999 (April 2000), at Part VI; hereinafter CIA Report.
92. A. Yasmine Rassam, " Contemporary Forms of Slavery and the Evolution of the Prohibition of Slavery and the Slave Trade Under Customary International Law," 39 *Va. J. Int'l L.* 303 (1999).
93. I.L. Oppenheim, *International law: A Treatise* 641 (8th ed. 1955).
94. Joint Human Rights Report, 43, 5.4.2 (where it was observed that "agents of trafficking are able to kill a woman who has been returned to Nigeria if they desire to do so and that agents have a strong network.)

95. Kant, 1996, 66 (italicized emphasis added, all other emphasis in original).
96. William Blackstone, *Commentaries on the Laws of England*, Book 1, Chapter 14 "Of Master and Servant."
97. H.H. Pyne, "AIDS and Gender Violence: The Enslavement of Burmese Women in the Thai Sex Industry" in J. Peters & A. Wolper, eds. *Women's Rights, Human Rights: International Feminist Perspective* (New York: Routledge,1995): 217.
98. Chigbo, 2005; (noting that "Queen Imotanyi Omoruyi, 25, used to be a hairdresser [in Benin, Nigeria] before she travelled to Italy two years ago for prostitution. Omoruyi, who had nothing before her trip seems to have hit it big in the sex trade . . . However, Omoruyi, will not be able to enjoy the fruits of her 'hard' labor peacefully. Omoruyi . . . came back in January with a strange ailment . . . Omoruyi's illness has deteriorated and now she is paralysed from waist down." (Emphasis in original). A medical doctor in Benin confirmed that Omoruyi's sickness was most probably HIV/AIDS infection. Id. See also Wallace, *supra* note 57, at 583 (recounting the story of Ana, a 26-year-old Nigerian woman who was forced into prostitution in Italy by her traffickers. Ana contracted AIDS thereafter).

Part III
Migration and Education

Chapter Ten

School Migration: A Major Concern in Historically Disadvantaged Schools in South Africa

Myra Maboya

INTRODUCTION

The research report by the Department for Education and Employment[1] shows that to some degree, however small, all schools have some level of pupils moving in or out. For the purpose of this study I chose the concept of school migration to refer to these movements. School migration is assumed to mean the movement by black learners away from the historically disadvantaged schools in search for better quality education elsewhere.[2] This movement appears to be influenced by the desegregation of schools that, for the first time in the history of South African education, has made possible the shift of learners across schools. School migration is contrasted with labor migration—the concept that dominates the literature. Labor migration is about adults while the former is about learners. However, a common terminology related to school migration that has been used by other researchers, for example, in England and Wales, is that of "pupil mobility."[3] Pupil mobility is defined by OFSTED as the total movement in and out of schools by pupils other than at the usual times of joining and leaving, (Mennell, 2005 and Pupil Mobility Guidance).

In essence, these terminologies mean the same thing, that is, the movement of learners from one school to another, though used differently according to context. For example, in the South African context, the movement of children that is "mostly common" and the focal point of this chapter is a movement that is planned well in advance, following the exit procedures where the school of choice or preference is selected and takes place after the whole process of applying, gaining admission and passing on essential information to the new school is completed. On the other hand, in the English context, literature concentrates on the impact that pupil mobility has in the receiving schools where pupils arrive at any time in all year groups, where schools are to continually begin afresh with new pupils, often arriving with no previous records.[4]

However, the study aims to elicit public views with regard to school migration, trying to understand the issue from the voices of those affected. Overall, the study aims to shed some initial light on the nature and causes of school migration and the implications this movement has for the departed schools in the following respects:

- What are the causes of migration?
- Does school migration really matter?
- What are the implications for the school reforms?
- What challenges does this present to schools or departments?

BACKGROUND TO THE PATTERNS OF SCHOOL MIGRATION[5]

It is significant to note that school migration is nothing new, although up until now it has not been recognized or studied systematically. However, it is increasingly recognized that migratory movements can no longer be defined narrowly as labor migration following the decontrolling of migration and the subsequent dismantling of the apartheid influx control policies.[6] Nor can it be defined exclusively in relation to Africans, as has also been the case in the past. During apartheid there was a system of highly restrictive influx control legislation that targeted blacks in particular, and which limited their entry and residence in cities and small towns including some so-called "white" areas in the so-called "homelands." These restrictive boundaries also applied in the educational sector, enforced through the education departments that were racially segmented.

Although people from rural areas or poor communities were forced to work in metropolitan areas as migrant laborers, the issue of school choice was far more complicated and was connected to apartheid group area legislation, demographic patterns and patterns of mobility.[7] Parents in the homelands would rarely send their children to township or city schools, even including those who worked there. Rather, they left their children behind for the purpose of schooling, and even those who happened to migrate to the cities with their families would send their children back to the boarding schools in the then Northern Transvaal, presently known as Limpopo Province. The Northern Transvaal was known for the institutions with boarding facilities.

These institutions were of missionary origin located in the three former Bantustans—Gazankulu, Lebowa and Venda—the migrants' home bases. Probably one other major factor that is also cited in Hartshorne and supported by Badat and Unterhaler is that during the period 1955 to 1966/67, the government paid very little attention to secondary education.[8] Hartshorne argues that: "Secondary education was artificially restricted by the regulation which laid down that the junior secondary schools (standard 6–8, presently known as grade 7–9) were to be paid for on the R-for-R system, this means that communities had to take initiative in erecting the school buildings and would then be paid fifty percent (50%) of the costs if funds were available. In addition, it was difficult to get secondary schools approved and registered in urban areas. Standard 9–10 were approved only in the new homeland areas as part of the separate development policy," (Hartshorne, 62–67.) The R-for-R system was used as a mechanism of pushing or encouraging communities to build their own schools with the hope that they would be refunded 50% of the cost as government subsidy, which in many instances had never been the case. Therefore it was not surprising that a considerable number of urban children found refuge in homeland high schools.

Whilst I support Souedien et al's argument that "the choice usually centred around issues of cost and social support, as well as stability,"(Souedien et al, 84). I would like to add that the major issues overriding all these factors were those of home language and culture, as parents still had to support their children financially whether in boarding school or living with relatives, which was also costly, and that children were sent to the schools of their language origin. Souedien et al cited one other issue that was held in common (as reported by the former students interviewed), that "when at particular times urban schools were sites of political activities, schooling in the rural setting was construed as being less disrupted and more stable," (Souedien et al, 84).

The pattern of movement took a dramatic change following the opening up of the school system in 1995. Since then, there is a high influx of black children enrolling in historically well-resourced schools where they had previously been denied access.[9] Again, it is sufficient to mention at this stage the influence of the growing awareness of the importance of basic literacy in 'information and communication technology' that would otherwise not be found in disadvantaged schools. Although this new influence is a challenge that needs to be perceived as positive and enriching, rather than to insist on traditional ideas of membership to society based purely on territory or descent as argued by Hartshorne, the envisaged loss of personnel in the near future, resulting from this migration, is one major aspect that needs to be considered.

GATHERING OF INFORMATION

Employing "surveillance" as a conceptual framework, school migration in Limpopo Province is unquestionably a general occurrence affecting almost all black communities as observed by the researcher who is a resident and a practitioner. For the purpose of this study a small sample was purposively drawn from within Mopani, one of the districts in Limpopo Province, which is comprised of three of the former apartheid government's Bantustans that are predominantly rural with some semi-urban areas. The sample comprised two informants who came to study in the then Northern Transvaal during the 1960s and 1970s, six families, six students in 'black' schools within the province; six students attending outside the province—three in high schools and three in tertiary; staff members (teachers) from one school who participated as a focus group and six school principals heading black schools. The balancing of the numbers of participants was not important for this study, as it was not intended for comparisons.

The six families had their children transferred from black to historically advantaged schools as follows: Two families, one from the village and another from the township bought flats in Polokwana and Gauteng (another province) respectively, hired maids to leave with all their children whilst they attend schools there; two families have their children in boarding schools within Mopani district; one family clusters with other parents from elsewhere to rent accommodation that is arranged by the institution in Polokwana; and the other family from the village has children commuting to the school in the township.

Data was collected through interviews, which were conducted with all informants using semi-structured questions. Interviews were chosen because of their nature of providing an opportunity to probe and expand the interviewee's responses.[10] With the consent of the participants, the interviews were tape-recorded and transcribed, with subsequent transcripts used confidentially for analysis. There was no time limit during the interviews as the focus was to achieve the main research objectives by getting as much information as possible. The informants were interviewed only once and I undertook full content analysis of the qualitative data.

The research began with two participants who came from Johannesburg and Rustenburg respectively in the 1960s and 1970s to study in the Northern Transvaal (the present Limpopo Province) institutions. The participants studied in two different institutions that were in different homelands/Bantustans. These participants were asked just one question each, 'why they preferred to come and study in the Northern Transvaal institutions during the 1960s and 1970s. For both, this question generated sufficient discussion to obtain the required information. The information from the two participants helped to shape the paragraph above about the traditional pattern of school migration.

DILEMMAS

What I considered a dilemma for the study was that in the new dispensation, the constitution allows everyone a right to decide on the school of choice for his/her children's education. Therefore, I thought asking people the question why they took their children to the far away schools would be regarded as a violation of their rights. However, this was not the case. All participating informants gladly welcomed the interviews as this enabled them to discuss the plight of education in black schools—their schools, of course.

RESEARCH FINDINGS

This research was set up to discover the importance that people attach to various factors that influence school migration. It might first be noted that all respondents appeared to hold very similar views. Almost all participants cited similar driving forces for school migration. The participants independently expressed similar opinions with those stated in the South African Broadcasting Co-operation (SABC) talk show on the causes of migration.[11] This inspires some confidence in the validity of the findings expressed in this chapter. Findings from the different groups of informants will be presented separately. However, lack of confidence in black schools was the first issue raised by all participants including teachers themselves.

INTERVIEWS WITH LEARNERS

High school learners who moved out of black schools expressed how committed their present teachers are, as compared to the teachers who previously taught them in black schools. One student mentioned that some teachers are not even as highly qualified as those in black schools and added that they commit themselves to their work. Students concur that: "Black schools do not have a future due to lack of discipline." They indicated that lack of discipline starts with teachers who do not come to school everyday. The students still enrolled in black schools who mentioned teacher absence as a problem in their respective schools supported this. All students said that, "even those who come to school, some of them do not come to the classes during their lessons; they sit and chat in the staff room and no one dares to call them because you can be in for it." When asked what the principals say about these, one said that the principals are afraid of some of the teachers. Learners appeared to be familiar with the pattern of teachers' absence. One learner remarked that "At my previous school, we knew in advance that teachers X and G would not come to school every 22nd of the month because it is their pay day and, where the pay day is Thursday we knew that teacher G would come back on Monday." One other learner states, "though I'm not a teacher, having teachers C & F (mentioning the names of the teachers) is just like having no teacher at all, and having to study on your own."

Regarding the question of perceived differences in education in general in their present and previous schools, learners in white led schools expressed satisfaction about the education they receive. They indicated that teachers are so enthusiastic with their work and that they stick to their programs. "Most importantly," one said, "there is no lesson disruption." The example cited for lesson disruption was that in black schools "it is common to be dismissed early when teachers are to attend the memorial services for colleagues, election meetings for their unions"—(the annual general meetings, I assumed)—and he gave examples of the successive meetings that were taking place before the schools closed on 19 March 2005 and after their reopening in different circuits. One student said, "Moving to this school does not mean that I am intelligent, but when I go to school I want to learn and because teachers are more responsible, they devote much time to helping us. For the few months that I have been here, I have learnt so many things in general that I don't regret that I'm in a good school."

However, students in tertiary institutions mentioned that job prospects are good in Gauteng (the six were all in different institutions in Gauteng) and that the job recruitment is non-discriminatory. They say that it is more industrialized and that one is already open to job opportunities as a student, and has increased accessibility in that one reaches out for interviews without many traveling expenses. One particular remarked that "it is possible to make your wish come true in Gauteng" and added that "chances of finding a job in Limpopo are limited if not poor." Another student exaggerated it by giving an anecdotal example that, "in Limpopo they do not consider skills, when 11 people have applied for the same job, the boss just say, 'let's take 2, 5, 6 and 8 and that is it." Moreover, other factors such as urban life and being exposed to mass media were mentioned by those from rural areas—the villages, as indicated earlier on. One student described his driving force as a desire for change in order to explore new possibilities and challenges that can enable him to realize his potential.

While I expected that students would mention something about facilities, they did not do so until I asked them. When asked, some indicated that computers, overhead projectors, laboratories and libraries were there at their schools. One even mentioned a TV set and video recorder, and that these things are not in use. "At times you can see teachers playing cards on the computers—some of them of course, not all," he remarked. This implies that there are facilities in some schools but without trained teachers to use them. But what about the TV that does not need training and which most families have? This was the question that I asked myself. Two students who said there were no laboratories at their schools indicated that science kits are there and kept in the staff room or principal's office, respectively.

FOCUS GROUP

During the focus group discussion, teachers truly expressed their lived experiences with their schools as follows: They said that school migration is caused by increasing deterioration of the state of education that results from lack of commitment, inadequate facilities, low teacher morale, and management incapacity that characterizes most of the black schools. On the other hand principals mentioned lack of support from senior education managers.

COMMITMENT

Teachers said that many of their colleagues (fellow teachers) are not committed to work, "they just report for work in order to get salaries for their own survival." One said, "teachers take advantage of the political transition for their deviant behaviour;" however, the union operations in some circuits can be partly blamed for this. Like the students above, teachers also referred to the current union annual general meetings that were held throughout the province and said that only black schools were affected while the other schools, those run by whites, functioned normally. "Surprisingly," as one teacher added, "a majority of the teachers never attended these meetings, instead they went about doing their own things. Don't you think there is something wrong with us?" He continued, "some teachers and principals are very involved in business and this makes them ineffective in their places of formal employment. They own taxis and some are moneylenders. Those with taxis first take loads of learners to various schools in the morning and arrive late at their workplaces, and on pay days, this means three times every month—the 15th for clerks, 22nd for teachers and the 30/31st for the police; money lenders have to get hold of their clients before they spend all their money. Is this not corruption?"

MANAGEMENT INCAPACITY

Teachers also blamed the incapacity of their school managers. One teacher remarked that "since the political wave that hit the schools in the 1990s, and attacked everything that was connected with management, some principals never recovered." He added, "I don't think some of them can ever effect change at their schools. Only their retirement will save those schools." In line with this response, Welten argues that "many of the teachers who support the process of social and educational transformation report that they lack role models for the new paradigm of management and learning, and that they are left feeling ill-equipped for their roles as agents of change."[12] He further explains that "they feel disempowered, deskilled and deprived of professional esteem and status by the pressure that they experience to both manage the present and build the future," (Welten, 175). Another teacher expressed his concern in this way: "One other issue of interest though very sad if deeply thought of, is that when we (black teachers) fail to come to school due to industrial activities, we first take our children to the private schools or those that were historically advantaged and then go to the meetings. I'm one of those who do that and this issue haunts me though I don't know how to help it out because I'm just a drop in the ocean."

TEACHER MORALE

Lack of incentives was cited as a de-motivating factor. The morale for many teachers is very low. One teacher expressed it as follows: "I already know that I'm going to get R4, 000 on the 22nd (the teachers' payday) no matter what effort I put [in], and so, hardworking does not make any difference." Another one said, "my work- performance exceeds what the department gives me, then what more . . . ? Teachers in private schools get high salaries and they are [driven] to work hard because parents pay a lot of money." This statement receives support from Souedien: when he argues about the commodification of education, he says, "more money buys a better education," (Souedien et al, 85).

INADEQUATE FACILITIES

Teachers unanimously expressed that their hopes were heightened with the inception of the new government through its emphasis on redressing inequality. One teacher said, "but nothing really changed in black schools. Black schools do not have facilities and the government insists that parents should pay school fees. Parents' money cannot equip schools with facilities; it cannot even buy the school enough toilet paper for one school term. The former white schools remain attractive as the apartheid government equipped them with the facilities that they are just adding on." This view receives support from Rebecca L. Weber.[13] "The government should not transfer its responsibility to parents," one added. Another one said, "this is not a joke, during the last elections (2004) our school wrote a letter to the Electoral commission and informed them that they could not use the school as a polling station because all classes leaked. Within two weeks, school renovation started, look at how beautiful it is now." They said that it is now one of the most attractive schools around even facility wise. As one teacher indicated, "other schools do not even have a duster, I'm telling you. Towards the next elections all schools should make similar demands as ours, to get their schools attended to."

LACK OF SUPPORT BY SENIOR EDUCATION MANAGERS (SEM)

The six principals independently expressed similar views regarding lack of support by SEM. One principal expressed it as follows: "You submit leave forms, no response, letters of misconduct, no response, and requests for substitutes for maternity leaves, no response. You find yourself faced with school problems alone."

Parents' responses could be embraced in one sentence, which is difficult to give its exact English interpretation. The Xitsonga words used by almost all parents were: "swikolo swa hina a swi nyawuli," the more related English interpretation is "our schools are rubbish." In addition to this, the issues of language and information technology emerged as crucial factors that four parents emphasized. Surprisingly, although English is taught in all schools, parents mentioned the acquisition of English as the main attraction in the alternative schools they chose for their children.

DISCUSSION: REALITIES AND CHALLENGES

From the information generated through the study, it comes out explicitly that there is urgent need for attention to the plight of education in black schools. These are the schools in rural areas and small towns in former homelands. While acknowledging that the opening up of schools has been one of the significant reforms after the inception of the democratic government in South Africa, one can argue that it also has caused the education system to be "instrumental in the distribution" of inequality among schools. On the other hand it appears to be a major influence on school migration. Evidence points to the direction taken by school migrants—moving from black schools to the historically privileged schools. The World Bank study by Leaver cited in Kallaway highlights the fact that "the poorest are always ignored in development programs."[14] One can argue that inequality is the consequence of the country's shift from the Reconstruction and Development Program (RDP) launched in 1994 as a reconstruction program to Growth Employment and Redistribution (GEAR) policy which came relatively suddenly and unexpectedly. RDP's main visible element was the increased state spending to improve delivery of key social services to promote equity.[15] Language of efficiency, competitiveness and fiscal austerity, which are the World Bank's ideology, enforced upon all countries in transition, were not within the context of the initial development of South Africa's education policy itself, hence the serious shortcomings since its ascendance, as it created constraints on state funding. This has defocused the government's social vision of education transformation as it intended to provide equality for all in the field of education. Therefore, insistence on equality and redress should now be considered a long-term imperative while it becomes necessary to develop short-term strategies to secure the already devastated black schools.

The introduction of user-fee, the policy requirement that school governing bodies (SGB'S) supplement state funds to improve education at the school level, worsened the disparity in resources and capacity between schools with the historically advantaged schools "maintaining the status quo."[16] The historically disadvantaged schools find it difficult to fulfill this legislated mandate to ensure quality education despite the schools' funding norms, which is said to direct most state allocations to schools serving the very poorest communities.[17] Chapman et al cited in Chaka and Dieltiens explain this as an act by government "to shift old problems to lower levels of the education system and to individuals even less capable of addressing them."[18]

SUGGESTIONS AND RECOMMENDATIONS

In this chapter I have posed questions in an effort to begin a conversation about the impact of school migration toward policy changes that are presented in the form of suggestions and recommendations: The plight of black schools poses a necessary challenge: the province has a major task of reaching out to the grassroots level—the schools—and to ensure that things are happening. David Cameroon, in his campaign for the Conservative Party leadership in the UK mentioned something very significant that can be applicable even to the context of this study. He said, "the government should go to those areas affected and address the problems."[19]

All major programs of re-skilling and re-empowerment that the provincial department has embarked on since the second half of 2003 as a response to the Revised National Curriculum (RNC) have to be accompanied by a well-developed strategy of implementation and regular monitoring based on the visionary system. It is perceived that there have been many attempts to transform education by the national department, for example the devolving of power to the level closest to those directly involved; the launching of Tirhisano[20] that emphasizes the return of Culture of Teaching and Learning Services (COLTS) in schools; the revised formula for school funding norms in favor of the poorest schools (Revision Norms and Standards for school funding, 1998) already identified, "the shift share allocation;"[21] and many others. However, based on my observation as a practitioner, these have not brought change in black schools due to the absence of monitoring. "Limited monitoring and evaluation of educational outcomes at all levels," is also included in Welton's list of problems experienced in implementing change, which is based on his research as part of the South African government and UNICEF program of work in South Africa, (Welton, 178).

Support for this prolonged transitional process of change from senior education management or consultants where senior managers lack expertise is more desirable. It should not be forgotten that the people who are now agents of change—principals, teachers and parents through school governing bodies (SGB's) were traditionally subjected to subordination by the system, and this makes them appear unprepared or uncommitted for their new role as agents of change, as suggested by responses of informants for this study. These people, I suggest, are very prepared and willing to act, but lack capacity and support to cope with change.

There is a dire need for management development programs for principals to be conducted concurrently with the teacher-development programs already receiving attention in the province. Robertson and Dale argue that successful organizations are the result of management practice.[22] They say, "whatever the social and economic context of the school, managerial practices are assumed to be able to determine school effectiveness not cultural explanations. Teachers, within this frame, are also viewed as managers of learning, managers of records and schemes, and managers of outputs (adding value)," (Robertson and Dale, 126). It is further suggested that in the near future, when principals would have been acting at full capacity, in-service training or staff development to improve subject knowledge and related pedagogical practices will need to be conducted at school level by principals and other teachers with expertise. A World Bank Review reveals that in-service training is most effective when it is linked directly to classroom practice and provided at the school level.[23]

RESPONSIBILITY OF THE STATE

Perhaps this is the time when the issue of capacity and incapacity should be looked at broadly, starting at the provincial level instead of ignoring the complexity of school life and reducing the very difficult social and political problems of schools to problems of school managers (principals), particularly during this transitional era. The Provincial Review Report highlighted the lack of capacity and skills, particularly in the area of financial management as a key problem hampering the delivery of a quality education in the provinces.[24] Therefore, it is clear that the state has a significant role to play to overhaul and remedy the whole system/structure. "The state has appropriate tools to deal with inequalities between schools."[25] Monitoring performance is the key and, above all, there should be a good strategy for evaluating progress, an endeavor that can push all schools at all levels to be competitive.

CONCLUSION

Things often happen contrary to the intentions of the education policy, whose aim has always been to redress access and equity by creating equality of opportunities to all. Nevertheless, there is no alternative in the development process but to build on this difficult foundation. In spite of all efforts identified so far, there are no visible reforms in black schools, which result in high school migration; it is telling that the trend may intensify and it will be rare to see anyone returning to the province that one already has low regard for. Kader Asmal, the former education minister, acknowledged that the scope is vast and that it is unclear how the problem of inequality can be resolved, Department of Education, 1999. However, I think setting short-term goals specifically to address problems faced and responding to the School Register of Needs could form part of the solution.

NOTES

1. J. M. Dobson, and K. Henthorne, *Pupil Mobility in Schools: Interim Report*, (Nottingham: DfEE Publications, 1999).
2. The purpose of this study was to look at the nature and causes of school migration in Limpopo Province which as observed is seen to be affecting

the historically disadvantaged schools. The interview participants were thus selected purposively from Mopani District in Limpopo District. Parents targeted were those whose children moved from historically disadvantaged schools to either private or former Model C schools. The six principals were drawn from various circuits within Mopani District. The focus group participants were teachers from one primary school and three high school students. The three students in tertiary level all attended the institutions in Gauteng Province and were interviewed during the Easter vacation when they were at their home in Mopani District. Most interviews with parents were carried out in their home except one parent who was interviewed at work (petrol filling station). Principals and teachers (focus group) were interviewed at their schools. Interview data were analysed according to Miles and Hurberman's framework for qualitative data analysis known as "transcendental realism" (Huberman, 1994), whose analysis has three main components: data reduction, data display and conclusion drawing and verification. During the analysis process issues were identified through which patterns emerged that were subsequently categorised. Quotations in the text represent examples of the issues that made up the categories. Due to the nature of the current issues this chapter addresses, the interviewees remain anonymous.

3. J. M. Dobson, and K. Henthorne, *Pupil Mobility in Schools: Interim Report*, (Nottingham: DfEE Publications, 1999); J. Mennell, *Breaking Point: Examining the Disruption Caused by Pupil Mobility,* (London: Association of London Government, 2005); DfES. *Managing Pupil Mobility: Guidance*, (Nottingham: DfES Publications, 2003); hereafter cited in text as Pupil Mobility Guidance, DfES. *Managing Pupil Mobility: Interim Report*, (Nottingham: DfES Publications, 2003); hereafter cited in text as Pupil Mobility Interim Report.
4. Dobson and Henthorne, 1999; Pupil Mobility Guidance; Pupil Mobility Interim Report; and Mennell, 2005).
5. The information to the background of study is based on my experience as a student of the apartheid time and a history teacher throughout my career. To update the information I interviewed two persons during November 2005 who came from Johannesburg and Rustenburg respectively, to study in the Northern Transvaal (the present Limpopo Province during the 1960's and 19970's.
6. J. Crush, and D. A. McDonald, "Transnationalism, African Immigration, and New Migrant Spaces in South Africa: An Introduction," *Canadian Journal of African Studies* 34 no. 1 2000: 1–19.
7. C. Soudien, H. Jacklyn, and U. Hoadley, "Policy Values: Problematising Equity and Redress in Education," in Y. Sayed and J. Jansen (eds.) *Implementing Educational Policies: The South African Experience*, Cape Town: UCT Press, 2001.
8. K. Hartshorne, *Crisis and Challenge: Black Education 1910–1990*, (Cape Town: Oxford University Press, 1992); S. Badat, *The Expansion of Black Tertiary Education 1977–90: Reform and Contradiction* in E Unterhalter, H. Wolpe, T Botha, S. Badat, T. Dlamini and B Khotseng,

Apartheid Education and Popular Struggles, (London: Zed Books Ltd. and Unterhaler ,1991).

9. S. Maile, "School Choice in South Africa," *Education and Urban Society,* 37 no. 11 (2004); 94 -116.
10. G. Hitchock, and D. Hughes, *Research and the Teacher: A Qualitative Introduction to School-based Research*, (London: Routledge, 1989), 93.
11. Morninglive Talk Show, South African Broadcasting Co-operation, 17 August 2005.
12. J. Welton, "Building Capacity to Deliver Education in South Africa," in Y, Sayed and J. Jansen, eds. *Implementing Education Policies: The South African Experience*, (Cape Town: Oxford University Press, 2001.
13. R. L. Weber, http://www.rebeccalweber.com accessed on 07 January 2006.
14. P. Kallaway, "The Need for Attention to the Issues of Rural Education," *International Journal of Educational Development*, 21 no.1 (2001), 21–32; 23.
15. K. Nicolaou, "The Link Between Macro-economic Policies and, Education Policies and the Education Budget," in E. Motala and J. Pampallis (eds.) *Education and Equity, The Impact of State Policies on South African Education*, (Sandown: Heineman, 2001).
16. Department of Education, *South African Schools Act, Government Gazette No. 84 of 1996,* (Pretoria: Government Printers, 1996); section 36.
17. Department of Education, *Norms and Standards for the Funding of Schools Regulations,* (Pretoria: Government Printers, 1998).
18. Chapman et al cited in T. Chaka, and V. Dieltien, "Stumbling Blocks in the Way of Democratic School Governance," *Quarterly Review of Education and Training in South Africa* 11 no. 2 (2004); 12.
19. BBC News 24, 29, Oct. 2004.
20. Department of Education, *Tirhisano: A Call to Action*, (Pretoria: Government Printers, 1999).
21. E. Motala, J. Perry, J. Aitchison, and T. Castle, "Access, Redress and Quality: Continuities and Discontinuities in Education Reform," *Quarter Review of education and Training in South Africa, 8 (1) January to March 2001.*
22. S. Robertson, and R. Dale, "Competitive Contractualism: A new Social Settlement in New Zealand," in D. Coulby, R. Cowen, and C. Jones, (eds.), *Education in Times of Transition.* (London: Kogan Page, 2000).
23. J. Lauglo, "Banking on Education and the Users of Research A Critique of: World Bank Priorities and Strategies for Education," *International Journal of Educational Development,* 16 no. 3 (1996), 221–233.
24. Department of Public Service and Administration. *The Provincial Review Report,* (Pretoria: Government Printers, 1997).
25. Dieltiens, 3; Chaka and Dieltiens, 13.

REFERENCES

Asmal, K. 1999. *A Call to Action: Mobilising Citizens to Build a South African Education and Training System for the 21st Century*. Statement by the Minister of Education, 27 July, Pretoria.

Badat, S. *The Expansion of Black Tertiary Education 1977–90: Reform and Contradiction,* in E Unterhalter, H. Wolpe, T Botha, S. Badat, T. Dlamini and B Khotseng, *Apartheid Education and Popular Struggles.* London: Zed Books Ltd., 1991.

Chaka, T. and Dieltien, V. "Stumbling Blocks in the Way of Democratic School Governance," *Quarterly Review of Education and Training in South Africa* 11 no, 2 (2004).

Crush, J. and McDonald D. A. "Transnationalism, African Immigration, and New Migrant Spaces in South Africa: An Introduction," *Canadian Journal of African Studies*, 34 no. 1 (2000), 1–19.

Department of Education. *Norms and Standards for the Funding of Schools Regulations*, Pretoria: Government Printers, 1998.

———. *South African Schools Act, Government Gazette No. 84 of 1996.* Pretoria: Government Printers, 1996.

———. *Tirhisano: A Call to Action.* Pretoria: Government Printers, 1999.

Department of Public Service and Administration. *The Provincial Review Report.* Pretoria: Government Printers, 1997.

DfES. *Managing Pupil Mobility: Guidance.* Nottingham: DfES Publications, 2003a.

———. *Managing Pupil Mobility: Interim Report.* Nottingham: DfES Publications, 2003b.

Dobson, J. M. and Henthorne, K. *Pupil Mobility in Schools: Interim Report.* Nottingham: DFES Publications, 1999.

Dieltien V. "Introduction," *Quarterly Review of Education and Training in South Africa*, 11 no. 2 (2004).

Hitchock, G. and Hughes, D. *Research and the Teacher: A Qualitative Introduction to School-based Research.* London: Routledge, 1989.

Hartshorne, K. *Crisis and Challenge: Black Education 1910–1990.* Cape Town: Oxford University Press, 1992.

Kallaway, P. "The Need for Attention to the Issues of Rural Education," *International Journal of Educational Development*, 21 no. 1 (2001), 21–32.

Lauglo, J. "Banking on Education and the Users of Research A Critique of: World Bank Priorities and Strategies for Education," *International Journal of Educational Development,* 16 no. 3 (1996), 221–233.

Maile, S. "School Choice in South Africa," *Education and Urban Society,* 37 no. 11 (2004); 94 -116.

Mennell, J. *Breaking Point: Examining the Disruption Caused by Pupil Mobility.* London: Association of London Government, 2005.

Motala, E.; Perry, J.; Aitchison, J and Castle, T. 2001. "Access, Redress and Quality: Continuities and Discontinuities in Education Reform," *Quarter Review of education and Training in South Africa, 8 (1) January to March 2001.*

Nicolaou' K. "The Link Between Macro-economic Policies and, Education Policies and the Education Budget," in E. Motala and J. Pampallis (eds.) *Education and Equity, The Impact of State Policies on South African Education.* Sandown: Heineman, 2001.

Robertson, S. and Dale, R. "Competitive Contractualism: A new Social Settlement in New Zealand," in D. Coulby, R. Cowen, and C. Jones, eds. *Education in Times of Transition*. London: Kogan Page, 2000.

Soudien, C., Jacklyn, H. and Hoadley, U. "Policy Values: Problematising Equity and Redress in Education," in Y. Sayed and J. Jansen, eds. *Implementing Educational Policies: The South African Experience*. Cape Town: UCT Press, 2001.

Unterhalter, E. "Changing Aspects of Reformism in Bantu Education 1953–89," in E Unterhalter, H. Wolpe, T Botha, S. Badat, T. Dlamini and B Khotseng, *Apartheid Education and Popular Struggles*. London: Zed Books Ltd., 1991.

Weber, R. L. (http://www.rebeccalweber.com) accessed on 07 January 2006.

Welton, J. "Building Capacity to Deliver Education in South Africa," in Y, Sayed and J. Jansen (eds.). *Implementing Education Policies: The South African Experience*. Cape Town: Oxford University Press, 2001.

Chapter Eleven

Pushing and Pulling: Western Education's Impact on Women's Subjugation in Ghana

Jamaine Abidogun

Ghanaian cultures have experienced changes due to Islamic and European trading contacts, European colonial presence and various internal interactions among its many indigenous societies. These experiences introduced a variety of institutional and ideological constructs to Ghanaian societies. The Western style formal educational institution (formal education) was one European construct that has continued into the current period to impact cultural change. Research conducted in southeastern Ghana at Medina and Legon was used to analyze interactions between the formal education institution and participants' ethno-linguistic societies.[1] Gender role formation was identified as one cultural aspect that demonstrated change as a result of formal education's interaction with indigenous cultures. Specific questions focused on elements of resistance, adaptation and transformation based on this interaction. A fluctuating model of gender role changes resulted from the findings that indicated a push-pull relationship between Western and indigenous concepts.

The cumulative effect was a transformative societal response regarding gender, that periodically and at times simultaneously moved closer to or farther away from Western models as transmitted through formal education or/and indigenous cultures. One common aspect shared by Western style formal education and across indigenous cultures was in incidents connected to family structure and employment patterns that produced disparities between female and male roles that resulted in the subjugation of female to male roles within Ghanaian society. This model reflected these incidents of resistance, adaptation, and transformation as well as other incidents regarding ongoing gender role changes based on Ghanaian experiences.

Ghanaian experiences came from multiple voices including students, teachers, school leavers, community members, curriculum materials and secondary documents. Student, teacher, and parent participants were selected from Madina #3 junior secondary school, while community members and school leavers came from the wider Madina and Legon communities. They represented various ethno-linguistic societies including but not limited to the Akan (Fanti and Twi), Ga-Adgangbe (Ada and Krobo), Ewe, and Mole-Dagbani (Dagomba, Nanumba, Mossi, and Mamprusi).[2] These voices were recorded through direct and written interview methods and through field observations. In this way participants provided descriptions of resistance, adaptation, and transformation in their identification, and formation of gender roles based on interactions with formal education and their indigenous cultures. Examples in this writing focus primarily on student, teacher, parent, and curriculum descriptions of such gendered incidents.

CONTEXT

Ghana has experienced formal education as an imposed institution in various forms and with various ethno-linguistic groups since the early 1800s. Western formal education was described by Rodney as "the transplantation of a version of European education into Africa."[3] This form of education in Ghana included four distinct periods: (1) formal schools introduced by English representatives of trade at Cape Coast; (2) mission schools instituted by English and Swiss Christian missionaries; (3) formal education implemented under British colonial policy; and (4) formal education experienced today in its neocolonial or postcolonial context.

While these periods of formal education contained unique characteristics and provided incidents of transition involving social resistance, adaptation and transformation, they were only one part of the educational structure in Ghanaian society. Indigenous education was another part of the educational structure. Indigenous education existed in Ghana before the arrival of Islamic education or Western education. Indigenous education, identified by Lar as "the traditional or natural education where ideas, norms, attitudes, values, beliefs and culture are original to the people," was interwoven into the fabric of each culture through such practices as age grade learning, gender-based training, cross-generational learning, and apprenticeships.[4] While Islamic education was located in Northern Ghana and some urban pockets in the South, its education system included only Moslems and for most participants has continued to compliment indigenous education practices rather than replace them. Western style formal education based on a European curriculum was experienced for several hours each day separate from participants' cultural milieu, and often conflicted directly with indigenous practices. This conflict resulted in cultural and/or educational incidents of adaptation, resistance and/or transformation.

CHANGING CULTURAL INSTITUTIONS

An awareness of Ghanaian cultural institutions and the formal education institution as interacting agents of change provided the baseline for interpretation. A postcolonial theoretical framework was used to collect, analyze and interpret the data. In particular, critical pedagogy maximized the potential for understanding through its attempt to represent all voices in the discourse among cultures and educational experiences. Young explained, "postcolonial discourse rewrites the relationship between the margin and the center by deconstructing the colonialist and imperialist ideologies that structure Western knowledge, texts, and social practices. Here, there are attempts to demonstrate how European culture and colonialism are deeply implicated in each other."[5] Giroux suggests more than rewriting or recovering the repressed stories and social memories of the Other; it means understanding and rendering visible how Western knowledge is encased in historical and institutional structures that both privilege and exclude particular readings, voices, aesthetics, authority, representations, and forms of sociality."[6] In-depth observations assisted an analysis based on critical pedagogy, as did participation and dialogue with members of the community as they interpreted cultural and educational interactions.

Freire's description of an "educand" or student also gave insight on the postcolonial implications of Western style formal education and its interaction with indigenous cultures. His description of an "educand" based on liberation education theory included: " . . . a recognition of oneself, the educand, as one of two agents here, each capable of knowing and each wishing to know, and each working with the other for an understanding of the object of cognition. . . . the educand really becomes an educand when and to the extent that he or she knows, or comes to know, content, cognoscible objects, and not in the measure that the educator is *depositing* in the educand a description of the objects or content."[7] All participants were viewed as "educands" within the context of Ghanaian society, though in this writing they were labeled according to their relationship with the formal education institution as listed previously. Freire's use of "*know*" indicated the "educand's" understanding or "reading" of knowledge's interrelation to the political, social, and economic contexts as manifested in their society's power structures.[8]

In order to integrate and apply these critical and liberation education concepts, a framework developed that also referenced Pan African and post-colonial discourses as they informed the historical and current contexts of Ghanaian cultures and their educational institutions. While critical pedagogy and liberation theory were specifically applied to critique formal education's interactions with indigenous cultures and the resulting effects on gender roles, each of these theoretical paradigms supported the position that formal education, as a formerly imposed Western institution effectively, had been and continued to act as an agent for neocolonial interests that, through interaction with indigenous cultures, resulted in various outcomes of cultural adaptation, resistance, and transformation.

GENDER ROLE CHANGE

In a review of gender studies research conducted in Ghana, some studies were used to establish a baseline of understanding regarding indigenous gender roles, for example, Greene and Bukh on women's roles in Ewe society, and Robertson (1975, 1984) on Ga society.[9] All of these studies focused on changes in the economic roles of women. Other studies provided more generalized descriptions of Ghanaian gender roles.[10] These studies profiled women's roles within the wider Ghanaian society by identifying common gender role assignments across indigenous cultures, as well as roles developed through postcolonial national formation. While these studies were referenced to aid understanding of participants' articulated experiences, in most cases participants' voices were allowed to stand for themselves as valid interpretations of their individual experiences regarding gender roles.

A few studies provided statistical and social formation information on gender and formal education in Ghana. These included Clarke, Dophyne, Hyde, Lloyd and Gage-Brandon, Folson.[11] Each of these studies focused on such issues as gender based disparities in educational access and attainment, and its relation to economic and occupational disparities. They looked at familial and societal causes for these disparities, which were culturally based and educationally based, respectively. All of these studies were taken into consideration alongside the participants' perspectives regarding changes in gender roles in relation to their formal education experiences.

Participants described a range of formal education experiences that often highlighted gender issues. Three major themes developed from the participants' narratives. These included formal education versus indigenous education in their impact on gender roles, formal education's impact on family and community gender role structures, and formal education's impact on gender based employment patterns. All of these themes demonstrated varying levels of adaptation, resistance, and transformation based on interactions between formal education and indigenous cultures.

FORMAL VERSUS INDIGENOUS CURRICULUM

Aspects of indigenous cultures were included in formal education's cultural studies curriculum but the physical separation of students from their home communities in order to participate in formal education resulted in loss of access to indigenous education and resulted in alienation from indigenous practices. For instance the cultural studies curriculum covered topics of rites of passage and marriage arrangements for Krobo, Akan, and "Northern" people. Initiation or rites of passage for females were described for Krobo and Akan ethnolinguistic groups. For example, a teacher asked if any student had experienced the Krobo initiation and a female student responded that she had. The teacher asked her to describe her experience and the student explained that the first week their breasts were exposed and a string was tied around their waist. A male student snickered at this description. The teacher interrupted and instructed this student and the rest of the class to "respect the girl's culture" and further explained that, "the exposure is to show that you are not pregnant."[12] During the description of female Krobo initiation rites a male student asked, "Do Akan perform initiates for boys?" and another male student responded, "Please," as if to indicate that the first student should know the answer. The teacher then explained that a boy's father just handed him a cutlass, a hoe, etc. to help with doing a "man's work."[13]

The teacher also used a female student to demonstrate that initiation rites for females continue to be practiced in Akan groups. As the teacher asked a female student to come to the front of the class to show her Akan woman's hair cut, "dansinkran," the teacher pointed out that this was a traditional mark of womanhood for the Akan people, (Observation #6). It was clear that many of the students had not participated in initiation rites, nor had they been informed of these rites through indigenous education. This was also indicated in a discussion with the headmistress as she explained that many of these students' parents had migrated from more rural areas for economic and educational opportunities, so many of them had no firsthand experience or knowledge, due to separation from their home communities.[14] Several students confirmed this observation by their indication that they did not live in their home communities.

This separation from their home communities coupled with exposure to the formal education curriculum resulted in adaptation to Western cultural mores in which age indicated adulthood versus participation in initiation rites. Information on initiation rites was often received as objectified pieces of knowledge rather than as part of the student's indigenous cultural norms and values. Contrastive incidents of resistance were indicated by those students who demonstrated continued participation in indigenous education and participation in these cultural practices. Transformation took place as most students indicated an acceptance that their culture included those members who followed indigenous practices and those who followed more Westernized practices without sanctions.

Another curriculum issue that informed gender roles was in the content of the cultural studies textbooks. When analyzed for gender balance in terms of representation of males and females this textbook series provided disproportional representation. Males were more often portrayed then females in active or authority roles in photos and drawings throughout the texts. The following is a breakdown of photos and drawings based on gender (Table 11.1 below).

The narratives also consistently described male roles in greater detail within Ghanaian national cultural roles and specific indigenous cultural roles as compared to their female counterparts. For example, book there contained a full chapter on chieftaincy roles (traditionally a male function) while there were only two paragraphs on the role of queen mother.[15] In addition, narratives on religion regularly used the terms "men" or "man" to represent people as a whole and all three textbooks invariably used male pronouns to represent God or Allah.[16] These incidents of gender imbalance in the formal education curriculum constitute instances of resistance to full recognition of significant female roles across indigenous cultures. It further distanced students from indigenous knowledge as this textbook series served as their primary resource for indigenous cultural content, since many of them, as stated previously, no longer resided in their home communities, and consequently, did not have direct access to indigenous knowledge through indigenous education practices.

TABLE 11.1 Female & Male Illustrations in Cultural Studies Junior Secondary School Series

Cultural Studies Book	# of Female Illustration	# of Male Illustration	# of Mixed Illustration	% of Female Illustration	% of Male Illustration	% of Mixed Illustration
Book 1	8	16	11	23	46	31
Book 2	7	20	12	18	51	31
Book 3	6	30	5	15	73	12
Total #	21	66	28			
Total %	18	57	24			

FAMILY AND COMMUNITY GENDER STRUCTURES

Formal education's interaction with indigenous cultures was also analyzed in terms of family structure and gender roles. Reported parental roles and student roles within the family were identified by gender and age divisions respectively. Parental roles were consistently categorized by gender. The father was usually credited as economically responsible for the family and the primary authority figure. While the mother was also valued, her role was not always as clearly described. For instance, CA commented about her father and mother in these terms, "My father tells us what we should do and I also bring up my mind . . . Whenever we are at home, he does his responsibilities that a father is suppose to do, . . . I'm proud of my father and I really loves him and my mom too."[17] KB, meanwhile, described family roles as, "My father is responsible of us. Everything that we need, we bring to him . . . My mom too, at times, whenever we do something wrong, they have to, they have to . . . they beat us. My mom for example need help in the kitchen, help us to prepare the meals. My father goes to work . . . My father doesn't stay at home," (Interview-A1997). In CA's case there was no role assigned to her mother, while KB viewed her mother's role as an extension of or support for her father's role as the authority figure in the house, as well as the one responsible for household duties. Even though 50% of the students reported helping their mothers to sell items in the market, when asked directly about parents' occupations, only students in single female headed households indicated their mother as being economically responsible for the household. Evidently their income was not viewed as the primary income in the family, which again reinforced their secondary status within the family structure.

Parent/guardian responses also indicated the male role as primary, with female roles identified through their relation to the male role. For example, parents/guardians were asked their relationship to the student on questionnaire forms. There was a list of family roles to circle that included "aunt" and "uncle" (in that order). In one instance the uncle circled "uncle" on his form, while the aunt circled "uncle" and modified it to "uncle's wife" on her form. It was confirmed that she in fact had completed the form on which she also identified her occupational background as "house wife" and described her educational experience as, "a middle school leaver and been a housewife" (KB Parent/Guardian Survey 1997). Similar responses by other female parents/guardians indicated in general a secondary status assigned to females within the participating indigenous cultures. Since often the same females that indicated these secondary roles also indicated some formal education experience and, further, that such terms as "housewife" did not have indigenous language equivalents, it could be summarized that such gender role assignments were in part an indication of adaptation and/or transformation based on interaction with formal education. These gender disparities were viewed as incidents of adaptation and transformation that combined indigenous cultures' aspects of gender disparities with Western gender disparities as presented in a formal education curriculum that described women in a supportive role within the extended and nuclear families (Abbiw et al. 1988, 9–10).

When it came to student roles in the family, both males and females were expected to assist in household chores, although this was often placed in the context of helping their mother, especially when participants referred to cooking or washing dishes. A few examples of responses to "Do you work after school?" included the following:

> AB: I go to the market and help my mother in selling. (Interview-A 1997)
>
> NQ: I help my mother with things in the house. When she's cooking I help her in cooking. (Interview-A 1997), and
>
> MS: I help my mom, when she's in the kitchen, when she's cooking I help her. (Interview-A 1997).

Such responses were expressed equally by female and male students. All except one student mentioned that they participated in household chores, such as sweeping, cooking and washing dishes or laundry. Only YM identified any of these chores with gender role assignment. When asked if he cooked, he responded, "I have sisters, so I don't cook," although he did indicate that he washed plates (Interview-B 1997). In identifying who students helped with cooking or helped with the washing, it was always a female adult of the household, that is, their grandmother, mother, aunt or an older sister. In descriptions of community activities, female and male students reported similar activities. Approximately 90 percent of students participated in communal labor, i.e. clearing gutters and weeding areas. Gender divisions were not apparent for youth in the home or in the community. This indicated that indigenous cultures' use of age divisions were maintained regardless of formal education experience. It was viewed as an incidence of resistance to formal education.

Conversely, incidents of formal education's adaptation to indigenous cultures' age division and gender role practices were in fact demonstrated. Even at the school site, age was considered over gender in students' role assignments. For instance, both male and female students regularly carried stacks of graded exercise books to the classroom and both were routinely asked to erase the blackboard. Gender role division did occur in education practices as without exception female students carried the purses and packages of female teachers to class, while male students assisted male teachers. This was also consistent with indigenous cultural practices that often separated males and females while maintaining age divisions that required younger people to serve older people, as demonstrated by Ewe practices as well as other Ghanaian indigenous cultures (EG Interview 1997).

When the institution of marriage was presented in the cultural studies course, the textbook and teacher's presentations described the structure of indigenous marriage arrangements along with some specific cultural norms and practices. For instance, when the teacher asked "What questions are asked before anyone decides to marry?" and a student replied, "Is he a drunkard?" Her question was understood as "Who will a female be allowed to marry?" As no other responses were forthcoming it was evident that this perception was shared across cultures. An example of Gonja marriage rites was also described by the teacher as, "the bride-to-be among the Gonja was asked three times, 'do you want him? Do you accept?'" While this indicated some consideration of the female's role in the decision to marry, the value of a female was also described based on any previous children she had conceived and her formal education status. The term "second hand girl" was explained as a female who already had a baby, so the groom may give only one cow, while a girl who had not had a child and was educated may ask for several cows (Classroom Observation #10 Oct 28, 1997). These cultural practices focused on the male's character and the female's economic worth.

When a male student in response to the decision making of the Gonja woman asked, "What if the girl loves both men very well?" the teacher replied, "By all means you'll love one better than the other" then she quoted the Bible stating, "You cannot serve two masters." This verse represented a Western concept of females' subordination to males. The disparate role for females was further reinforced by the teacher, who explained that the parents may force the marriage of a female, so she may have to marry an older man with other wives. She did explain that the girl may run away, although if she did, she would have no legal or moral recourse, so any bride wealth would likely be forfeited by her family if she left (Classroom Observation #10 Oct 28, 1997). This classroom observation demonstrated cultural transformation. As stated in the earlier case involving marriage roles, a combination of indigenous and Western gender roles was demonstrated through incidents of cultural transformation.

Males and females came under scrutiny in the Akan description of marriage rituals in the text which the students read aloud, that indicated both were investigated for any criminal or immoral behavior and to make certain the male and female were not related. The teacher also stated that the bride wealth went to the bride's mother's family in the Akan system, as they followed inheritance patterns through the female lineage (Classroom Observation #10 Oct 28, 1997). However, in a teacher focus group discussion, P2 commented, "We, Ghanaians, saw that the disadvantages of belonging to the mother's side outweighs that of the patrilineal society. So when we, teachers, discuss it with students, we found out that they weren't happy. Those who inherited matrilineally, say that they were not going to sit down for their cousins, that is the nephews of their fathers, to come and inherit," (Educator Focus Group, Nov 20 1997). This teacher went on to the change in attitude to knowledge that the students had gained through the formal education cultural studies curriculum. The curriculum provided an opportunity to compare cultural content, so that while Akan bride wealth remained with the mother's family, the challenging of inheritance patterns resulted in incidents of adaptation to patrilineal cultural patterns.

The impact of formal education interaction on indigenous cultures created a varied response. In the maintenance of family and community gender role structures, incidents of cultural resistance were evident. This resistance included the maintenance of age divisions along with separation by gender in social interactions. While information about marriage roles and rites demonstrated combining or incidents of cultural adaptation and transformation that most often reinforced gender status inequities that relegated females to subordinate positions, the exception was the Akan example that indicated less indigenous predisposition to gender inequities, but still had experienced some degree of adaptation to Western norms.

GENDERED EMPLOYMENT PATTERNS

Gender was analyzed in terms of reported types of employment, as desired by the student and as reported by parental occupations. Initially, students were asked how their education fit in with community standards and expectations. An overwhelming 93 percent of students responded, "So I can be someone in the future." This response indicated cross cultural incorporation (adaptation) of formal education as a necessary experience to gain status. Due to this response a follow up question asked them what they meant. Many offered a desired occupation that they perceived as fitting in with community expectations. Female students included the following as occupations that they would hold in the future: seamstress, hairdresser, caterer, accountant, secretary, policewoman, and computer operator. Only one female indicated that marriage would limit her employment experience: as SB stated, "To get married or finish school, then I'll marry." A discussion followed about how the community saw her education as a benefit to her marriage, and she explained, "If I finish work before, then I reach about twenty . . . then I go for somebody to marry . . . they know that because I'm attending school . . . I will advise." (Interview-A 1997). Female student responses demonstrated some amount of adaptation to traditional Western female occupations, in relation to their formal education experience.

Male students also demonstrated this type of adaptation, although in later responses as recorded below, they also indicated a degree of cultural resistance. Male students planned to attain the following occupations: engineer, auto mechanic, manager, firefighter, teacher, pilot, minister of government, electrical engineer, mechanical engineer, cartographer, bank manager, and accountant. There was consistent movement away from (and in resistance to) traditional indigenous occupations. While a few students had previously mentioned helping to raise livestock or working on their parents' farm, none of them indicated in this initial response that these occupations would be a part of their future. For instance, RE earlier stated his home responsibilities as "I go for leaves for our goats . . ." and "A farm, yeah I have a farm . . . my parents raise goats." He informed us that they grow onions, but when asked about his own future, RE replied, "I want to be a manager. Fire service manager. . . ." (Interview-A 1997). He indicated an incident of resistance to indigenous occupations based on formal education experience.

These participants also indicated gender-based differences in their parents' occupations. Female parents' occupations were reported as: trader, seamstress, farmer, raiser of poultry and goats, caterer, and hairdresser. Male parents' occupations were reported as: electrician, policeman, farmer, raiser of poultry and goats, clan chief, accountant, and cocoa market board member. There was evident disparity in the economic status of occupations held by females as compared to males both in the students' occupation goals and in their parents' occupations.

An example of this disparity was that of trader for the female parents as reported by almost 50% of students. Again, as mentioned earlier, not one female or male student mentioned trading as their future occupation. This aversion to trading was demonstrated in DN's interview as follows:

ME: So you don't plan to be a trader when you finish school, though you plan to go on to vocational school?

DN: Yes.

ME: Is that all right with your family?

DN: Yes.

ME: And will you help them trade when you finish school?

DN: No, no because my mother even she says if I can continue in school to even the university level she likes it so if I can even go far then what I'm now thinking of [a caterer] they like it.

(Interview-A 1997)

JA also indicated a trend away from traditional occupations. As JA explained, "Yeah, if they've finished JSS then they will like to do that [trading] so when it is time for them to go to school (SSS), they will go and they will stop the marketing" (Interview-A 1997). These exchanges provided examples of educational resistance to traditional indigenous occupations since the preferred occupations were directly linked to participation in formal education.

Formal education equated to jobs that required some literacy, thus indicating incidences of cultural adaptation to formal education. Even occupations that had been traditionally attained through indigenous education forms, such as apprenticeships, were perceived as requiring formal education. This demonstrated transformation, by including some preparation within formal education. For example, LK explained, "I like school because if you are not educated and if you want to be a seamstress or hairdresser I don't think you know how to, I mean how to measure the things or be a hairdresser, that is to know about names of the creams for it" (Interview-A 1997).

When students were asked what they had learned from family and community they often responded with occupation related answers. The occupations mentioned by female students included airhostess, hairdresser, farmer, caterer, seamstress, accountant, trader, and secretary. The addition of airhostess to the earlier list of female occupations provided one more example of resistance to indigenous occupations and adaptation to formal education's occupational expectations. By contrast, male students mentioned occupations that differed significantly from earlier responses. They included occupations such as farmer, raiser of goats, carpenter, printer, sandal maker, seamstress [tailor], and drummer. These responses indicated resistance to formal education, as they could all be attained through indigenous education practices. For instance, AB described his apprenticeship experience as follows:

AB: And I've learned how to print.

ME: Print, to use a printing press?

AB: Yes.

ME: Who taught you that?

AB: At Vantage Press, the man have been teaching me.

ME: At Vantage Press?

AB: Yes.

ME: How long have you worked there?

AB: Every pleasant day, I've worked.

ME: Since when, for how long, two months? A year?

AB: About four or five years.

ME: Four or five years?

AB: He teach me when I was nine years old. I'm now fourteen.
(Interview-B 1997)

Similar experiences were shared by other students although more often described by male rather than female students. This indicated a greater maintenance of male indigenous occupations across cultures than female occupations. Female indigenous occupations were limited to trader, raiser of goats and/or poultry, hairdresser, and seamstress.[18] The differences in identification of female and male occupations conformed to stereotypical Western gender role assignments that demonstrated again a degree of cultural adaptation to formal education that, as a historically imposed institution early on, replicated such inequitable gender assignments. The historical reality of limited European female presence in Ghana bears this out, as European men were the bearers of formal education and so contributed to the invisibility of female roles. The only shared occupations between the sexes were farming and raising goats, most likely because these occupations were family based with no one person is completely responsible for the work. These two indigenous occupations demonstrated resistance to formal education in maintaining the occupation's value and in maintaining male and female roles within it.

When questioned whether they would continue to senior secondary school (SSS), all students, female and male, responded in the affirmative, even though statistics indicated that up to a third of these students would not continue. Teacher comments confirmed these statistics, that while students held formal education-based occupational goals, their occupational realities were more closely tied to indigenous occupational patterns. In representative comments, EG noted that many students worked while attending school due to economic hardship. She stated, "Many of the children go home. They go to sell and come back tired and may not be able to read. So they sleep and other children who are in this school are fending for themselves" (Interview 1997). As a result, many students left school in order to earn a living. Student interviews aligned with teacher comments, as the majority of students reported helping a relative after school or on weekends to sell in the market. This was borne out by researcher observations of many of these junior secondary students, who were employed in the markets or as "any work" boys on the university campus.[19]

Another teacher, PA, viewed this pattern as particularly true for male students, as she explained her perceptions of community and school standards: "The home is the first factor and the primary school. The foundation there is not good because some of the homes the parents are in the market . . . so the boys, some of them go to work and . . . the girls too, they go and follow the boys for money and all those things" (Interview 1997). This indicated cultural resistance to formal education as parents' actions demonstrated that formal education may be desirable but was not a top priority.

Her comments also reinforced the perception of female employment opportunities as limited in comparison to male employment opportunities, thus leaving them dependent on relationships with men for economic security. Even though it was demonstrated that the attainment of formal education did not align with many of the students' cultural occupational practices, the concepts of Western style occupational gender divisions had been communicated to these students and reinforced incidences of cultural adaptation and transformation that served to maintain gender disparities in an indigenous context. This disparate gendered employment pattern combined with the gender roles within marriage as further indicators of cultural adaptation and transformation, because formal education did not remedy these disparities but appeared to reinforce and increase these gender disparities in employment patterns.

CONCLUSION

The above descriptions of gender role adaptation, resistance and transformation based on formal education interaction with indigenous cultures are only representative samples. The actual number of incidents recorded regarding gender is illustrated in 11.2 and 11.3 tables below:

As indicated in the (tables) below, incidents identified under gender were labeled as representing cultural adaptation, resistance, or transformation in relation to interaction with formal education, and as representing formal education adaptation, resistance, or transformation in relation to indigenous cultures. Some of these incidents have been highlighted through the examples provided, under the themes of formal versus indigenous curriculum, family and community gender structures, and gendered employment patterns. Incidents of cultural adaptation to formal education varied from males and females being educated together, to the de-emphasis of female puberty rites for formally-educated females.

Cultural and formal education adaptation to gender roles included the continued gender assignment of traditional indigenous and Western occupations along with an acceptance of a legal trend away from matrilineal

TABLE 11.2 Gender Incidents as Related to Western Education

	Adaptation	Resistance	Transformation
Gender	XXXXXXXXXXX XXXXXXXXX	XXXXXXXXXX XXXXXXXXXX XXXX	XXXXXXXX XX

TABLE 11.3 Gender Incidents as Related to Indigenous Cultures

	Adaptation	Resistance	Transformation
Gender	XXXXXXXX XXXXXXX	XXXXXXXX XXXX	XXXXXXXXX X

inheritance patterns that moved family gender structures closer to Western models. Formal education adaptation to indigenous cultures varied from no demonstrated expectations that male and female students should interact outside the classroom, to female teachers and educators that retained their family surnames upon marriage, even though Western Christian based models of taking the husband's surname existed in the formal education content.

Incidents were identified under gender as cultural resistance and as formal education resistance. Incidents of cultural resistance varied from the continued practice of initiation or puberty rites to students' identified preference for Ghanaian literature over Western literature. Formal education resistance included instances ranging from the alignment of higher income occupations with increased formal education attainment, to the separation of students from access to indigenous education in order to attend formal education, and the lack of scheduling accommodations for students or teachers to participate in indigenous cultural practices, such as puberty rites or traditional festivals.

Moreover, incidents of transformation were identified under gender. These ranged from the incorporation of formal education into indigenous occupations preparatory to marriage, to gender roles that reflected both indigenous and Western aspects of female roles as subordinate to male roles. Finally, the overall demonstration of increasing participation of males and females in the formal education system was viewed as an ongoing transformation of formal education and indigenous cultures.

These incidents for each individual moved periodically closer and further away from formal education norms, values, and beliefs, and periodically closer and further away from indigenous cultural norms, values and beliefs. At times the interaction of various gender issues, as equilibrium was sought between both contexts, resulted in transformations that were not solely identifiable by Western formal education standards, nor by indigenous cultural standards. These changes occurred as each member of the society was influenced by both Western formal education and by indigenous cultures, and also as each member acted in both Westernized and indigenous cultures. The cumulative effect was a push-pull and transforming societal response that periodically and at times simultaneously moved closer to or further from Western formal education gender roles and/or indigenous cultural gender roles. As a continual process with infinite variation in influence and response, the dynamic aspect of culture was effectively represented by the constant movement and change in gender roles with the ultimate possibility that either or both of the original contexts, that is, indigenous or Western, would be rejected or transformed at their core.

Even though it was not possible to predict what incidents of resistance and adaptation would continue to be negotiated, it was possible to suggest an agenda. Part of this agenda would be the use of critical pedagogy to critique the above incidents with the intention to provide for indigenous cultures and the national culture's overall stability. While gender role divisions may be based on Western and indigenous assignments, the formal education system could become a forum to renegotiate disparities found in these gender roles. This model demonstrated the dynamic aspect of cultural change and it recognized the ability consciously to mold incidents of adaptation, resistance, and transformation in order to create more equitable outcomes regarding gender as related to the themes represented above and other gender issues impacted by formal education and cultural interactions.

While it is understood that such research results are unique to the location and people who participated, this experimental procedure is easily transferable to other locations and people, in order to assess systematically the interaction of formal education and indigenous cultures. This systematic approach would provide education policy makers and community members, within the framework of critical pedagogy and liberation education theory, a way to aid formal education so that it at once supports indigenous cultures by incorporating indigenous knowledge, and maintains and promotes their dynamic qualities to redress gender disparities found in formal education and indigenous cultures.

As a final note, even though some data contradicted current theoretical frameworks, such as Pan-African theory, critical pedagogy theory, liberation theory and postcolonial theory, all data was utilized to develop the model. While all of these theories assumed some level of conflict in the form of an oppressor-and-oppressed dichotomy, some participants at times explained incidences of Western influence or transformation as a way to maintain their culture within a global reality. The fact that the global reality was Western dominated was understood, but their cultural transformation was often viewed as self-initiated and self-directed, even when there was evidence to the contrary. It has been argued that this type of perception indicated that the oppressed had not yet learned "their world," as Freire explained in the following:

> In general, a dominated consciousness which has not yet perceived a limit-situation in its totality apprehends only its epiphenomena and transfers to the latter the inhibiting force which is the property of the limit-situation. This fact is of great importance for the investigation of generative themes. When people lack a critical understanding of their reality, apprehending it in fragments which they do not perceive as interacting constituent

> elements of the whole, they cannot truly know that reality. To truly know it, they would have to reverse their starting point: they would need to have a total vision of the context in order subsequently to separate and isolate its constituent elements and by means of this analysis achieve a clearer perception of the whole.[20]

As this study aimed through the implementation of critical pedagogy to provide a vision of the whole, it was argued that the allowances of Western accommodation, and incidents of transformation toward a Western norm or value through formal education, could be demonstrations of participants' unawareness of their reality. In order to respect the validity and integrity of the participants' perceptions, it was also necessary to consider that there were those participants who understood their reality. For these individuals, their movement toward Westernization or a transformation within their cultural milieu would be self-initiated and self-directed independently of the oppressor/oppressed dichotomy.

In order to take participants' perspectives one step further in the process of critical pedagogy, Ghanaian education policy makers, through support of their educators, should provide Ghanaians with the complete historical, political, economic, and social contexts of the formal education structure and process, so that they may consciously negotiate incidences of adaptation, resistance, and transformation. Then, as Giroux suggested, education would serve as a direct link "to the creation of alternative public spheres, . . . an ideal and a strategy in the service of struggling for social and economic democracy. . . . based on a commitment to the elimination of forms of class, racial [ethnic], and gender oppression," in order to transform cultures, and, as in this case, gender issues, to the benefit of all its members—female and male.[21]

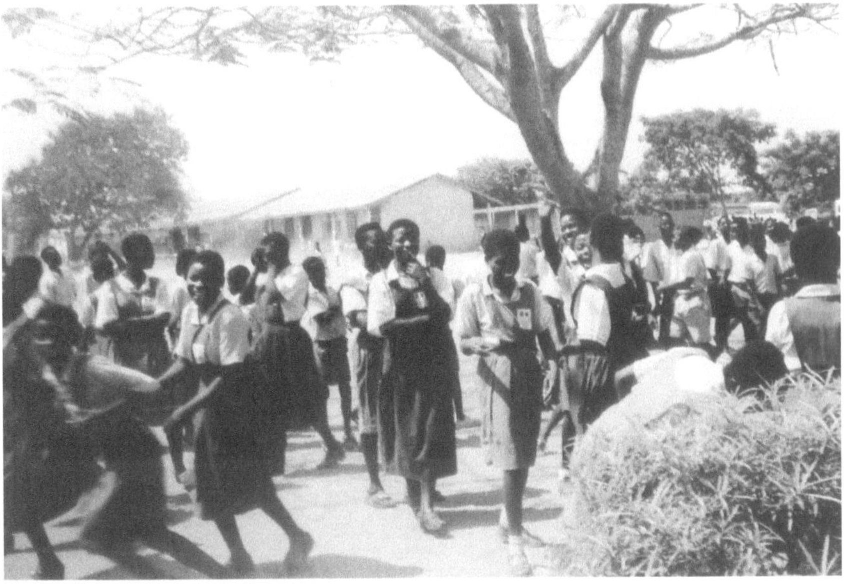

Figure 1. Madina, Ghana: Junior Secondary School #3 students on break, 1997. Photo taken by Jamaine Abidogun

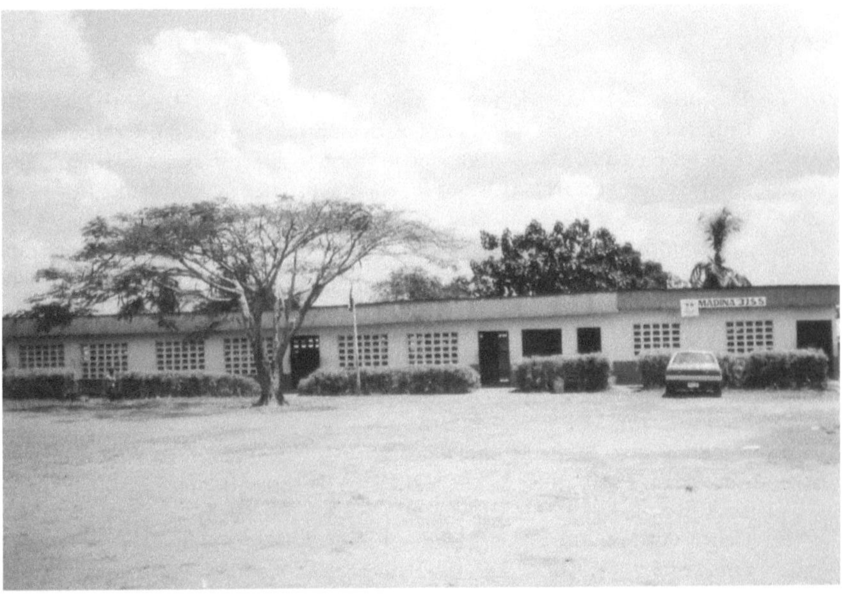

Figure 2. Madina, Ghana: Junior Secondary School #3 (1997). Photo taken by Jamaine Abidogun

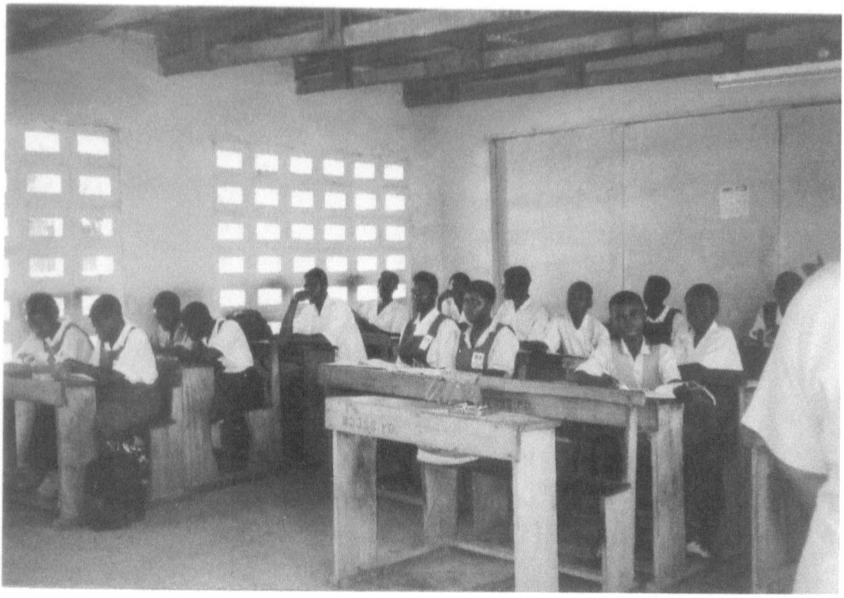

Figure 3. Madina, Ghana: Junior Secondary School #3, Year 3 class, 1997. Photo taken by Jamaine Abidogun

NOTES

1. The original fieldwork was conducted in 1997 with support from the University of Ghana, Institute of African Studies at Legon. Gratitude and recognition go to Dr. George Hagan, former director and Mr. Joseph Tettah, graduate research assistant for their assistance in completing this fieldwork.
2. The majority of participants were Twi from the Akan ethnolinguistic group, no one identified as Fanti, with other participants representing the rest of the ethnolinguistic groups as listed.
3. W. Rodney, *How Europe underdeveloped Africa*, (Washington DC: Howard University Press, 1982), 246.
4. M. Lar, *Aspects of nomadic education in Nigeria*, (Jos: FAB Education Books, 1990), 34.
5. Robert Young, *White Mythologies: Writing History and the West* (London: Routledge, 1990), viii. As cited in Henry Giroux, *Border Crossings* (New York: Routledge, 1992), 27.
6. Henry Giroux, *Border Crossings: Cultural Workers and the Politics of Education*, (NY: Routledge. 1992), 27.
7. Paulo Freire, *Pedagogy of Hope: Reliving Pedagogy of the Oppressed*, Trans. by Robert R. Barr, (New York: The Continuum Publishing Co., 1994), 46.

8. Paulo Freire, 1994, 48–49; Paulo Freire, *Teachers as Cultural Workers: Letters to Those who Dare to Teach*, Trans. by D. Macedo, D. Koike, and A. Oliveira, (Boulder, CO: Westview Press, 1998), 20–21.
9. S.E. Greene, *Gender, Ethnicity, and Social Change on the Upper Slave Coast: A History of the Anlo-Ewe*, (Portsmouth: Heinemann, 1996); and J. Bukh, *The Village Woman in Ghana*. (Uppsala: Scandinavian Institute of African Studies, 1979); A.F. Robertson, "Composition and Procedure in Ahafor Councils," In *Changing Social Structures in Ghana*, ed. J. Goody, (London: International African Institute, 1975), 229–244; A.F. Robertson, *Sharing the Same Bowl*, (Bloomington: Indiana University Press, 1984).
10. D. Pellow, *Women in Accra: Options for Autonomy*, (Algonac, MI: Reference Publishing Co. 1977); Toyin Falola and Steven J. Salm, *Culture and Customs of Ghana*, (Westport, CT: Greenwood Press, 2002); Yao Chachah and John Kuada, *Ghana: Understanding the People and Their Culture*, (Accra: Woeli Publishing Services, 1999).
11. G. Clarke, "The Plight of the 'Girl Maid,'" *The Ghanaian Child* 1, (1997): 9; F.A. Dolphyne, "The Girl-Child and School," *The Ghanaian Child*, 1, (1997): 6–8, 22–23, 30–32; K.A.L. Hyde, "Sub-Saharan Africa. King," in *Women's Education in Developing Countries*, ed. E.M.and M.A. Hill, (Baltimore: John Hopkins University Press, 1993), 100–135; A.J. Gage-Brandon and C.B. Lloyd, "High Fertility and Children's Schooling in Ghana: Sex Differences in Parental Contributions and Education Outcomes," *Population Studies* 48 (1994): 293–306; Rose B. Folsom, *The Contribution of Formal Education to Economic Development and Economic Underdevelopment Ghana as Paradigm*, (Frankfurt/Main: Peter Lang,1995).
12. Classroom Observation #5 Oct 7, 1997. All classroom observations were conducted at Madina #3 Junior Secondary School, Madina, Ghana by the author during 1997.
13. Classroom Observation #6 Oct 9, 1997; hereafter cited in text as Observation #6.
14. Interview A, Oct 30, 1997. All interviews reflected formal interviews where a consent form was completed. The consent form indicated that all participants unless they stated in writing that they wanted their identity to be revealed would be kept confidential. As no participant indicated that they wanted their identity to be revealed a two alpha character was used as an identification code for each participant. For student participants two interviews were conducted, so Interview-A or Interview-B may appear in the references.
15. Abbiw, Ampene, Asamoah, Braimah, Essel, Kyei-Anti, & Oparehene *Cultural Studies for Junior Secondary Schools: Pupil's Book 3*, (Accra: Ghana Education Service, Curriculum Research and Development Division, 1989), 63–68 and 70–71 respectively.
16. Abbiw, Ackumey, Ampene, Amusah, Essel, & Kyei-Anti, *Cultural Studies for Junior Secondary Schools: Pupil's Book 1*, Reprinted 1993, (Accra:Ghana Education Service, Curriculum Research and Development Division, 1987), 75–94; Abbiw, Ampene, Asamoah, Braimah, Essel, Kyei-Anti, & Oparehene, *Cultural Studies for Junior Secondary*

Schools: Pupil's Book 2. Accra: Ghana Education Service, Curriculum Research and Development Division, 1988), 91–120; Abbiw et all, 1989, 120–129.

17. Interview-A, 1997.
18. While seamstress and tailor were originally a Western occupation brought in by missionaries, they were adopted early into the indigenous apprentice systems.
19. "Any-work" boys were titled such because university students would yell outside of their dorm rooms for "any-work" and these boys would come and work for them for a few cedis. The types of work most often involved cleaning the room, washing laundry, running errands, or hauling heavy loads. Females were not allowed to participate although they may work for the formal laundry or cleaning operations on the university campus.
20. Paul Freire, *Pedagogy of the Oppressed*, Trans. by M. Bergman Ramos, New Rev. Ed., (New York: The Continuum Publishing Co., 1993), 85.
21. Henry Giroux, *Theory and Resistance in Education: Towards a Pedagogy for the Opposition*, Revised and expanded edition, (Westport, CT: Berginand Garvey, 2001), 239.

REFERENCES

Abbiw, Ackumey, Ampene, Amusah, Essel, & Kyei-Anti. *Cultural Studies for Junior Secondary Schools: Pupil's Book 1.* Reprinted 1993. Accra:Ghana Education Service, Curriculum Research and Development Division, 1987.

Abbiw, Ampene, Asamoah, Braimah, Essel, Kyei-Anti, & Oparehene *Cultural Studies for Junior Secondary Schools: Pupil's Book 2.* Accra:Ghana Education Service, Curriculum Research and Development Division, 1988.

———. *Cultural Studies for Junior Secondary Schools: Pupil's Book 3.* Accra: Ghana Education Service, Curriculum Research and Development Division, 1989..

Bukh, J. *The Village Woman in Ghana.* Uppsala: Scandinavian Institute of African Studies, 1979.

Chachah, Yao, and John Kuada. *Ghana: Understanding the People and Their Culture.* Accra: Woeli Publishing Services, 1999.

Clarke, G. "The Plight of the 'Girl Maid.'" *The Ghanaian Child* 1: 9, (1997).

Dolphyne, F.A. "The Girl-Child and School." *The Ghanaian Child* 1: 6–8, (1997). 22–23, 30–32.

Falola, Toyin, and Steven J. Salm. *Culture and Customs of Ghana.* Westport, CT: Greenwood Press, 2002.

Folson, Rose B. *The Contribution of Formal Education to Economic Development and Economic Underdevelopment Ghana as Paradigm.* Frankfurt/Main: Peter Lang, 1995.

Freire, Paulo. *Pedagogy of the Oppressed.* Trans. by M. Bergman Ramos. (New Rev. Ed.), New York: The Continuum Publishing Co., 1993.

———. *Pedagogy of Hope: Reliving Pedagogy of the Oppressed.* Trans. by Robert R. Barr. New York: The Continuum Publishing Co., 1994.

———. *Teachers as Cultural Workers: Letters to Those who Dare to Teach*. Trans. by D. Macedo, D. Koike, and A. Oliveira. Boulder, CO: Westview Press, 1998.

Gage-Brandon, A.J., and C.B. Lloyd. "High Fertility and Children's Schooling in Ghana: Sex Differences in Parental Contributions and Education Outcomes." *Population Studies* 48 (1994): 293–306.

Giroux, Henry. *Border Crossings: Cultural Workers and the Politics of Education*. NY: Routledge, 1992.

———. *Theory and Resistance in Education: Towards a Pedagogy for the Opposition*. Revised and expanded edition. Westport, CT: Bergin and Garvey, 2001.

Greene, S.E. *Gender, Ethnicity, and Social Change on the Upper Slave Coast: A History of the Anlo-Ewe*. Portsmouth: Heinemann, 1996.

Hyde, K.A.L. "Sub-Saharan Africa. King." in *Women's Education in Developing Countries*, ed. E.M. & M.A. Hill, 100–135. Baltimore: John Hopkins University Press, 1993.

Pellow, D. *Women in Accra: Options for Autonomy*. Algonac, MI: Reference Publishing Co., 1977.

Robertson, A.F. "Composition and Procedure in Ahafor Councils." in *Changing Social Structures in Ghana*, ed. J. Goody, 229–244. London: International African Institute, 1975.

———. *Sharing the Same Bowl*. Bloomington: Indiana University Press, 1984.

Part IV

Refugees, Displacement, and Re-Settlement

Chapter Twelve

Peoples Without Homes: Displacement and the Security Situation in Africa[1]

Bukola Adeyemi Oyeniyi

INTRODUCTION

While inter-state conflict in Africa has diminished greatly in recent years,[2] a disturbing escalatory trend exists in the total magnitude and in the occurrences of violent conflicts within African States. Reports from different African countries like DR Congo, Somalia, Eritrea, Rwanda, Burundi, Liberia, Ethiopia, Ivory Coast and Nigeria, to mention but a few, reveal that Africa is witnessing an increasing incidence of socio-economic and political conflict. These conflicts have decimated large areas, reduced fragile socio-political and economic relations within states into hostility and chaos, and led many newly emergent and long-established states to the brink of structural collapse.[3]

Although an overwhelming number of reasons could account for the violent conflicts that abound in Africa,[4] scholars and policy makers have devoted so much attention to identifying the causes and impact of inter and intra-state conflicts that the fate of people who are displaced before, during, and after a war has remained largely untreated. One wonders if a whole community of displaced persons who have been bred (but survived) in a system of violence, but lacking the needed skills for handling conflicts, and whose moral development may have been limited by their immersion in these conflicts, can be said to have little or no impact on conflict resurgence and escalation.

Either serving as foot soldiers in regular combat or in guerrilla situations, or as victims of wars, displaced persons are, unarguably, the victims of most conflicts.[5] They have witnessed the death of loved ones, been denied access to food, education, and are forced away from the comfort of homes and parental security to become refugees and victims of war in places other than their homelands.

Whether pressed into "service" by coercion, intimidation, false inducement, or ignorance, (Albert, 2002, 6) those who served as combatants in wars became pitted against their own communities through "military training," early exposure to violence and the possession of firearms.[6] Their lives are consequently reshaped such that the bond of trust between them and their communities is destroyed, (Albert, 2002, 7). The situations of those who escaped "service" are not much better. They become security risks to themselves, their host communities and the international community at large.

From the Atlantic to the Indian Ocean, Africa is broken in the middle by a dense area of conflict. The belligerents and non-belligerents as well as those who have not directly experienced war at all, all bear the burden of conflict.[7] While the scars of combat bear witness to those who have experienced it, others have borne the burden of conflict as refugees and displaced persons, suffering by-products such as food and nutrition insecurity, economic disruption, climate change and the spread of HIV/AIDS.[8]

This chapter, while not pretending to be a 'tour de horizon' of conflicts and displacement situations in Africa, uses the examples of the Democratic Republic of Congo and Nigeria to examine the intersection between displacement and the security situation in Africa.[9] It must be noted that the two variables involved in the study of displacement are refugees and internally displaced persons (IDPs). Stated differently, displacement can be divided into two categories: Refugees and the Internally Displaced People. Therefore, while the DR Congo is used to explain the displacement situation in countries-in-conflict, Nigeria, on the other hand, is used to explain displacement in countries where there is relative peace. This division into countries-in-conflict and countries-out-of-conflict is borne out of the fact that not all African States are experiencing conflict and war at the present moment. While nations like the DR Congo, Sudan, Rwanda, Sierra Leone, Ivory Coast, Eritrea, Ethiopia, Somalia, etc have had or are still experiencing one form of conflict, other African nations like Nigeria, South Africa, Togo, Egypt, Libya, Guinea, etc have witnessed relative or at least limited peace. Hence, the use of the DR Congo is but a representation of nations wracked by many years of strife, while Nigeria represents nations that have experienced limited or relative peace over the years. This case study method is aimed at showing, in a sharp relief, that problems associated with displacement in Africa have reached an alarming state for countries-in-conflict, for countries-out-of-conflict and even for those countries in Africa where relative peace pervades.

Among other things, the study interrogates the intersection between conflict resurgence and displacement situations, and posits that conflict resurgence in Africa today results, in part, from pockets of unresolved displacement problems. To solve African socio-political and economic problems, therefore, the study submits that efforts must be made to solve the numerous problems faced by both the externally and the internally displaced, to foster the urgently needed environment for sustainable peaceful development.

This study adopts a thematic approach. It discusses displacement as a national security imperative and as one of the yet unconsidered factors in conflict resurgence and as a continuing security problem in Africa. The impact of displacement on the displaced persons, their hosts and Africa at large, can only be examined judiciously through a survey of the various factors necessitating displacement. Although different factors account for displacement in different African states, the results of displacement are the same in all African states and so also are their future implications. The first part of the study reviews the numerous literature on displacement, and progresses to examine the identifiable lapses in the current understanding of the term and the implications that these have had on policy direction in Africa. Having identified the two types of displacement, the study examines with examples drawn from the refugee situation in the Democratic Republic of Congo to bring to the fore the specific security implications of displacement in countries-in-conflict. With the example of Nigeria, the study also examines the nexus between national security and internal displacement, in countries where there is relative peace.

Moving from the specific to the general, the study progresses to illuminate the nexus between national security, displacement, conflict resurgence, and the plethora of socio-economic problems bedeviling and causing underdevelopment in Africa. The study concludes that in order to end violent conflict, and to ensure sustainable development in Africa, the issue of displacement must be given an urgent attention.

LITERATURE REVIEW AND THEORETICAL DEFICITS IN THE STUDY OF DISPLACEMENT

To attempt a review of available literatures on displacement in Africa is not an easy task, especially in a study like this. One reason for this difficulty is the volume of literature dealing with displacement. Another reason deals with the peculiar nature of these literatures. From the subject-specific to the country/regional-specific, most works focus wide-ranging issues like health, relief assistance, food and nutrition, and several other aspects of the problems associated with displacement. Some have even gone as far as to establish a linkage between displacement and the spread of HIV/AIDS. A review of all these works would only result in a jumble and a tangled skein. Only a thematic description and analysis can impose order on the tangled web that the available literature has created.

In order to achieve a meaningful review, the study begins by examining the definition and the nuances involved in our understanding of displacement and security. It then examines the available works on displacement in the DR Congo and the Federal Republic of Nigeria, which are the case studies used in the overall examination of displacement problems in Africa.

To begin with, what is displacement? Who are refugees and IDPs? If any, in what ways are IDPs different from refugees? This section seeks to proffer answers to these and many other questions. The cachets of meaning and relevance associated with internal displacement and refugee status are multidimensional and eclectic, such that to many scholars and policy makers, the two explain and describe one thing, from victims of wars and violence to people fleeing from conditions that threaten human rights. The two have become separate identity tags that differ only in the context in which they are used. The International Committee of the Red Cross (ICRC) defines "Internally displaced persons," "internally displaced," "displaced persons," "displaced population," "displaced," and "IDPs" as "persons displaced within their own country."[10]

Francis Deng, the United Nations Secretary-General's Representative on Internally Displaced Persons in a paper titled *Guiding Principles on Internal Displacement* defines it as, "persons or group of persons who have been forced or obliged to flee or to leave their homes or places of habitual residence, in particular as a result of or in order to avoid the effects of armed conflict, situations of generalized violence, violations of human rights or natural or human-made disasters, *and who have not crossed an internationally recognized state border*," (Francis, 1995, Para.2, 1), (emphasis mine).

Most international and non-governmental organizations, borrowing from this accepted definition, limit their understanding, policy focus and relief assistance mainly to the refugees while the internally displaced persons, who have not crossed an internationally recognized state border, are left at the mercy of the very government that caused the displacement in the first place. This, in part, arose from the acceptance that displaced people needed emergency assistance mainly as refugees. Those who are displaced within the borders of their native country are considered the responsibility of their state government. This affects policy orientation and policy direction of these organizations, especially in their response to complex emergencies regarding those still in the country-in-conflict.

Gunther Beyer, on his part, sees little or no difference between refugees and internally displaced persons. His differentiation is limited to mere nomenclature, daubing one as international refugee and the other as national.[11] He maintains that a refugee and an internally displaced person are either victims of both war and human-rights-threatening situations, or natural and man-made disasters. In his definition, he asserts that: "any persons or categories of persons who have left the territory of the state of which they are nationals; and they become refugees as a result of their relationship with the existing government (ruling class). National refugees are defined as people fleeing under pressure of persecution from one part of a nation state to another in search of protection under national legal norms," (Beyer, 1981, 27).

Explaining the dichotomy between an international and a national refugee, Gunther Beyer maintains that the difference in the two is only in name and not in identity, experience or station, especially as conditions alien to the normal situations that could guarantee continued existence in their places of habitual residence. While it is incontestable that there is congruence in their experiences of, among other things, fear, deprivation, loss of limbs and loved ones, their experiences differ in terms of access to basic life saving necessities like home, shelter, health facilities, and food. While the definition of refugees, according to the UN, imposes considerable limitations on donor agencies in their endeavors to reach-out to those "national refugees," just because they have not crossed any internationally recognized border, their lack of identity, wars and conflicts by their very nature impose great limitations as they remove or shift the responsibility for the "upkeep" of displaced persons to a collapsed state.

On the other hand, most definitions of "refugee" are based on the 1926 Arrangement of 12 May and 30 June 1928, the Protocol of 14 September 1939, and the 1951 convention, which is quoted *in extensio* below:

> A refugee is any person who:
>
> (a) has been considered a refugee under the 1926 Arrangement of 12 May and 30 June 1928, the Protocol of 14 September 1939, or the constitution of the International Refugee Organisation;[12]
>
> (b) as a result of events occurring before 1 January 1951 and owing to well-founded fear of being persecuted for reasons of race, religion, nationality, membership of a particular social group or political opinion, is outside the country of his nationality and is unable, or owing to such fear, is unwilling to avail himself of the protection of the country; or who, not having a nationality and

> being outside the country of his former habitual residence as a result of such events, is unable, owing to such fear, is unwilling to return to it. In the case of a person who has more than one nationality, the term "the country of his nationality" shall mean each of the countries of which he is a national, and a person shall not be deemed to be lacking the protection of the country of his nationality if, without any valid reason based on well-founded fear, he has not availed himself of the protection of one of the countries of which he is a national, (Intergovernmental Committee, 383).

The convention went on to analyze the obligation that the state has to refugees within its borders, including with the provisions of refuge, shelter and basic services. The Convention, drafted in 1951 by a panel, defined persecution based on race, religion, and nationality, membership in political groups or political opinions. A conception of which individual identities can be presumed excludes the internally displaced as well as gender-based violence not only as unacceptable reasons for seeking asylum but also for denying them access to relief assistance. The convention, on a closer analysis, recognized claims to asylum of people who, for one reason or the other, were in another country when war or conflict forced them to remain in such country. This category of refugees is called "sure-place" refugees.[13]

It must be noted that the causes of displacement have shifted over time. At the time that the convention was drafted, the emergence of the Cold War between the Soviet Union and the US was high in the minds of Western supporters of the convention, who were eager to protect and support political dissidents from communist regimes that had been established across Central and Eastern Europe. During the 1960s, the era of anti-colonial struggle in Africa generated new and significant refugee flows, and was part of the rationale for the inclusion in the OAU's convention of 1969 on "external aggression" and "foreign occupation" as potential causes of flight in the refugee definition.[14] Subsequently, the superpower rivalry and proxy wars fought by the Soviet Union and the US have given ways to a more diffuse set of conflicts in the post-Cold War era, each of which has generated new refugee flows.

All available definitions of refugee emphasize not only the condition necessitating flight and its attendant life-threatening situations, but also the need to cross an internationally recognized state boundary. From this, it is clear that the difference between a refugee and an internally displaced person deals primarily with having crossed an internationally recognized state border. This deficit in our understanding and definition of displacement is a security concern that has reached a state of emergency, especially with the recent spate of displacement-inducing situations in Africa, in which we have about four or five internally displaced persons to every refugee.

In spite of the limitation imposed by this definition, the UN, in its *Guiding Principles on Internal Displacement*, recognized two basic elements common to displaced persons, either as refugees or IDPs. Basically, all displaced persons were coerced to move and their movement was involuntary. The document also mentions some of the most common causes of involuntary movements, such as armed conflict, violence, human rights violations, and disasters, (Deng, 1995, principle 1, para. 2). These causes, it must be stated, give neither notice nor choice to people but compel them to leave their homes and deprive them of the most essential protection mechanisms, such as community networks, access to services, and livelihoods. Displacement severely affects the physical, socio-economic, and legal safety of people and should be systematically regarded as an indicator of potential vulnerability.

The UN also recognizes the fact that such movement takes place within national borders, especially given the difficulties of reaching a border between land mines and warring factions. Those living far away from border areas can, at best, hope to get as far as they can to safety and can only depend on the generosity of relatives and friends who are also living in constant fear, as well as eking out a living through the barest product that they can garner from the land. However, unlike refugees who have been deprived of the protection of their state of origin, IDPs remain legally under the protection of national authorities in their country of habitual residence.

The UN and donor agencies maintain that IDPs should enjoy the same rights as the rest of the population. As stated in *The Guiding Principles on Internal Displacement*, the national authorities and other relevant actors in their country of habitual residence should assume responsibility to ensure that IDPs' rights are respected and fulfilled, despite the vulnerability generated by their displacement, (Deng, 1995, principle 3, para. 1 and 2).

Although everyone suffers who is affected by conflict and/or human rights violations, the policy focus and definition of displacement by international and donor organizations fail to note that displacement from one's place of habitual residence may make the internally displaced particularly vulnerable. The fact that the internally displaced persons may be in transit from one place to another, may be in hiding, may be forced toward unhealthy or inhospitable environments, or may face other circumstances that make them especially vulnerable, is in itself a condition that should warrant a redefinition and reassessment of their need for relief assistance. Again, it is important to note that the social organization of displaced communities may have been damaged or destroyed by the act of physical displacement; family groups may be separated or disrupted; women may be forced to assume non-traditional roles or face particular vulnerabilities.[15]

In the same vein, internally displaced populations, especially groups like children, the elderly or pregnant women, may experience profound psychosocial distress related to displacement, and the removal from sources of income and livelihood may add to physical and psychosocial vulnerability for displaced people. Schooling for children and adolescents may be disrupted. Internal displacement to areas where local inhabitants are of different groups or are inhospitable may increase the risk to internally displaced communities, especially when they are faced with language barriers. Internal displacement may lead to hatred and suspicion, especially when the hosts and the displaced people have to contend for scarce resources. It may also cause or lead to abuse by armed combatants or other parties in the conflict. Internally displaced persons may lack identity documents essential to receiving benefits or legal recognition. In some cases where such documents exist, the fear of persecution has forced many of the displaced persons to get rid of such documents.

Today, although several countries, like Azerbaijan, Bosnia and Herzegovina, Colombia, Croatia, Georgia, the Russian Federation, Nigeria, the DR Congo, and other African nations, have adopted legislation providing for the creation of a national status for IDPs or selected groups of IDPs (those displaced by a particular conflict, for instance), such a status usually provides for the registration of those entitled to the status and provides beneficiaries with social, economic and legal assistance to safeguard rights endangered by displacement and to support the implementation of durable solutions. These statuses ought not to deprive IDPs of their rights under human rights and humanitarian law, but as seen in the case of Nigeria and the DR Congo, the reverse is the case. For instance, the refugees in Nigeria are quartered in the two camps (Ogun and Kano States), and there is no institutionalized residence for IDPs. In the DR Congo, adequate attention is given to the care of the refugees in camps at Ituri and Kivu, but only a tacit recognition is so far accorded the IDPs who were mostly in the forest and in homes of relatives and friends in different parts of the country.

From the foregoing, it is pertinent to note that the both the refugees and the IDPs are victims of conflicts, war, human-made or natural disaster, and human–rights-threatening situations. Therefore, for the purpose of this study, a displaced person can be either a refugee or an IDP. Hence, displacement means forced migration, movement, or flight from a place of habitual residence to another place, which may or may not involve the crossing of an internationally recognized state boundary. The merit of this definition lies in removing the constraints imposed by the UN definition, which insists that the displaced persons must cross an internationally recognized boundary to qualify as refugees and people in need of urgent relief assistance from the international and donor agencies. This also removes the misunderstanding and seeming insensitivity in our understanding, response, and policy imperatives of international and donor agencies whose policies favored only the refugees while the IDPs were left at the mercy of the very state that turned them to a community in perpetual flight.

After many years of autocratic, dictatorial, and military misgovernance in Africa, the fall of the Berlin Wall in 1989 and the emergence of the third wave of democracy, Africans in the last two decades have witnessed or experienced new opportunities to express long-suppressed democratic aspirations after many years of repressive military rule. Therefore, conflicts of one form or the other have dotted the African landscape. As earlier noted, it can be safely argued that colonial rule sowed the seed of war in Africa while military rule fertilized it. With the end of military rule, new opportunities to act out aggressive behavior were opened for the various the ethnic groups that formed nation-states in Africa, and, as the new political leadership failed to use the new wave of democracy to foster unity, they became engaged in sectarian agendas, which polarized their nations. The point is that with the third wave of democracy in Africa came a new opportunity not only to rebuild the various African states, but also for the various ethnic groups to act out their pent-up angers and frustrations, which were repressed under military rule. As each group jostled for coveted resources, opportunities, and positions, conflicts arose that served as the needed triggers to let out these pent-up feelings. In consequence, Africa has become a home to millions of displaced persons—a situation that has no parallel anywhere in the world.

The return to democratic rule in Africa has come with a mixed bag of accomplishments and challenges. While it serves as a new window of opportunity to satisfy the need for sustainable development, to renegotiate ethnic relations, and to restore hopes, it also serves as a release-valve for pent-up feelings, which has now allowed for the development of fissiparous tendencies that are gradually pulling Africa apart at the seams. The first leg of the paradox has produced genuine transformations including the end of apartheid in South Africa and the quelling of violent conflicts in Mozambique, Angola and Sierra Leone. The other, based largely on unmet aspirations, has produced near-genocidal situations in countries like Rwanda, Burundi, Ethiopia, DR Congo, Somalia, Liberia, Sudan, Eritrea and Ivory Coast, and wrecked nations like Nigeria, where old conflicts and new ones suddenly reared their ugly heads. In a recent report on Nigeria, 252 conflicts occurred in 2003 alone.[16] The situation is no different in other parts of Africa, as one form of conflict or another dots the landscape from the Atlantic to the Red Sea, from the West to the East and from the North to the South.

Having considered displacement and its nuances, the second important concept in this study is security. As a concept, security is rather an eclectic subject to define. Many have defined it based on their subject area. Put differently, it means different things to different people.

Security has been defined as a property that a creditor can claim in case a debtor defaults on obligation. It can also be a formal declaration that documents a fact of relevance to finance and investment. It could be the state of being free from danger or injury. It could also mean anything from a guarantee that an obligation will be met to the protection of oneself or one's property from harm. Alternatively, freedom from anxiety or fear, the same as feeling the presence of a watchdog or a police dog gives. It could mean a defense against financial failure or financial dependence. It has been defined as a precaution against theft or espionage or sabotage etc.; or as simply as freedom from risk or danger; freedom from doubt, anxiety, or fear or something that gives or assures safety, or measures adopted by a government to prevent espionage, sabotage, or attack. It could also be any measures adopted, as by a business or homeowner, to prevent a crime such as burglary or assault, or measures adopted to prevent escape or something deposited or given as assurance of the fulfillment of an obligation.[17] It could also mean safety from harm, a term that has different dimensions in psychology, public safety, defense and military matters, and information access. In finance, a security is a document representing an investment.[18]

In the organization, for example, the computer industry, security refers to techniques for ensuring that data stored in a computer cannot be read or compromised by any individuals without authorization. Most security measures, in this case, involve data encryption and passwords. Data encryption, which is also a security measure, is the translation of data into a form that is unintelligible without a deciphering mechanism. A password is a secret word or phrase that gives a user access to a particular program or system.

As an academic field of inquiry, security has come to assume different meanings other than the mundane. Depending on the specific area, security can be economic, political, national, and international, etc. As far as this study is concerned, security is used in terms of national security. Just as there are a plethora of meanings for security, national security has been defined in different ways. Each academic discipline has defined national security in their narrow disciplinary terms. While this narrow perspective does not remove the shine from national security, it has nevertheless led to a situation in which issues that are not of particular interest to the discipline are regarded as intruders and not strictly security issues. For instance, when national security began as an academic field, it was defined as any measures taken by a military unit, an activity, or installation to protect itself against all acts designed to, or which may impair its effectiveness.[19] In yet another definition, it is conceived as a matter of a state's military or a state's defense by military means.[20] Another definition states that it connotes the effort to protect a population and territory against organized force or forces while advancing the state's interests through competitive actions, (Geoffrey and David Dabelko, 1995, 3). It has also been conceived as measures taken as a precaution against theft, espionage, or sabotage, etc.[21] It important to state that these state-centric or state-centered definitions of security became popular immediately after World War II and this results from the belief that the state is the sole entity capable of deploying violence as well as guaranteeing security. These state-centered definitions of security not only dominated discussions in international relations, diplomatic, and other related studies, but also led to a conception of threats and crises as mainly military challenges, which have elicited police or military actions.

As earlier noted, this narrow perspective to national security treats issues that are not strictly military in nature as non-security issues. However, with the oil crises of the 1970's, this jaundiced view changed to a more inclusive view of security. As a fall-out of the crisis, issues of economic, environment and resource scarcity became acceptable as security issues. Further advancement in security scholarship came with the collapse of the Soviet Union, as Western economies began to focus on trade and economic competition, thereby making economic competition one of the security considerations of the 21st century, (Geoffrey and David Dabelko, 1995, 3). This refocusing was hinged primarily on the fact that anything capable of increasing the stress-level of any society and cause panic could affect a people's well-being and cause insecurity within the populace. In the same vein, situations in post-colonial Africa made it more germane for the Western powers to redefine security to include threats other than immediate military ones. One of the contributions of this modest improvement in security scholarship is the realization of the fact that focusing exclusively on military threats carries the potential cost of neglecting other, more menacing dangers. Therefore, it was widely accepted that issues such as population growth or decline in developing nations, competition over scarce resources, and Trans-boundary migration could result in severe security-threatening situations like conflicts, wars, displacement, etc.

Resultant from this development, security, especially national security, has come to assume different meanings, each bordering on specific perspective of (1) the author and (2) the subject of discussion. One of such definition sees security largely as an: action or sequence of events that (1)threatens drastically and over a relatively brief span of time to degrade the quality of life for the inhabitants of a state, or (2) threatens significantly to narrow the range of policy choices available to the government of a state or to private, nongovernmental entities (persons, groups, corporations) within the state, (Geoffrey and David Dabelko, 1995, 3).

Moving beyond the strictly state-centric definition of security, Myers, Mathews, Mische, Renner, and Prins suggested: "security applies most at all level of the citizen. It amounts to human wellbeing: not only protection from harm and injury but access to water, food, shelter, health, employment, and other basic requisites that are the due of every person on Earth. It is the collectivity of these citizen needs—overall safety and quality of life—that should figure prominently in the nation's view of security."[22]

For the purpose of this study, security can be defined as policy choices, institutional responses and measures taken or that are to be taken by an individual, organization, or state, to increase the available options for preventing real or perceived danger. Security, defined in this way, removes all the constraints imposed by disciplinary persuasions. It also shows that issues like displacement, population dislocation, etc qualify as national security issues.

Many works on refugee and IDP problems in Africa have drawn attention to the magnitude and composition of the people involved.[23] The figures reveal a peculiar pattern, especially when compared with other regions of the world, which indicates that there is an astronomical rise in the number of people involved. Aside from the increasing number, another issue raised is the demographic aspect of the problem. In most African states, 80 percent of the displaced are women and children.[24] Some scholars have devoted attention to the general condition of displaced persons.[25] Some have examined institutional responses of different African states to the plight of the displaced and have submitted that, in most African countries, hesitant attention if any is given to the care of the IDPs while, to some extent, attention has always been devoted to the care of refugees. Aside from recognizing this, none has established a link between our understanding of displacement and policy directions of most governments and international agencies. For instance, in the West African sub-region, only Nigeria has refugee camps; others in the region have treated the issue of displacement like a non-issue.

Most works have succeeded in establishing the fact that most countries in Africa have neglected the IDPs and left them to the mercy of the very governments who could not prevent their displacement in the first place. As could be seen in our examination of the UN paper on displacement, the understanding is that the government of a country should be responsible for the upkeep of its citizens and that a citizen becomes an international burden only when he or she may have crossed an internationally recognized state boundary.

Issue-specific works also abound and their interests intersperse health-care, child-care, demobilization and debriefing, conflict resolution, capacity building, education and a host of others. In the main, aside from examining their topics in relation to specific countries or regions on the continent, some have made useful contributions to our understanding of the enormity of the problem by establishing linkages between the problems associated with displacement and other socio-political and economic problems. A good example is the linkage between displacement and the spread of diseases like HIV/AIDS. Others have devoted their search to other, inter-related issues, such as food and nutrition insecurity, crop-losses and environmental or climate change.

In a paper titled "Exiles in Their Own Home: Conflicts and Internal Population Displacement in Nigeria,"[26] O. Okechukwu Ibeanu examines the growing problem of internal population displacement in Nigeria. He argues that a central causal variable in population displacement in Nigeria is state violence. Aggression of the state towards certain groups appears as inter-group conflicts. The paper locates the socio-economic and political basis of state violence in Nigeria in military rule, crude oil production and communalism, three factors that also give rise to the three most important displacement-generating conflicts in Nigeria. An analysis of these conflicts shows the deepening link between state violence, insecurity and population displacement. The paper also addresses issues of humanitarian assistance and protection for displaced people. It concludes that the management of internal population displacement in Nigeria calls for the elimination of state violence and the transformation of the state into an instrument of equitable resource allocation and conflict management among groups. The key to these, the paper argues, is the democratization of the state.

In a 2005 report by the Global IDP Project, Norwegian Refugee Council / Global IDP Project, entitled "Internal Displacement in Nigeria: a Hidden Crisis," the author examines the IDPs' situation in Nigeria and argues that with a history of ethno-religious conflict in Nigeria, the past year has witnessed an alarming upsurge in the level of violence and its impact on civilians. Almost one year after spiraling violence between mainly Muslim cattle herders and Christian farmers in central Plateau state left possibly more than 1,000 people dead and 258,000 temporarily displaced; many of those who fled are still too scared to return. This paper assesses the causes and consequences of such mass displacements. It looks at obstacles preventing the return of people to their homes, and weighs up the humanitarian response to the situation. The paper therefore concludes that while the immediate needs of the IDPs were adequately addressed, their long-term needs have been given scant attention. It also recognizes that assistance for return and reintegration is the most pressing need of IDPs in Nigeria, and that relief assistance should include not only physical rehabilitation of homes, public buildings and infrastructure, but also support for peace and reconciliation initiatives, especially at the grass-roots level. The paper therefore calls for improved emergency response and a strong initiative to address the root causes of conflict-induced displacement, thus avoiding the types of humanitarian crises currently plaguing several of Nigeria's neighbors.

In another paper, "Ecology, Identity, Developmentalism and Displacement in Northern Nigeria," Kole Shettima examines the significance of the state and of multilateral institutions in the political economy of irrigation schemes in northern Nigeria. He argues that one of the major initiatives of the state and of multilateral institutions after the drought and famine of 1972–1974 was the building of dams for irrigation. Official discourse justified large-scale mechanized irrigation schemes as "development." Although those who discuss the importance of the state and of multilateral institutions in the agricultural sector have contributed to the analysis of the politics of drought and irrigation, there has been less analysis of their social dimensions. First, there is little discussion of irrigation schemes as developmentalism, and their consequences on displacement. Two case studies of irrigation schemes as development projects (Bakolori and Kano) show massive displacement of communities and other negative consequences, including rural-urban migration and urban social conflict. The case study of urban social conflict in the Maitatsine uprising in Kano and other parts of northern Nigeria illustrates some of the consequences of developmentalism and displacement. However, peasants do not always resist development and displacement by migrating to urban centers: in some cases, they became involved in other forms of resistance, such as civil disobedience as seen in the case of the Bakolori uprising in 1980. Secondly, while the literature on irrigation has thrown light on technical and economic problems, the paper attempts to deepen the technical and economic debates, as well as to throw light on other social dimensions of irrigation, such as subjectivity and identity. Throughout, this essay analyzes the connections between developmentalism and displacement, and their relation to subjectivity and identity.[27]

William Pat Ama Tokunbo in "Religion, Violence and Displacement in Nigeria," examines the role of religion as a critical factor in the study of displacement in Nigeria and the current controversy generated by the Mohammed cartoon and the reported 500,000 people already displaced is bearing out his argument.[28]

Leo Dare, in "Political Instability and Displacement in Nigeria," examines displacement and political instability during and after military autocracy. He argues that political instability usually produced scores of displacement both within and outside Nigeria. Some have fled the country for fear of persecution and repression to foreign countries, while others remained under extreme fear in the different parts of the country where they could best guarantee their safety.[29]

It is important to state that none of the existing literature has ever established a linkage between conflict resurgence and displacement, not because there is no such linkage, but because either their focus is on something else or it escaped their notice.

Just as works abound that discuss displacement in Nigeria, quite a lot has been done on the DR Congo, and, like the case of Nigeria, they have found no serious correlation between displacement and conflict resurgence. For instance, in a work titled "Crisis of Government, Ethnic Schisms, Civil War, and Regional Destabilization of the Democratic Republic of Congo." Paul Orogun examines the internal and external factors that precipitated the war in the DR Congo. He analyzes the effects of post-Cold War international politics on the regionalization, ethnicization, and militarism of internal socioeconomic and politico-cultural tensions in the Great Lakes region. A review of the immediate triggers of the conflict and a discussion of the nature and evolution of the persistent internal rebellion will provide the relevant historical framework of the study. To illustrate the complexity of the crisis, the work focuses on the problems, obstacles, and constraints that have pre-empted the possibility of a credible, peaceful, diplomatic resolution of the DRC conflict. Congo's civil war, he argues, centered squarely on the perceptions of ethnic marginalization, citizenship, land, regional security, democratization, and the quest for good governance. Other relevant issues include the National Sovereign Conference for Congo's political and economic dispensation, commercial imperatives, and military opportunism, which help to underscore the intricate nexus between domestic and the external dimensions of the conflict. The role of regional, continental, and international organizations, with regard to the process of peacemaking, peacekeeping, and post-conflict peace maintenance in the Great Lakes region is also critically examined. In all this, the writer failed to place any significance on the contributory role that displacement played in conflict resurgence in the DR Congo, despite the fact that he mentioned that land scarcity between the hosts and the IDPs remain a constant headache.[30]

On her part, Esther van der Velde, using examples from UNICEF field projects, concentrates on the effects of displacement on children in the DR Congo. After examining four important variables, i.e. advocacy, assessment, care, and protection, she argues that children in flight are at greater risk for malnutrition and disease, physical danger, and psychological trauma. In addition, she claims that this explains why many of these children do not survive. When they do, their ability to lead normal lives is greatly impaired, as many have no access to education and health care.[31]

In "Does a Man Die at your Feet . . . : Gender, History, and Representation," in *The Catastrophist (Critical Essay)*,[32] Patricia Coughlan examines the issues of masculinity, roles among the different genders, children and the effects of displacement in the Belgian Congo, now DR Congo. Although it critiques a literary work, the article underscores the important roles played by displacement in, among other things, conflict situation in Africa. It is ironic that the literary work put in perspective the interplay of displacement and one crucial factor in conflict escalation, resurgence, and the peace building process.[33]

From these examples and many more on displacement situations in both Nigeria and the DR Congo, it appears that while existing literatures have underscored the various problems associated with displacement, they have however failed to show the interconnectivity between displacement and incessant conflict in Africa; this study aims at bridging this obvious gap. It will now turn to a proper examination of the displacement situations in the Democratic Republic of Congo and Nigeria.

As is common in scholarship on organized violence, conflict has been separated into "high intensity" and "low-intensity" categories. High intensity conflicts include countries or areas engaged in civil war or experiencing continuous armed violence, while "low-intensity" conflicts include countries or areas where there is high tension but only sporadic clashes of arms. The last category deals with countries or areas that have recently emerged from violent conflict and may be experiencing low tension, if any. The DR Congo topped the list of countries with high intensity conflict, while others in the category include Sudan, Burundi, Angola, Uganda, and Somalia. On the lower threshold, Namibia topped the list while others like Zimbabwe, Eritrea, Ethiopia, Republic of Congo, Chad, Cote d'Ivoire, Morocco, Central African Republic, and Algeria followed in ranking. Out-of-violence countries include Mozambique, Sierra Leone, Angola, South Africa, Lesotho, Rwanda, Liberia, Malawi, and Nigeria. In so far that our analysis of displacement oscillates between refugee situations and internal displacement, DR Congo and Nigeria offer us useful instruments of measurement in the analysis, as the two occupy "important" positions in their respective groupings.[34]

DISPLACEMENT IN THE DEMOCRATIC REPUBLIC OF CONGO

Since the mid-1990s, millions of people from the Democratic Republic of Congo, formerly Zaire, have fled their homes to escape fighting between rebel groups and the national government in a complex conflict that has involved as many as nine neighboring countries. Close to four million people are believed to have died because of the conflict, which was accompanied by widespread human rights violations. Displacement peaked in 2003, with an estimated 3.4 million people forced from their homes, most of them in the eastern DRC. The UN estimated that over 2.3 million people remained displaced as of mid-2005.[35]

Hundreds of thousands of IDPs returned home in the wake of the establishment of a transitional power-sharing government in June 2003 and following the strengthening of international peacekeeping operations. The situation deteriorated in the second part of 2004, however, when clashes among armed groups and against civilians escalated in eastern DRC, and large numbers fled their homes, particularly in Ituri District and the Kivu Provinces, and the return process was consequently slowed down. Displacement has been accompanied by the killing of civilians, widespread sexual violence against women, child recruitment, looting and burning. Aid organizations have responded to the renewed crisis by bringing assistance to the displaced, but fighting and attacks on aid workers and peacekeepers by armed groups have prevented access to the most vulnerable. According to the UN, the humanitarian crisis in eastern DRC is the most serious in the world, (IDP Project, 7).

ORIGIN OF DISPLACEMENT IN THE DR CONGO

While the eastern province of North Kivu was the location of ethnic clashes and the displacement of thousands in the early 1990s, internal displacement spread throughout the DRC during fighting in 1996 and 1998. The underlying causes of displacement have been the disintegration of the state, which started long before the 1996 demise of President Mobutu Sese Seko's regime, and the subsequent competition among various ethnic groups for political and economic power in their respective provinces. A series of rebel groups, more or less closely linked to outside powers such as Uganda and Rwanda, have competed to control large areas of the eastern DRC. These groups have repeatedly clashed among themselves, as well as with the Kinshasa government and foreign troops. Civilians have suffered the worst of this violence, often being targeted for ethnic or political reasons. Their meager resources have been seized, children have been conscripted into the armed forces, and combatants have used women and girls as sex slaves, (IDP Project, 7).

Following an upsurge of violence by militias in Ituri in mid-2003, the UN Security Council authorized the UN Mission in the Democratic Republic of Congo (MONUC) peacekeeping force, under "Chapter VII" of the UN Charter, to use all necessary means to protect civilians under imminent threat of physical violence, in Ituri and in the Kivus. MONUC was also tasked with monitoring compliance with the arms embargo imposed by the UN Security Council in July 2003 on armed groups operating in eastern DRC. With the establishment, in mid-2003, of a Transition Government, which included the main armed groups and the political opposition, violence decreased until mid-2004.

In the second half of 2004 and in 2005 however, a series of crises caused heightened insecurity and displacement, and the Congolese government struggled to affirm its authority in the east of the country, particularly in Ituri and in the Kivus. One major problem was that while in theory former belligerents who joined the transitional government should have integrated their armed groups into a new national army, in reality most of the combatants were still controlled by the same military hierarchies as before the transition.[36] Also, the looting of DRC's natural resources by various armed groups continued, and those responsible for their illegal exploitation had not been held responsible.[37] Weapons continued to be channeled to various armed groups in DRC from neighboring countries, despite the establishment of an arms embargo.[38] National elections planned for June 2005 were delayed, notably due to insecurity and to the logistical challenge of registering 28 million voters in a country with limited infrastructure.[39] The voter registration process started on June 20, 2005 (IRIN, 26 July 2005).

In March 2005, the UN Security Council noted that the situation in the DRC continued to constitute a threat to international peace and security in the region.[40] The Hutu Rwandan Armed Liberation Forces (FDLR), Mai Mai factions, and other local armed groups were still attacking the local population. Unruly and unpaid Congolese military personnel were also reported to terrorize farmers, steal livestock, and pillage local plantations.[41] According to the UN Secretary-General, reports have shown that there was collaboration between Rwandan Hutu rebels and Mai Mai militias, and between Rwandan Hutu rebels and elements of the Congolese army.[42] Despite the presence of UN peacekeepers, militias in Ituri attacked the population, collected revenues from gold-mining, and smuggled goods and weapons to and from neighboring Uganda.

From February 2004, dissident officers from the former rebel movement Rassemblement Congolais pour la Democratie-Goma (RCD-G) sparked clashes in North and South Kivu which resulted in the displacement of tens of thousands in May/June 2004, particularly of ethnic Tutsis.[43] Many also fled after the fighting, out of fear of ethnically based reprisals, since the dissident commanders were Tutsi.[44] Years of war have contributed to hostility against the Congolese Tutsis, as they are increasingly identified as "Rwandan" by other Congolese.[45] Over 150 ethnic Tutsi refugees from DRC were also massacred across the border in Burundi, in August 2004.

Following the targeting of ethnic Tutsis, Rwandans being predominantly Tutsis, the Rwandan government mobilized its troops along its border with the DRC, interpreting the violence as a threat against all Tutsis. The military mobilization, as a response to the massacre, played on the fears of many people in the DRC that Rwanda might still be planning a large-scale intervention. In response to threats by Rwanda in December 2004 to enter the DRC to disarm Rwandan Hutu rebels by force, additional Congolese troops were sent to North Kivu. Since then, different segments of the Congolese army in the region, members of the former Congolese Army and members of the former rebel group RCD-Goma, all of them[?] reportedly backed by Rwanda, have repeatedly clashed. In December 2004, fighting and soldiers' looting of homes and shops in North Kivu caused the displacement of more than 180,000 people, many of them into the forest areas.[46]

The peacekeeping mission, MONUC, has over 16,000 troops, who are mainly tasked to facilitate and assist the transition process. In September 2004, the UN and the Congolese government started to disarm and reintegrate ex-combatants in Ituri. Delays and a slow disarmament, demobilization, reintegration, and rehabilitation process, however, led to the remobilization of militias and widespread insecurity, according to the UN Office for the Coordination of Humanitarian Affairs (OCHA).[47] Still, some 10,000 combatants, 3,000 of them children, had put down their weapons as of April 2005, either voluntarily or by force.[48] One of the biggest clashes involving MONUC troops in eastern Congo occurred in early March 2005, when peacekeepers killed at least 50 militiamen a few days after nine Bangladeshi UN troops were killed in an ambush in Ituri.

While Congolese living near the borders easily crossed into neighboring countries to become refugees, most were not so lucky and they were forced to live with different host communities or hide in forests in the DRC. Following massive influxes of people, IDP camps were set up, particularly in Ituri, North Kivu and Katanga. The latest IDP estimate from OCHA is some 2.3 million Congolese. This figure is to be taken with caution, as the IDP estimates of several provinces have not been updated since 2003, and while new IDPs figures are usually added, those IDPs who return are not always taken off the lists. About 95 percent of IDPs are in six provinces: Orientale, North Kivu, South Kivu, Maniema, Equateur, and Katanga.[49] While some returned, many others were displaced in 2005.

From mid-2003 to mid-2005, according to OCHA, an estimated 900,000 IDPs returned to their homes in eastern DRC, particularly in the provinces of Ituri, Maniema, Katanga, and the Kivus, (OCHA UN Office Reports). Most of them returned home with little or no assistance. As earlier noted, the pace of returning slowed down in the second half of 2004, due to heightened insecurity in eastern DRC.

Hundreds of thousands were displaced in the region in the first half of 2005. From the end of December 2004 to March 2005, some 100,000 ethnic Hema Congolese fled the attacks of ethnic Lendu militias in Djugu, a territory to the north of Ituri's main town, Bunia. Over 80,000 of them are now living in IDP camps. During their attacks, Lendu militias burnt down homes, looted food and animals, and destroyed crops that were growing in the fields.[50] UN observers and NGOs reported that the Lendu militias' objective was to change the ethnic composition of Djugu.[51]

Mai Mai militias continued to destabilize eastern DRC, despite having signed an agreement that incorporates them into the new national integrated army. In May 2005, for example, at least 1,700 people fled attacks by Mai Mai in Katanga Province, during which the militias raped women and girls and burnt houses.[52]

In June 2005, members of the Congolese army caused the displacement of 190 families from villages, of at least five people per family, close to Bukavu, South Kivu Province, following looting, extra-judicial executions, and rapes. In the same month, the Congolese army, supported by the Rwandan Hutu militia FDLR, caused the displacement of populations in Bukavu, South Kivu, during fighting against another Hutu group called Rastas.[53] The FDLR signed an agreement at the end of March 2005, under which it would demobilize and return to Rwanda, but it continued to attack civilians nevertheless, causing the displacement of thousands in North and South Kivu.[54] In July 2005, the UN Security Council reported and condemned the massacre of some 50 people, most of them women and children, who were reported to have been burnt alive by Hutu militias in South Kivu.[55] Following this gruesome event, many took to their heels into the bush. The International Rescue Committee estimates that 3.8 million people have died, while about 10 million became internally displaced because of the war since 1998.[56]

PHYSICAL SECURITY

The protection of the displaced and other civilians remains a serious concern throughout the DRC, particularly in the Kivus, Katanga, Maniema and Ituri. In June 2005, the UN Inter-Agency, Internal Displacement Division reported continuing widespread human rights violations by armed groups, including killings, rape, sexual exploitation, abductions, forcible conscription of children, looting, plundering of crops, illegal taxation and general harassment of civilians. It also said that the illegal exploitation of natural resources (gold and diamonds), and the smuggling of goods and weapons, added to the violence.[57]

Rape has been used extensively as a weapon of war by virtually all the forces involved in the conflict.[58] Soldiers and rebel fighters have engaged in acts of sexual violence in the context of fighting, to attack the fundamental values of the community, to scare the civilian population into submission, to punish them for allegedly supporting enemy forces or to provide gratification for the fighters.[59] Thousands of women have also been abducted and kept as slaves in the militias' camps to provide sexual, domestic, and agricultural services. Often, the combatants seize the women's clothes so that they cannot run away.[60] From 1998 to 2004, according to a World Health Organization representative, over 40,000 women were raped in eastern DRC alone.[61] In July 2004, the UN reported that 70 percent of the women interviewed in the town of Kalemie, Katanga Province, and in neighboring IDP, camps had been victims of rape.[62] In the first half of 2005, armed militia raped over 200 women and girls in Walungu territory, South Kivu.[63] Men and boys in increasing numbers are also reporting having been sexually assaulted by combatants.[64] The UN agency, UNIFEM also denounced sexual mutilation and cannibalism by various armed groups against Pygmy women.[65] Members of the MONUC peacekeeping force have also committed abuses against displaced women and girls. The highly publicized scandal over UN peacekeepers and child prostitution led to an investigation by the UN Office of Internal Oversight Services. The office identified a pattern of sexual exploitation by uniformed personnel involving women and girls and asked the concerned troop-contributing countries to take swift disciplinary action. In a report to the UN Security Council, the UN Secretary-General noted that the reputation of MONUC had been severely damaged by acts of sexual exploitation and abuse committed by some peacekeepers against the local population.[66]

Many displaced children have been forcefully conscripted into the ranks of the armed groups. Although the total number of children associated with the armed forces and groups is unascertainable, estimates vary from 20,000 to 40,000.[67] In 2003, *Save the Children Alliance* claimed that it was difficult to escape the impression that the town of Bunia, Ituri District, had been taken over by children, who were used by local militias to terrorize its residents.[68] According to UNICEF, by mid-2005, at least 3,000 children were still in the hands of militias in Ituri and an even greater number remained in armed groups in the rest of the country. Girls too are recruited, and often suffer both sexual abuse and forced labor, (Save the Children Fund, 2003). Up to 12,500 girls were estimated to be in armed groups as of early 2005.[69]

HUMANITARIAN CONDITIONS

Despite the establishment of the Transition Government, civilians continue to live in crisis conditions in many parts of the DRC. Millions lack access to basic infrastructure (health centers, schools and roads), potable water, food, seeds, tools, clothes and straw to build houses. With the DRC's healthcare structures collapsing, displaced people are particularly vulnerable to infectious diseases. In Maniema Province, for example, 80 percent of healthcare structures have been destroyed during the fighting or in subsequent looting.[70] In Ituri, over a thousand people were believed to have caught the Bubonic Plague in 2004. A DRC Health Ministry official attributed the upsurge to incessant population displacements caused by the continued fighting between rebel groups.[71] Also in Ituri, overcrowding and poor sanitation were killing some 25 IDPs every day in just one camp in early 2005.[72] In March and April 2005, aid workers were unable, due to insecurity, to reach thousands of the displaced in camps in Ituri, where cholera had broken out.[73] Displaced people are also disproportionately exposed to HIV/AIDS infection, as they usually lack the means to protect themselves and do not have information about its transmission. In eastern provinces, up to 20 percent of the population may be infected with HIV.[74]

The displacement of farmers, the burning of fields and food stocks, and the destruction of infrastructure has caused widespread malnutrition in eastern DRC, an area with considerable agricultural potential. According to the UN, an estimated 1.9 million children suffered from acute malnutrition as of mid-2004.[75] *Save the Children Alliance* also reported that in the first four months of 2005, 59,000 children died as a direct and indirect result of the conflict in the DRC, the vast majority of them from easily preventable and curable causes such as diarrhea, malnutrition, and malaria.[76] Without food, medicines, and shelter, displaced people have also been denied a range of other essentials. Few attend school in the current war-damaged education system, reducing their prospects for a more secure future. Only

40 percent of children in eastern DRC are enrolled in school, and in some areas, such as in North Kivu, only a third of girls go to school.[77]

INADEQUATE RESPONSE TO THE NEEDS OF IDPS AND RETURNEES

At the national level, both the Ministry for Solidarity and Humanitarian Affairs and the Ministry for Social Affairs have responsibility for responding to the needs of IDPs. While the first focuses on protection and assistance during displacement, the second is the focal point for return.[78] Other ministries also have some responsibilities towards IDPs, which complicates their coordination.[79]

In November 2004, the UN Secretary-General appointed Ross Mountain, a national of New Zealand, as his Deputy Special Representative for the DRC. In this capacity, he also serves as Resident Coordinator and Humanitarian Coordinator for the DRC and is responsible for ensuring a strategic and coordinated response to internal displacement in the country.[80]

UN agencies, national and international NGOs and the ICRC are providing IDPs with food and non-food items, seeds and tools, health care, and emergency education. However, according to the Internal Displacement Division, while a number of agencies are involved in activities related to return and reintegration, there is yet no overall strategic framework. As a result, in most cases humanitarian and development actors operate in separate worlds.[81]

Humanitarian activities related to the return of IDPs have, up to now, been focused on transport assistance and the distribution of return packages, mainly because of lack of funding for other projects, such as the rebuilding of infrastructure and basic services in return areas. In 2005, the UNDP, in partnership with the Congolese Ministry of Social Affairs, launched a Pilot Project on Return and Reintegration of IDPs in the DRC. Close to 1,600 IDPs were helped to return to their villages in Equateur and Orientale Provinces.[82] The project, according to the Internal Displacement Division, demonstrated that many IDPs in the DRC are ready to return to their homes if minimal support is provided. It also showed that for returns to be sustainable, improved collaboration between a wide range of government authorities, humanitarian and development organizations is needed.

The worsening security situation since mid-2004 slowed down assistance to IDPs, particularly in Ituri. Armed groups in Ituri killed several peacekeepers, and repeatedly attacked, looted and took hostage humanitarian staff operating in that region.[83] In June 2005, several humanitarian

NGOs suspended their assistance activities in certain part of Ituri, like the *Solidarity* in the IDP camp of Gina.[84] Other factors hampering the response to the needs of displaced people and returnees include the sheer size of the country, the absence of roads and the high degree of geographical dispersal of IDPs.

Funding has also been inadequate. In order to address this question, the DRC has been chosen as a pilot country for the *Good Humanitarian Donorship* initiative. Under this initiative, 18 donors have pledged to improve the flexibility of their financing, to provide funds based on need, to reinforce local capacities to prevent crises, to respond rapidly and to support the transition from emergency to development through appropriate funding.[85] Still, the level of funds committed to respond to the humanitarian needs of IDPs has remained disappointing. The 2004 UN Consolidated Appeal, which requested $163 million compared to $268 million for the 2003 Appeal, received just 73 percent of the requested funds. For 2005, the humanitarian community has requested some $185 million for essential life-saving assistance of which no more than 40 percent has been received.[86]

DISPLACEMENT IN THE FEDERAL REPUBLIC OF NIGERIA

In specific terms, Nigeria is, unarguably, the most populous nation in Africa. It has a population of between 100 and 120 million people and more than 350 ethnic groups. Given these, the nation is also saddled with a multiplicity of religious, ethnic, and political fault lines, which periodically erupt into violent conflicts.[87] These conflicts situations have created a sizeable yet fluctuating number of deaths and displacements, particularly since the return of democracy in 1999. Conservative estimates put the number of both the displaced and those who have lost dear ones or their lives in these conflicts since 1999 at about 10,000 (internally displaced) and 1,000 (dead) while some government figures stand at more than 50,000 (internally displaced) and 3,000 (dead) for central Plateau State alone.[88]

Prior to now, the various military regimes, most especially the rule of General Sanni Abacha (1993–98), kept the underlying tensions in check, and, since the attempted secession of the Eastern Region under the name of the Republic of Biafra in 1967, any separatist aspirations were brutally suppressed. Almost three decades after the civil war, Nigeria returned to a democratic rule with the election of President Olusegun Obasanjo in 1999. This opened up new opportunities for people to express their grievances and new areas of conflict were created by the competition for political spoils. The resulting rise in violent conflicts can be attributed to various factors, including: ethnic rivalry (as seen in Izon-Urhobo, OPC (Yoruba)-Hausa, etc conflicts), religious violence (generally between Christians and Muslims), land conflicts (Ife-Modakeke, Uhumuleri-Aguleri, the Mambilla Plateau, Adamawa-Gombe); conflicts related to the demarcation of administrative boundaries (Ife-Modakeke, Cross River-Akwa Ibom) and political elections (Kwara State, Delta State, Ondo State), and conflicts linked to oil production in the Niger Delta (Ogu-bolo in River State, Nembe in Bayelsa State; the Bakassi Boys and Egbesu Boys activities are notable examples of this kind of conflict).[89]

While some of these conflicts may appear to be caused by a single factor, such as religion or ethnicity, the reality in Nigeria is that their causes are usually more complex. For example, the introduction of the Islamic Sharia law in 12 of Nigeria's 36 States in recent years has caused tensions, but when Muslim and Christian groups in these parts of the country clashed, this has usually been caused by other factors, for example pressure on land or unequal access to social services, as seen in the Jos crisis has since daubed as Christian/Muslim and Hausa/Tiv conflicts. However, the polarization that follows is often along religious lines, and the conflict is easily stereotyped as a "religious war." The same dynamic is often observed with regard to "ethnic conflicts." Perhaps the most significant cause of violent conflict in Nigeria is the entrenched division, throughout the country, between people considered indigenous to an area, and those regarded as settlers.[90] Even though settlers may have lived in an area for hundreds of years, they are consistently discriminated against in terms of land ownership, control of commerce, jobs, and education. For example, in predominantly Christian Plateau State, the majority of "settlers" belong to the northern Hausa-Fulani ethnic group who, as nomads, gradually moved southwards as the expanding Sahara desert dried up their traditional grazing lands. The Hausa-Fulani Muslims have long complained that the predominantly Christian farmers steal their cattle and prevent them from grazing, whilst the farmers countered that the cattle encroached on their land. At the same time, there are indigenous Muslim ethnic groups who are fiercely opposed to the perceived expansionist tendencies of fellow Muslim Hausa-Fulanis.

"The crux of the problem is that a lot of people are coming to this part of the country and trying to stake a claim to land that is not rightfully theirs," notes Sheikh Yusuf Gomwalk, an Islamic scholar of the Jama'atu Nasril Islam organization in Jos, the Plateau State capital. "It is only the politicians who play the religious card," the cleric concludes.[91]

This argument is widely repeated in different areas of the country. "Whatever the historical justifications, the conflict is always and everywhere about access to scarce resources . . . Many observers in Nigeria believe that the roots of the violence across much of the country are not religious or cultural. They say the conflicts are created and stoked by politicians both at a local and national level who seek to gain advantage from social division . . . Once triggered, the violence has its own momentum."[92]

Conversely, major towns in northern Nigeria, such as Kano and Kaduna, have, in recent years, been the scenes for violent clashes between Muslims (again, mainly Hausa-Fulanis) and Christian minority populations, often considered "settlers" in these areas. The 2004 Plateau State crisis, which culminated in May 2004 in the massacre of several hundred Muslims by Christian militia in the town of Yelwa, in turn sparked deadly reprisals in Kano, where Muslims rampaged against the Christian minority. About 30 people were killed and some 10,000 people, mostly women and children, were displaced.[93]

In November 2002, more than 30,000 people may have been temporarily displaced during the "Miss World riots" in Kaduna.[94] Violent conflicts have also forced residents, mainly Hausas, of the commercial capital Lagos to flee. Even though Lagos is not geographically linked to the northern region, these two conflict areas are indirectly related as populations from both areas are involved. There have been several occasions in which violence in the north has triggered revenge/reprisal attacks in the South West (Lagos) and vice versa.[95] While the Hausa-Fulanis have been seen as the main perpetrators of violence in some of the conflicts in the North, the same group has equally been victims and targets when violence erupts in Lagos. Clashes in Lagos in October 2000 and February 2002 were both reported to have caused the displacement of between 3,000 and 5,000 people both out of Lagos and out of many Northern States.[96]

Displacement has also been closely linked with oil production in the southern Niger Delta. While environmental degradation and lack of benefits from oil revenues appear to have been a catalyst for many of the conflicts during the 1990s, the more recent transfer of money back to local communities has become a reason for violence. One reason for this paradox is that community development programs funded by the oil companies have made political positions increasingly attractive. Furthermore, the demarcation of new administrative boundaries and the creation of new political constituency areas have become, in many cases, the focus of violent disputes between communities, between different political parties and even between factions of the same party. The violence triggered by these disputes has frequently forced people in the oil-producing states to flee their homes, and want on destruction of property has occurred. In September 2004, it was reported that at least 6,000 people were displaced in several weeks of violence between local militia and security forces, as well as by in-fighting among ethnic militias.[97] Hundreds of foreign oil workers were evacuated after direct threats by the leader of the Niger Delta People's Volunteer Force, Asari Dokubo. Amnesty International reported that between January and August 2004, between 670 and 1000 people had been killed in the Niger-Delta region.[98]

LESSONS FROM THE DR CONGO AND NIGERIA

It is important to state that from the two examples here considered, two important points must be noted i.e. institutional responses and treatment of the displaced persons. Institutional responses to displacement have always tilted towards the refugee alone. For instance, in Nigeria while there were two refugee camps (in Oru, Ogun State and Kano State respectively), there exists no institutional abode for the internally displaced. At best, the IDPs are usually quartered in Police/Army barracks, churches, mosques and with friends and relatives. In all these places, no adequate care is given and when the IDPs had to stay for more than a week, food and medical supplies soon thinned out and competition soon arose over these and other basic needs. As seen in the Jos crisis, the Tivs soon began to see the Jukuns as responsible for their economic woes and they were regarded as having 'over-stayed' their welcome and therefore were forced to return to their original state in Taraba. In the case of the DR Congo, it is on record that the peace process has been halted, as incessant crises broke out over the returnees (refugees and IDPs alike). In all the examples in the DR Congo, competition over land between the displaced people and those who remained often generated conflict as the displaced were considered as having left the country in a time of need and were therefore cowards not deserving of land or other resources.

In terms of the treatment received, efforts have been concentrated on the care and treatment of the refugees, and not until recently has attention been shifted in the direction of the IDPs—and even this, on an *ad hoc* basis. While the refugees are provided with basic life-saving infrastructure like health care centers, schools, vocational institutes and others, the IDPs are left to the mercy of the various charity groups who occasionally visit them, mostly on Fridays and Sundays. While records have shown that most IDPs are either in need of immediate medical attention, counseling services and/or life-support; these are usually beyond the meager facilities available to churches, mosques, and police/army barracks. In Nigeria, 500,000 people have recently been displaced because of the Jyllands-Posten cartoon in Denmark. Most of these Nigerians are today in churches, mosques and barracks and may remain in these places for the next year or more.

DISPLACEMENT IN AFRICA IN GENERAL

Displacement of people, whether within their countries of birth and habitual residence or in neighboring ones, is one of the most neglected, least reported, and most grossly misunderstood factors in conflict resurgence. Experiences from all over Africa have shown that displacement brought about crop-losses, as people who ought to till the soil are often forced to flee their farms for safety elsewhere. In most cases, when they get to these new places, they often have to contend with equally impoverished relatives and friends over scarce land and waterways in their bids to eke out a living. In Nigeria, the IDPs have to depend on relatives and friends for cultivable land (in Jos and Ile-Ife), waterways (in Niger-Delta), or pasture (Northern States). In most cases, the IDPs pose serious challenges to the hosts, who soon find out that the available resources are not enough to cater for the ever-increasing number of IDPs. The resultant situation gradually metamorphoses from joyful reception to regret and persecution, especially where the available resources are stretched thin, threatening food insecurity in the host communities.

The common result of this is that the hosts soon start to see the IDPs as unwanted guests, and, as the economic decline worsens, hatred soon boils over to open confrontation. As mutual trust becomes eroded, conflicts soon break out between the hosts and their guests. Where natural resources are involved, chances are good that conflicts tend to escalate as the hosts see the guests as encroaching on what rightly belongs to them.

In 1979, it was noted, "the number of refugees in Africa has increased rapidly during the past ten years, and African refugees pose today the largest refugee problem the world has to face."[99] Today, the refugee situation, one leg of the displacement problem in Africa, has increasingly assumed a disturbing dimension in terms of the number and composition of the persons involved,[100] the causes, and the limited success obtained thus far in the search for a permanent solution, (Beyer, 1981, 31). As earlier noted, the refugee problem is but one leg of the displacement problem, the other leg being those of the war and/or conflict who are internally displaced, numbering three to every refugee. Taken as a whole, Africa today is home to about 15 million refugees (out of the world's 27 million) and about 45 million internally displaced persons.[101]

In 1967, there were no more than a quarter of a million refugees and IDPs in Africa. However, by 1979, the figure had risen to 4 million. This deteriorating situation has been adduced to political crises that erupted in several African countries, notably DR Congo, formerly Zaire, Ethiopia, Somalia, Angola, Chad, and Uganda, as well as the liberation struggles in

Nigeria, Zimbabwe Namibia, and South Africa.[102] This disturbing escalatory trend in the total magnitude and occurrences of violent conflicts within societies in Africa continues, in spite of the much-orchestrated democratic experiment that was believed to hold the Midas touch for African peace and development.

Although it is extremely difficult to estimate the total number of the displaced persons in Africa, the enormity of the problem, no doubt, calls for emergency action, as, by the end of 1979, there were 56,000 Angolan refugees, 20,000 DR Congolese, 35,000 Namibians, and 1,000 from South Africa. The number of the internally displaced during this period was double the figure for the refugees, (Internal Displacement, 5). With increasing tension in Namibia and the racist regime in South Africa, the displaced population increased from a low of 10,000 at the end of 1977 to 40,000 by the end of 1980, 70,000 by the end of 1990 and a cumulative total of 45 million in 2005, (Internal Displacement, 5). Thousands of refugees flocked to Angola in the wake of the disturbances in the Shaba Province in DR Congo, though most have since returned home. Most of the refugees in Djibouti were Ethiopians. The number increased from 12,500 in 1978 to 14,500 in 1979 and by 1995, it had risen to 45,000. The estimated 12,000 refugees in Ethiopia in 1980 are mostly from the southern Sudan. In contrast, about 800,000 Ethiopians were displaced during the disturbances in the Ogaden; these now live in Somalia.[103] Conflicts in Ethiopia and in the Eritrea region have resulted in thousands of refugees fleeing to the Sudan.

Refugees in Kenya, numbering about 7,000 in 1980, consist mainly of Ugandans, Ethiopians and a few from Rwanda and Mozambique, (Aderanti, Dimension of the Refugee Problem). The nationalist struggle in Zimbabwe forced thousands of people to flee their places of habitual residence to neighboring countries as refugees. In 1975, an initial stream of 20,000 refugees entered Mozambique while about 65,000 or so Kenyans were scattered in different bushes and forests. By 1981, the number of both the refugees and the internally displaced persons in Kenya rose rapidly to about 120,000, and to about 160,000 by the end of the year, (Aderanti, Dimension of the Refugee Problem, 28). These refugees were settled in five organized camps.

The tension in the Horn of Africa between Ethiopia and Somalia, especially because of the war in the Ogaden region in early 1978, led to a large influx of refugees and internally displaced people, mainly of Somali origin. Government estimates for the number of the internally displaced and the Somali refugees are 1000,000 IDPs, and 650,000 registered refugees. About 800,000 unregistered people were said to be living with the local people and other nomads who continue to roam the country, (Aderanti, The Refugee Situation, 35).

Sudan, christened as 'a land of asylum for 400,000 refugees,'[104] has been receiving refugees from Ethiopia since the late 1960s, but with the increasing brutality of Idi Amin in Uganda, the number of refugees in Sudan rose from a low of 300,000 in 1980 to about 1.2million by 1985. By the end of that year, the number of registered refugees in Sudan stood at 40,000 Ugandans, 450,000 Ethiopians, 800,000 Chadians, and 8000 DR Congolese. Today, Sudan is again enmeshed in conflict, especially western region of Darfur, which has produced over a million deaths and an equal number of refugees while the IDPs were tentatively reckoned between 4 and 5 million people.[105]

The bulk of refugees in Tanzania are from Burundi. The struggle between the farmers and cattle herders in Burundi, which started in the late 1960s and early 1970s, climaxed in 1972; because many farmers fled to Tanzania where they now constitute about 500,000 of the estimated 800,000 refugees in that country, (Rogge and Akol, Reparation, 184–200). Moreover, there were about 30,000 Rwandese refugees at the beginning of 1979, and a total of 250,000 refugees in Tanzania, out of which about 6,000 Ugandans have since voluntarily returned home. By the end of 1980, the internally displaced in Uganda totaled about 650,000. The refugees in Uganda today include Rwandese (300,000), DR Congolese (100,000), and about 100,000 more from an assortment of African nations, (Beyer, 1981, 30). It must also be noted that the DR Congo received thousands of Angolan refugees prior to the latter's independence and, at this time, most of the refugees settled among the local people, especially in Bas-Zaire. A large number of Angolan refugees again entered the DR Congo between 1977 and 1982; the number consisted of 300,000 Angolans, 100,000 Ugandans, 30,000 Burundians, 40,000 Rwandese, and 10,000 Zambians, (Gould, 1974, 413).

The figure for the Southern Africa dramatically increased in Zambia between 1979 and 1983. Early in 1978, there were 80,700 refugees–mostly Angolans, Zimbabweans, South Africans, Namibians, and the DR Congolese. However, by the end of 1983, the number had fallen to 25,000 Zimbabweans, 26,000 Angolans, and 6,800 Namibians due to both voluntary and spontaneous repatriation. Botswana, Lesotho and Swaziland also received refugees continuously from South Africa, Zimbabwe and Namibia. Since 1977, over 50,000 refugees have entered Botswana, mainly en route Zambia. By mid-1978, there were more than 30,000 refugees, including 20,000 Zimbabweans. The number rose to 25,000 by the end of 1978, and to 28,500 a year later. The number of registered refugees in Swaziland totaled 10,500 by the end of 1980, (Gould, 1974, 414).

Other African countries host refugees to varying degrees. For examples, in Burundi, there are about 500,000 refugees, mainly Rwandese who fled Rwanda in the 1960s and during the genocide of more recent years. Nearly half of this number live in Bujumbura, the country's capital. Now, an estimated 1,000,000 refugees from Burundi live in Rwanda, while an almost equal number of Rwandan refugees reside in Burundi.[106] By 1980, an estimated 10,000 Senegalese, and 5,000 Chadian refugees had entered Nigeria and the Central African Republic, (Rogge and Akol, Reparation, 200). The number of refugees in Gabon, which had earlier stood at 50,000, dwindled to about 30,000 by the end of 1980 after the repatriation of about 30,000 from Equatorial Guinea, (Rogge and Akol 1989, 198). The latest wave of refugees and IDPs today are coming from Darfur and spreading like wildfire all through Africa.

As the various examples considered above have shown, no place in Africa is insulated against either the waves of IDPs or the burden of refugees. In fact, the situation today in Africa has become so complex that almost, if not every country in Africa, serves as both the countries of origin of refugees and IDPs as well as hosting them.

FACTORS LEADING TO DISPLACEMENT IN AFRICA

What are the factors responsible for so much displacement in Africa? Without gainsaying the facts, factors occasioning widespread displacement in Africa are many and multifarious, but the most talked about are conflicts and war. While several scholars have looked at the numerous factors and causes of conflicts and war in Africa, one aspect which has not received adequate attention, is the role of displacement, especially internal displacement.

Scholars and policy makers have identified, among other things, poverty and economic benefits accruing to both combatants and their counterparts-in-evil, the arms dealers, (Collier, 1999) as some of the major factors responsible for conflicts and war in Africa. Other factors considered include Africa's colonial heritage and the fact that the past colonial masters partitioned Africa among themselves and divided it into nation-states without considering Africa's various and unrelated ethnic cleavages, which today bedevil integration and peaceful coexistence.[107] In their inter-group relations, conflicts often arose among the various ethnic groups that make-up modern African states and, as new conflicts arise or escalate (as in Chad, Nigeria, etc) or as existing ones deteriorate (as in the Rwanda/Burundi, Somalia, Sudan, Ethiopia/Eritrea conflicts), the successive African elite often resort to the use of brute force and coercion (via the instrumentality of the Police and other state agencies), just like the colonial leaders before them.[108]

The resultant situation is even more exacerbated by the duo of the emerging world politics that polarized the entire world, and the autocratic, military dictatorship that took-over from the political elite after coups and counter-coups shortly after Africa's political independence. The implication is that Africa's fortune is in no way made better whether under the colonial administration, the African political elite, or the military. If anything, the military stifled opposition and opponents were treated as renegades. Some were hounded to death as others were cowed into silence. Following the fall of the Berlin Wall in 1989 and the end of the Cold War, world power support for autocratic government in Africa collapsed and military governance became an aberration. Africa was forced to democratize by the very forces that colonized, encouraged, and supported its militarization, and, from the 1990s; the continent began its third wave of democratic governance. In spite of this, armed conflict has become a major cause of displacement, death, and destruction of property in Africa.[109] The wave of armed confrontations in an increasing number of African countries is related mainly to increasing struggles for domination and contests over resources between persons or groups with religious, racial, ideological, or ethnic differences.

Chad offers a pertinent example of how struggles for leadership between groups or individuals in independent African states can snowball into a big crisis, (Aderanti, The Refugee Situation, 29–34). The fratricidal intransigence in Chad, which has claimed thousands of lives and made thousands more homeless, escalated initially in large part because of the struggle for leadership between the country's President and the Minister of Defense. The same situation had once played itself out in Nigeria, when personal squabbles between Gen. Yakubu Gowon and Gen. Odumegwu Ojukwu plunged the entire nation into a needless, costly, but avoidable civil war between 1967 and 1970.[110] Recall the clash of interests between the former Osun State governor, Chief Bisi Akande and his Deputy (now Senator) Chief Iyiola Omisore. Witness also the ongoing conflicts between Governor Chris Ngige and Chris Uba and the on-going one in Oyo State between the incumbent governor, Senator Rasheed Ladoja and Chief Ariyibi Adedibu, who was described by the president, Chief Olusegun Obasanjo as "the strongman of Ibadan politics."[111] As is frequently the case in such conflicts, external forces have complicated the confused situation, which involved about twelve factions in the case of Chad and many unknown forces in the case of Nigeria. In DR Congo, aside from the underground involvement of many actors, about nine African states were, at one time, involved in the conflict that ended to up to a million lives. In all these cases, properties worth billions of naira and countless number of lives were lost, as groups and individuals engaged one another in war.

In spite of the fact that this multitude of factors is responsible for conflicts and war in Africa, current literature is bedeviled with "the tyranny of the single-cause" syndrome. This is the tendency to explain a problem from the mono-causal perspective. In an essay titled "The Theoretical Deficit in the Study of War," Cusak reminds us that although "war remains a major social problem, it is reassuring to know that in the last few decades a significant number of political and other social scientists have devoted considerable effort to the study of its causes and consequences."[112] As if reporting the result of these "considerable efforts," Kalevi Holsti maintains, " . . . there is no single cause of a conflict. Nor is there any single precondition for sustainable peace. Different factors vary in importance, and reinforce or neutralize each other. The analysis of the situation must therefore include assessing the relative importance of the different indicators and their interrelationship."[113]

In fact, Holsti and Cusak are rebelling against the tyranny of the single-cause in the explanation of causes of both war and lower-level conflict. The same argument goes for displacement. This study represents an exception to the tyranny of the single-cause syndrome, which has dominated studies on causes of conflicts and violence in recent times. Nevertheless, the study does not lay claim to having found the "philosopher's stone" or the "magic formula," which, mechanically applied, will produce the desired result and thus substitute sustainable peace for the uncertainties and risks of conflict and war. Rather, the study, backed by extensive data, illuminates the role played by displacement, among other variables, in provoking conflict, conflict resurgence, and conflict escalation.

As already noted, conflict is one of the primary factors necessitating flight and displacements in Africa. September 1961 marked the beginning of an era in African history, as it was at this time that massive movements of refugees began in the continent.[114] While it is absolutely easier to date when refugee movement began in modern African history, it is difficult to state in precise terms when internal displacement of persons began in Africa. This is because of the fact that prior to the colonial intrusion, Africans have had one reason or the other to flee their places of habitual residence to find refuge in other lands. A good example of this case can be found among the Yoruba where a hundred year internecine war destroyed a whole civilization, the Old Oyo Empire, causing population dislocation and demographic change over the entirety of Yorubaland.[115]

During this period, the various Yoruba groups lived under their different kings and chiefs, and the entire Yoruba country was never considered as a nation-state. During the 100-year war, intra-ethnic displacement, i.e. the displacement of different peoples but with similar ethnic alliances, arose among the Yoruba ethnic group resulting from the destruction of the Old Oyo Empire, with the Oyo Yoruba people fleeing to other Yoruba towns and villages like Osogbo, Ile-Ife, Ogbomoso, etc. They were to dominate and change the ethnic mix of Osogbo, the Ijesha town, to that of Oyo. Those who fled to Ile-Ife and who were later named the Modakeke went through what Samuel Johnson described as "untold mystery of the refugees," the mystery that remains until today in the Ife-Modakeke conflicts of the past two centuries. The numerous wars of Shaka Zulu of South Africa, the Buganda and Bunyoro wars in Uganda, etc., produced intra-ethnic displacement, i.e. the displacement of people of different ethnic backgrounds to territories claimed by other ethnic groups.

From this African experience, intra-ethnic displacement is synonymous with the current IDP situation in modern Africa while inter-ethnic displacement is synonymous with the current refugee situation. In colonial Africa, measures were taken to integrate the displaced into the socio-political and economic fabric of the host society. In some cases, for example, in Osogbo-Nigeria, hosts have capitulated, yielding places to the displaced. In some other cases, displacement and re-integration have led to conflict and war.

Displacement, be it intra-ethnic or inter-ethnic, as noted above, is not a new thing to Africans, as conflicts and war have led to population dislocation during both the pre-colonial and colonial periods. However, internal displacement, as currently understood by the United Nations, donor, and international agencies, is novel to Africans. The precise dating of when internal displacement began in Africa can be traced to the experience of Rwanda, where the first case occurred in 1961. Despite this, Africa experienced the first refugee problem when several thousand refugees crossed the border from Rwanda to Tanzania to escape the ravaging civil war. In this particular case, as with nations like the DR Congo (1960–77), Sudan (1970s and 1980s), Angola (1977–78), Somalia (1970s), Ethiopia (1979), Eritrea (1979), Chad (1960s and 70s), Nigeria (1967–69), and other African countries, conflicts and wars arising from factors as diverse as agitation over mineral resources, competition over land, waterways, boundaries, etc., was the major cause of the influx of refugees and internal displacement.[116]

In the mid-1970s, oppression, characteristic of the foreign-dominated areas of Africa, especially in Zimbabwe (then Rhodesia), Mozambique, Angola, Namibia, and South Africa (all in southern Africa), and Guinea Bissau in West Africa, was a major cause of population dislocation, (Aderanti, Dimension of the Refugee Problem in Africa). Sadly enough, the attainment of independence in these countries, instead of solving this problem, in some cases exacerbated it, as in the case of the civil war in Angola (1977–78) and the DR Congo's Shaba Province (1977); the boundary disputes between Somalia and Ethiopia; the oppressive regime of Idi Amin in Uganda, secessionist moves in Ethiopia's Eritrea; fratricidal civil war in Chad, the Biafra's secessionist bid in Nigeria; and scores of pro-democracy activists, which forced many Nigerians to flee during the Sanni Abacha era in Nigeria, to mention a few examples.

Another factor is natural disaster, such as famine,[117] drought,[118] fire,[119] Tsunami,[120] hurricanes,[121] etc. In Ethiopia, for example, famine and drought intermixed with war in both Eritrea and the Ogaden province to produce about two and a half million displaced persons inside the country. This led in turn to the destruction of homes, food reserves, grazing land in Sidiamo, Bale, and Harrarghe regions, while close to an estimated two million people fled as refugees to Somalia, Sudan, Kenya, Uganda, and Djibouti, (Aderanti, The Refugee Situation, 32). Another example worth mentioning here is the Somali shortage of water and the deterioration of existing water supplies because of the prolonged drought of 1980. Nigeria, in a similar manner, received thousands of refugees from Niger Republic in 2005.[122] Several other West African countries became producers of refugees and displaced persons as locust invasion and drought made their nations uninhabitable and their people had to negotiate with their feet, (OCHA, The Eight Plague).

In all these examples, many people either were forced by circumstances of war, civil conflict, natural disaster, and other human-rights-threatening situations to relocate from their place of habitual residence, to seek refuge in other places in their countries of birth or to cross international boundaries to other nations as refugees. As noted already, when civil war broke out in Rwanda in 1961, millions of Rwandese were displaced within the borders of their country while thousands were forced to seek refugee in Tanzania. An estimated 40,000 Rwandese refugees were said to be in Tanzania, while about 150,000 were believed to have been displaced within Rwanda, (Aderanti, Dimension of the Refugee Problem in Africa). As noted by D'Souza, "the Horn of Africa is no longer in the headlines, but it indisputably remains the area with one of the largest refugee populations in the world."[123] With about 1.3 million refugees and about 5 million internally displaced persons in the area in 1980, Africa's share of refugee and displacement problems is undoubtedly the largest and fastest growing in the world today.[124] In 1967, there were not more than 750,000 refugees with a little above 1 million internally displaced persons.[125] The number rose to 1 million refugees and about 3 million IDPs in 1975, 3.7 million refugees and 10 million IDPs in 1977, 4 million refugees and about 15million IDPs in 1980, 5 million refugees and about 16 million IDPs in 1981, (UNHCR, *The Last Ten Years*, 4). Today, Africa is home to about 35 or 45 million refugees, with IDP populations tripling the figure for refugees.[126]

DIMENSIONS OF DISPLACEMENT IN AFRICA

A rather curious dimension to the displacement problem in Africa is the gender-age factor. D'Souza, earlier quoted, states, "more than 50 percent of all refugees are children and young people of school age; four-fifths come from developing countries," (D'Souza, 7). The Global IDP Project informs us that most internally displaced persons, like the refugees, are women and children of between age 6 months and 15 years. This age and sex-composition reflects the prevailing demographic structure in developing countries where about one-half of the population consists of children under school age. It is also associated with the major causes of displacement in Africa, which, in recent years, are related to war and conflict within sovereign states.

As noted by Adepoju, data on the demographic characteristics of the displaced persons, especially their age, sex-composition, education, and skills is severely limited, (Aderanti, Dimension of the Refugee Problem in Africa, 22). As also noted by Joshua Dariye, Governor of Plateau State, Nigeria, figures are in most cases exaggerated and there were a few basic generalizations from reports even from organizations like the United Nations High Commissioner for Refugees, the news media, and various other sources, especially in Africa where no conscious effort was made to register both the refugees and the IDPs.[127] In spite of this, there appears to be a consensus, especially when one visits refugee camps and displaced people's settlements, that the majority of the displaced persons are indeed women and children, (Norwegian Refugee Council, 6). It should be noted, however, that the age-sex composition might as well be slightly biased, as women and children constitute the most needy among the internally displaced and refugees in these camps, and therefore of the greatest concern to these international organizations and bodies.

In the major centers of conflict in Africa, notably Sudan, Somalia, Rwanda, Burundi, Liberia, Ivory Coast, DR Congo, Ethiopia, Eritrea, etc., the majority of refugees and the IDPs were women and children. In Somalia, and Burundi, for instance, more than 75 percent of the families there have female heads.[128] In the Sudan, of the estimated 4 million refugees and about 10 million IDPs, 45 percent were women and girls; 60 percent were children, (D'Souza, 8). In Swaziland, where refugees from

South Africa during the apartheid era congregated, more than 50 percent of the estimated 8,000 were women and girls, (Aderanti, Dimension of the Refugee Problem, 31). Also in Tanzania, 19,000 or 51 percent of the 37,000 refugees in Mishamo Camp were women and girls while 25 percent of the entire refugee populations have women as family heads, (Patterson, 2003, 30).

One other feature of displacement situations in Africa is the predominance of children under age 15. In general, between 40 and 60 percent of the displaced in Africa consist of children under age 15, (Machel, 2004, 73). In Sudan, more than 50 percent from Darfur are children; indeed, as of 1979 in Botswana, children make up more than 60 percent of the population in refugee camps at Francistown and Selebi Pikine, (Gould, 1974, 422). In Somalia, 80 percent of the total population of the displaced were children under age 14, (Gould, 1974, 426). The situation is the same in other African countries like Nigeria, where more than 5000 refugees were airlifted to the Republic of Benin during the civil war, (Norwegian Refugee Council, 26). Of this figure, more than 80 percent were children. The same applies to Burundi, Rwanda, DR Congo, Djibouti, etc, (Gould, 1974, 435).

While explaining this age-sex composition, the UNHCR notes, "Since armed conflicts are often the cause of their flight, the children escape while the men (and in some cases, the women) are killed, imprisoned, or stay behind to fight," (Vincent, 1999, 48). As noted by Albert, women and children are now deliberate targets of hostilities by combatants; hence, they are the most hit whenever conflicts snowball into full-scale war, (Albert, 2002, 5). Most families, having realized this, have previously sent their families, mostly women and children, to cross the borders or flee to neighbors and friends in other parts of the country, which were believed to be insulated from the war for one reason or another.[129] For instance, in Chad, the combatants encouraged their families to cross over to Sudan and settle with friends and relatives; they later visit their wives and children there. The situation in Zimbabwe and South Africa is similar to this. Although the age-sex composition is startling, this is not to say that the displaced are mainly women and children, as the law of war pays no respect to sex, age or name.

The situation of this vulnerable group is better encapsulated by the UNHCR in "The Refugee Child" as follows:

> Refugee children are an especially vulnerable group both physically and psychologically. The constant stress of separation, the exhaustion of travel during and after the refugees' escape, the initial residence in

> cramped, overcrowded condition enhances the spread of epidemics . . . Psychological problems greatly enhance the vulnerability of refugee children to the vicissitudes of life. They start-off with a significant disadvantage. They are doubly dependent: dependent on life, nourishment, and sustenance on parents or other adults who are themselves dependent on the protection and assistance of others. It is not difficult to imagine the traumatic effect on a young child of an abrupt uprooting from a place he has always called home; of flight, often preceded or accompanied by violence, of being thrust into a new, unfamiliar environment . . . These psychological problems are further complicated by a breakdown in communication between refugee parents and their children, and a resulting alienation, which may be exacerbated by the parent's attachment to the home country conflicting with the children's speedier adaptation to conditions in their new world . . . [130]

The circumstances and processes of flight from home could be as devastating as the living conditions at the place of refuge. This is lucidly described in a 1981 article in *Refugee*; "Some leave their homes accompanied by parents, usually mothers, others get separated from relatives during long and often hazardous journeys, while still others depart alone or are dispatched to provide a human anchor for their families to join them later . . . Child refugees represent a particularly vulnerable and unhappy minority in need not only of food, shelter and education, but succor to help them overcome the emotional deprivations and physical abuse experienced by so many."[131]

Equally important is the fact that the situation of a displaced woman has a multiplier effect on the displaced people in general. This is so because what affects the woman, affects the rest of her family, especially the children. In spite of the displaced situation in which the women might find themselves, they are still expected to perform their various roles to care for children, fetch firewood and water, etc. In an unfamiliar terrain, especially where the land is awash with landmines, as is the case in most African countries, these tasks expose her to needless but costly risks, while at the same time they impose additional strains on her and her household.

To situate this and other problems related to displacement situation in Africa, the study will consider two examples of displacement problems. The first example is that of the Democratic Republic of Congo, which has been described as Africa's First World War, (Lind and Sturman, 2002, 2) while the second considers the Federal Republic of Nigeria, which experienced a 4-year civil war followed by long years of internal crisis. It is instructive to note that, at one time or the other, almost all African countries have witnessed internal and inter-state conflict. Some have experienced limited internal peace; for example Nigeria, when compared with other African nations. The reason mostly adduced to this situation is the plural nature of African societies, which has the in-built mechanism of producing war, internal strife, and socio-political and religio-economic conflict.

DISPLACEMENT AND ITS IMPLICATIONS FOR NATIONAL SECURITY IN AFRICA

Just like security in general, the concept of national security is a fluid one whose conceptualization changes in accordance with the social, economic and political transformation of a society. Nwolise made a distinction between the old, traditionalist conceptualization of security and the new, more inclusive one. A critical look at the concept of security examined above shows that it would be better to look at national security from different perspective in order to gain an informed view of the concept.

We live in an era when national security is considered a highly ambiguous interdisciplinary research item, and gradually it is becoming an issue of global concern. The focus on security is shifting towards the individual from the old state-centered definition. There are emerging efforts in reshaping and reappraising the security sector. Such efforts relate to the question of who should be a target of security reforms and for what. This could translate to the question of the implications of displacement on national security. Central to this security debate is the UNDP approach that focuses on health, economic, food, environmental, community and political threats,[132] while at the same time reiterating such questions as security for whom. Security for which values? Security from what threats? Security by what means?[133] Mahbub ul Haq[134] responded to the question of "security for whom" succinctly. He suggests that the world is "entering a new era of human security in which the entire concept of security will change dramatically." In this new conception, security will be equated with the "security of the individual, not just security of nations." Put differently, "security of people, not just security of territory." He went further by stating that, "we need to fashion a new concept of human security that is reflected in the lives of our people, not in the weapons of our country." In fashioning this new concept, we may ask ourselves, what values will we seek to protect? Although Haq is not explicit on this issue, clearly the prime values are individual safety and well-being in a broad sense. Whereas the traditional conception of security emphasizes territorial and political integrity as primary values that need to be protected, human security pertains above all to the safety and well being of "all people everywhere—in their homes, in their jobs, in their streets, in their communities and in their environment," (Haq, 1).

From the above, there is no gainsaying the fact that displacement is a security issue not only for Africa, but also for the rest of the world. The sheer number and total magnitude of displaced people in Africa either as refugees or IDPs indicates that Africa may as well be on the verge of structural collapse.

Before going into the negative implications of displacement on Africa, it is important to state that although displacement carries quite a lot of negative connotations, yet it has a few blessings in disguise, which must not escape the notice of this study. Whether in nations that have witnessed major conflicts like the DR Congo or those that have experienced relative peace like Nigeria, experiences of both the returnee IDPs and refugees have shown that as people move from one clime to another in search of safety from the vagaries of nature, pestilence and war, they move with their language, customs, culture, and economic activities. Therefore, these ideals are transported from one community to another, albeit indirectly. In the refugee camp at Oru, Ogun State, Nigeria; refugees from the West African countries of Liberia, Togo, Ivory Coast, and Sierra Leone who were quartered there introduced quite a lot of trade and trading activities to the local community. A good example of these trades includes hairdressing. Before the establishment of the refugee camp, the town was largely a sleepy town devoid of most modern facilities like regular electricity, good roads, pipe-borne water, and superstores. With the establishment of the refugee camp, most of these facilities became available and local markets developed in the area, thereby changing the economic activities and thereby the accruable revenue to the state. Of utmost importance in the development of Oru is the opening up of vocational centers, health clinics, passable roads and well-structured primary schools for the community.

The same is true of the refugee and IDPs camps in Orientale, North Kivu, South Kivu, Maniema, Equateur, Katanga and at the Ituri division in the DR Congo, where community schools, health centers, and a host of modern facilities hitherto unknown in these areas prior to the setting up of camps suddenly developed, which have revolutionized life in those areas.

In spite of these paradoxes of displacement, nothing is comparable to the evil of population dislocations caused by displacement. For instance, as of February 2004, the United Nations reported that over 45 million people in the world were either experiencing or recovering from conflict and that these millions of people were in dire need of food and other emergency humanitarian assistance.[135] Of this number, 48 percent were said to be refugees and internally displaced persons native to sub-Saharan Africa alone. In yet another report, an estimated refugee population from the Central and Great Lake Region stood at 1,267,700; 770,500 from East and the Horn of Africa, 245,100 from Southern Africa while the figure for West Africa stood at 465,100. By this, an estimated 2,748,400 refugees came from sub-Saharan Africa alone.

The estimated number of IDPs currently triples that of the refugees. In mid-2005, an estimated 2.3 million IDPs were said to be in the DR Congo alone. As the table below shows, there are 15,757,691 IDPs and 4,444,569 refugees in 23 African countries, whose total population stands at 51,701,000.[136]

Aside from the large number involved, the age-sex composition of people involved calls for serious concern. As noted by D'Souza more than 50 percent of both the refugees and the IDPs are women and children. In most parts of Africa, children and girls of school age, i.e. under the age of 15, constitute about 80 percent of people involved. This has considerable implications for the future development of Africa. As already noted, both the refugees and the IDP population everywhere in Africa are exposed to serious inhumane conditions like lack of food, clothing, and shelter. Where humanitarian assistance exists, it is, almost in all cases, inadequate; and where not, the displaced people settle for the meager ones provided by friends and relatives who are also in perpetual fear of death resulting from conflict and war.

One of the fundamental problems facing Africa today is food and nutrition insecurity. The brutal query in the mouths of the over 200 million people living in sub-Saharan Africa is how long will food and nutrition insecurity plague Africa? This teeming populations are victims of undernourishment and are increasingly hungry, scratching out a living of less than a dollar per day on subsistence farming in an area littered with landmines and lacerated by internal strife, conflict and war.

As Graça Machel had noted, aside from natural disasters, "Among the main reasons for food and nutrition insecurity in Africa are civil strife, which leads to refugees and internal displacement of people as well as economic disruptions; climate change, which has provoked droughts or floods; deforestation; and more recently, the impacts of HIV/AIDS on households and communities," (Machel, 2004, 70–74).

As already noted, conflicts and wars are the highest producers of displaced persons. While displacement has led to a number of problems, none has had more effect on Africans than missed crops. In countries-in-conflict, countries-out-of-conflicts, and countries that have experienced limited or no conflict, the problem of missed crops is common in Africa. In March 2003, most countries in areas of dense conflict have recorded a number of

TABLE 12-1: African Countries and their Estimated Refugees

AFRICAN COUNTRIES	ESTIMATED REFUGEES	ESTIMATED IDPs	ESTIMATED TOTAL POPULATION (IN MILLION)
Algeria	1,000,000	10,691	32,85
Senegal	8,332	5,000	11,65
Guinea	4,782	82,000	9,40
Liberia	335,467	450,000	3,28
Ivory Coast	23,655	500,000	18,15
Nigeria	23,888	200,000	131,53
Sudan	730,612	6,000,000	36,23
Congo	462,203	100,000	57,54
DR Congo	28,152	2,330,000	3,99
Eritrea	131,119	59,000	4,40
Ethiopia	63,105	132,000	77,43
Somalia	389,292	400,000	8,22
Kenya	3,847	360,000	34,25
Uganda	31,963	1,600,000	28,81
Rwanda	63,808	2,000,000	9,03
Burundi	485,764	170,000	7,5
Zimbabwe	9,568	150,000	13,01
Angola	228,838	340,000	15,94
Central African Republic	31,069	200,000	4,03
Liberia	335,467	66,000	3,28
Guinea Bissau	1,018	350,000	1,58
Sierra Leone	41,801	250,000	5,52
Togo	10,819	3,000	6,14
TOTAL	4,444,569	15,757,691	51,701,000,000

Sources: Figures for Refugee population are based on the United Nations' High Commissioner for Refugees report of June 2005. Those for the Internally Displaced Persons as well as population per country are obtained from the Internally Displaced Monitoring Center's Global IDP Project Report of August 25, 2005.

missed crop situations. For example, Sudan reported that 40,000 households have experienced missed opportunities either to plant or to harvest because of conflicts, wars, and displacement. Angola recorded a similar number. Rwanda, Burundi, Ivory Coast, Togo, and Niger, etc., have all recorded cases of loss of land, crops and vital life-saving activities during their respective conflicts. With over twenty years of conflicts in most countries in sub-Saharan Africa, food and nutrition crises are only a matter of time.

In Mozambique, Angola, DR Congo, Niger Republic, Sudan, the Congo, Sierra Leone, Madagascar, Central African Republic, Liberia, Somalia, Guinea, Angola, Cape Verde, Ethiopia, Eritrea, Kenya, Rwanda, and Burundi, (Machel, 2004, 72) over 50,000 square kilometers of land in each of these countries has remained uncultivated since the past ten years. Almost all this land may remain uncultivated in the next two decades or more. This is because when conflicts and wars are over and the arms are silent, landmines continue to kill, maim, and thereby prevent agricultural activities. In some of these nations, droughts, floods, and pest-invasion have made life even more brutish and short.

In another vein, Isatou Jallow of the National Nutrition Agency, The Gambia, noted that while slavery and colonialism underdeveloped Africa prior to now, "the lack of adequate food, the lack of adequate health services, inadequate caring practices, and an unsanitary environment, which combine to make up nutrition insecurity, are under-developing Africa now," (Machel, 2004, 18–21).

In the same paper, she also noted that one-third of African population live in abject poverty, as a direct consequence of conflicts and wars, which dried up food and water supplies. One-third of African countries are now living below the recommended calorie intake of 2,100 per diem. With 200 million people, i.e. 27 percent of African population, and almost 33 percent of sub-Saharan Africa's population, lacking access to the minimum amount of calories, Africa, in the next few years, may be facing the worst security crisis in recorded history.

As it is today, stunting, understood as low height-for-age, is gradually becoming a normal African phenomenon. Stunting is caused by chronic malnutrition and is an outcome and measure of nutrition insecurity prevalent in an area. However, this is not to say that all short people are malnourished. Stunting and being underweight are two indicators of inadequate access to food, health care, and a sanitary environment. They are therefore a two-pronged barometer to measure a nation's measure of socio-economic development and indicator for poverty reduction strategies.

In 1990, there were an estimated 32.8 million stunted children in Africa. This figure jumped to 45.1 million in 2000, and increased to 46.5 million by 2005. A breakdown of this figure reveals that North Africa, the region least disturbed by internal strife, conflicts and wars, has 6.2 million stunted children in 1999, 4.6 million in 2000, and 7 million in 2005. Southern Africa followed with 1.3 million in 1990, 1.5 million in 2000 but with a slight increase to about 2 million by 2005. For East Africa, the figure shows 12 million in 1999, 19.4 million in 2000, and 25 million in 2005. Central Africa has 4.5 million stunted children in 1999, 6.8 million in 2000, and 12 million in 2005. West Africa has an estimated 8.8 million stunted children in 1990, 12.7 million in 2000, and 20 million in 2005.[137] With an estimated 46.5 million stunted children with more than 65 percent being girls, Africa is no doubt facing the greatest security challenge since the slave trade era.

Where are these children and who are they? What are their names and where do they live? How does this affect you? How does this affect me? Answers to these and many more that the figures above may generate are better illustrated with concrete examples than explained in abstract terms.

It is common knowledge that a malnourished pregnant woman, with low-weight during the pregnancy, can only give birth to an equally malnourished, low-birth-weight child. Such a child, raised under similar circumstances that made the mother malnourished, is disadvantaged right from birth. The newborn grows into a stunted child with frequent infections, inadequate care, and inadequate health services. The child grows with reduced or low mental capacity to stunted adolescence with reduced physical labor capacity and low educational attainment. What are his or her chances? Africa is notable for its adolescent and teenage pregnancy; she probably gets pregnant and under the circumstance, gives birth to an equally low-birth-weight baby, and the cycle continues.

The implications here for Africa are ominous in that whatever the investment in education in Africa, malnourished schoolchildren stand no chance in life. If we invest in agriculture, increased agricultural productivity cannot be attained if we have malnourished farmers that have lowered productive capability. What chances do they stand? This, no doubt, is as a crucial factor in the underdevelopment of Africa.

As noted above, 65 percent of the displaced population in Africa are women, girls, and children. In fact, recent statistics from UNICEF reveal that 60 percent of the displaced in Africa, either as refugees or IDPs are girls between the age of 3 and 15, and that this population is currently facing serious threats of infection from various sexually transmitted diseases. Marda Mustapha and Aiah Gbakima told the story of a 16-year-old, Mary, a Sierra Leonean girl who not only witnessed the death of both parents in the hands of rebels but also lost her virginity when two of the armed men raped her. After her escape, the doctors told her she needed surgery and that she had contracted HIV.[138] The same was the story of Hawa, 17, who became pregnant through rape by combatants and was forced to become a rebel's wife. She was denied medication, forced to use cocaine, denied food, and became infected with a sexually transmitted disease, (Physician for Human Rights, 2002, 68).

Recent study has shown that conflicts and displacement facilitate the spread of HIV. It has also been argued that civil wars and conflicts account for much of the spread of HIV in Africa. This argument is buttressed by regression analysis that shows a strong correlation between wars, conflicts, and disease. Lynellyn Long shows how the phenomenon of sexual violence seems to be part of the pattern of civil conflict in Africa. She examines regional examples throughout sub-Saharan Africa and discovers that there seems to be a systematic perpetration of sexual violence against women and girls in particular. Studies have shown that there are two or more types of sexual violence perpetrated against females during wars, conflicts, and displacement, i.e. status or statutory rape and war-related sexual violence and rape.

By status or statutory rape, it means sexual violence, not necessarily rape, but sexual relations "condoned" and often "solicited" by women and girls in exchange for protection either by the combatants or by relief agencies and international forces, and this has been found rampant not only among combatants but also among donor agencies, relief workers, rebel forces, government armies, and international forces. From Sierra Leone to Rwanda, Burundi to Eritrea, Ethiopia to Nigeria, cases of such practices have been reported. According to the Associated Press, some of the victims that have opened up on this claimed, "If you escape death, you cannot escape rape. If you reject them, the soldiers will either maim you and afterward rape you or kill you after they have used you."[139]

Some IDPs also reveal to Associated Press, "Some girls said . . . it is better to love and survive than keep your pride and die of hunger. If you look at the need to survive during a civil war, you can conclude that a lot of girls were affected by the practice."

In "Our Bodies . . . Their Battleground,"[140] the Integrated Regional Information Networks reported that in all conflicts in Africa, sexual violence against women has become the new weapon of mass destruction. The women interviewed maintained that most of them were gang-raped in the presence of their families, husbands, and children. Some of the combatants interviewed revealed that sex is indeed a weapon to break the resolve to resistance and to instill fear in the mind of the populace.[141] This reasoning is premised on the ground that such practice would have traumatized, removed the will to resist, forced the people to flee, and made available to the combatants enough resources to carry on the war. Aside from committing sexual abuse against the mothers, their daughters, and, sometimes, infants as young as three years, the combatants sometimes either maim them or take them away to their camps as sex-slaves. Only one soldier so far, however, has been tried, found guilty, and jailed!

Most sexual violence, be it statutory or status rape or war-related sexual abuse, occurred in places and circumstances where medical facilities are hard to come by, nor were the victims screened for sexually transmitted infections. The likelihood of being infected during gang rape or unprotected/forced or induced sexual escapades increases dramatically, especially if the rapist is HIV positive.

The Associates for Global Change reported in 2000 that 36 of the 82 civilians working for the 176 Sierra Leonean soldiers during the conflicts and wars in the country tested positive for HIV. Of the 80 female soldiers in the contingent, 40 percent tested positive. In the same report, 89 percent of Nigerians that participated in the ECOMOG mission in the West African sub-region tested positive to HIV and about 50 percent of them had full-blown AIDS by 2000. This was reported in the two refugee camps in Nigeria, as well as in others in the Horn of Africa, the Great Lakes Region, and other parts of the continent. The inference from these figures are that these soldiers either engaged in unsafe sexual practice among themselves, with the workers assigned to them, or with the people they went there to protect.[142]

The above scenario directly points the way of the future for Africa. While conflicts and wars would provide teeming millions as refugees and IDPs, displacement will lead people away from their farms and make their land unsafe for cultivation, thereby leading to food and nutrition insecurity, which in turn would ensure a rapid decline in Africa's population. HIV/AIDS, for its part, will ensure that the rest of the active population is doomed through unsafe sex, mother-child transmission, and other accidental blood transfusions. This is the security imperative facing Africa today, and nowhere is insulated from its impact!

NOTES

1. This chapter would not have taken this shape if not for the invaluable assistance from my indefatigable student and assistant, Miss Ogunbowale Mopelola Oreoluwa of the Department of History and Strategic Studies, Redeemer's University, Nigeria, Saheed Aderinto of the Department of History, University

of Texas at Austin, USA; the Integrated Regional Information Network whose generous contributions to the study of Displacement is really commendable. I acknowledge here the three Documentaries sent by IRIN to enhance and widen my knowledge on the subject. The invaluable contribution of the Norwegian Refugee Council, especially the inexhaustible data available in their archives on Displacement is commendable.

2. T. R. Gurr and M. G. Marshall with D. Kholsa, *Peace and Conflict 2001: A Global Survey of Armed Conflicts, Self-Determination Movements and Democracy.* Center for International Development and Conflict Management (CIDCM), University of Maryland, 2000. The report can also be obtained in www.bsos.umd.edu/cidcm/peace.htm
3. Jao Gomes Porto, "Contemporary Conflict Analysis in Perspective" in Jeremy Lind and Sturman Kathryn (eds.) *Scarcity and Surfeit: The Ecology of Africa's Conflict.* African Centre for Technology Studies and Institute for Security Studies, South Africa, 2002, 1–9.
4. Works abound that discuss the causes of wars and conflicts in Africa. While some argue that conflicts in Africa deal largely with Africa's colonial past, some have argued that reasons as varied as political, economic, ethnic, religious etc account for conflicts in Africa. For economic factors, see Paul Collier, *"Doing Well Out of War," The World Bank*, April 1999; Paul Collier and Anke Hoeffler, *"Greed and Grievance in Civil War" The World Bank*, October 2001; Bartos Otornar and Paul Wehr, *Using Conflict Theory,* Cambridge University Press, Cambridge, UK, 2002. For works that discuss ethnicity as factors necessitating conflicts, see Charles P. Cozic (ed.) *Nationalism and Ethnic Conflict.* Greenhaven Press, Inc., 1994; H. B. Haruna, O.B.C. Nwolise, D. Oluyemi-Kusa, (eds.), *A Guide to Peace Education and Peace Promotion Strategies in Africa: The Nigerian Approach,* African Refugee Foundation (AREF), Lagos, Nigeria, 2003, Okpu Ugbana, "Ethnic Minority Problem in Nigerian Politics: 1960–1965., *Acta Universitastis Upsaliensis*, 1977, E.G. Osaghae, I. Toure, N. Kouame, I.O. Albert, Jinmi Adisa, (eds.) *Urban Violence in Africa*, Institut Francais de Recherche en Afrique (IFRA), Ibadan, 1994, etc. Ecological factor was considered by Jeremy Lind and Sturman Kathryn (eds.) Scarcity and Surfeit, *The Ecology of Africa's Conflict.* African Centre for Technology Studies and Institute for Security Studies, South Africa, 2002. etc.
5. I.O. Albert, "Child-Soldiers and Security Pitfalls in Africa" in *Africa Notes*, Nov/Dec., 2002, Institute for African Development, Cornell University, USA, 5–11.
6. Michael Renner, "Curbing the Proliferation of Small Arms," in *State of the World*, A Worldwatch Institute Report, 1998, 131–149.
7. The burden includes having to cater for the refugee population, IDPs, HIV/AIDS orphans, and cases of female-headed families that have become rampant in Africa today.
8. Graça Machel, *Mitigating, Preventing, and Ending Conflicts in Africa* in IFPRI, "Assuring Food and Nutrition Security in Africa by 2020: Prioritizing Actions, Strengthening Actors, and Facilitating Partnerships," International Food Policy Research Institute, Washington, DC, 2004, 70–74).

9. The two variable involved in the study of displacement are the refuges, which for the purpose of this study, the example of the Democratic Republic of Congo will suffice; and the Internally Displaced Persons, which the example of Nigeria represents.
10. Francis M. Deng, "The Guiding Principles on Internal Displacement," United Nations Document E/CN.4/1996/52 Add.2 of Dec. 1995.
11. Gunther Beyer, "The Political Refugee: 35 Years Later," in *International Migration Review*, Vol. 15, No. 1 / 2, *Refugee Today* (Spring—Summer, 1981), 26–34.
12. Intergovernmental Committee on Refugees, *International Organization,* Vol. 1, No. 2 (Jun., 1947), 382–383; hereafter cited in text as Intergovernmental Committee.
13. W. T. S. Gould, "Refugees in Tropical Africa," in *International Migration Review*, Vol.8 No.3, (Autumn, 1974), 413–430.
14. United Nations, Economic Commission for Africa (UNECA), "Report of the Conference on the Legal, Economic and Social Aspect of African Refugee Problems," Addis Ababa, (Document E/CN 14/442), 1969.
15. Evidence from different parts of Africa suggest that women-headed family are now on the increase and cases of kid-headed family have also tripled what obtained in the past.
16. Peace and Development Projects and Friedrich Ebert Stiftung Foundation, *Annual Report on Violent Conflicts in Nigeria, 2003,* Sot Print Productions, Lagos, Nigeria, 2004.
17. For the plethora of definitions of security, see http://www.webopedia.com/TERM/S/security.html.
18. Microsoft ® Encarta ® Reference Library 2005; 1993–2004 Microsoft Corporation.
19. http://www.its.bldrdoc.gov/fs-1037/dir-032/_4740.htm
20. Geoffrey D. Dabelko and David D. Dabelko, "Environmental Security: Issues of Conflict and Redefinition," in *Environmental Security Debates: An Introduction*, Woodrow Wilson Center, USA, Spring 1995, 3.
21. http://www.wordreference.com/definition/security.
22. Norman Myer, "Not Far Afield: US Interest and the Global Environment," World Resources Institute, Washington D.C., 1989; Michael Renner "National Security: The Economic and Environmental Dimension," Worldwatch Paper, No. 89, Worldwatch Institute, Washington, USA; Mische Patricia. "Ecological Security and the Need to Reconceptualize Sovereignty," *Alternatives* 14 (4): 389–427.
23. Adepoju Aderanti, "The Refugee Situation in the Horn of Africa and Sudan," In *Issue: A Journal of Opinion*, Vol. 12, No. 1 / 2, African Refugee and Human Rights (Spring—Summer, 1982, 31; hereafter cited in text as The Refugee Situation. See also, United Nations High Commissioner for Refugees (UNHCR), *Refugees, Geneva,* 1979, 64, Adepoju Aderanti, "The Dimension of the Refugee Problem in Africa" in *African Affairs*, Vol. 81, No. 322, January 1982; hereafter cited in text as Dimension of the Refugee Problem. Others include John R. Rogge and Joshua O. Akol, "Reparation: It's Role in Resolving Africa's Refugee Dilemma" *International Migration*

Review, Vol. 23, No. 2 (Summer, 1989), 184–200; Beyer, 1981, 30. See also Gould, 1974, 413.

24. Almost all works on Displacement, whether on refugees or the IDPs emphasize the fact that most of the displaced are women and children. The numbers reveal that more females, most girls with the age of 7 to 25 are involved. The implications of this are quite bad for Africa.
25. See among others, Albert, 2002.
26. O. O. Ibeanu, "Exiles in Their Own Home: Conflicts and Internal Population Displacement in Nigeria," in *Journal of Refugee Studies*, Oxford University Press, 1999; 12: 161–179.
27. Kole Ahmed Shettima, "Ecology, Identity, Developmentalism and Displacement in Northern Nigeria," in *Journal of Asian and African Studies*; 6/1/1997
28. Pat Ama Tokunbo Williams, "Religion, Violence and Displacement in Nigeria," in *Journal of Asian and African Studies*; 6/1/1997. For update on the displacement of Nigerians because of the Mohammed cartoon riots, see "The Comet," Vol.7, No. 2356, Feb 24, 2006.
29. Leo Dare, "Political Instability and Displacement in Nigeria," in *Journal of Asian and African Studies*; 6/1/1997.
30. Paul S. Orogun, "Crisis of Government, Ethnic Schisms, Civil War, and Regional Destabilization of the Democratic Republic of Congo," in *World Affairs*; 6/22/2002.
31. Esther van der Velde, "The Rights of Internally Displaced Children: Selected Field Practices from UNICEF's Experience," in *Refuge*; 2/1/2002.
32. *The Catastrophist* is Ronan Bennett's 1998 novel that takes place in an African milieu at a key historical moment of decolonization and of cynical neo-colonial manipulation. Set principally in 1959–60 in the then Belgian Congo, The Catastrophist (which appeared in the year of the Belfast Agreement) also contains, within its representation of international history, an important if tactically muted Irish sub-text. (1) The explicit mentions of Ireland are infrequent: Ireland's English question forms a partially submerged and barely spoken part of the book's thematic structure, which is shown in its staging of geopolitics and history, and clearly amounts to an anti-colonial proposition of a more general kind. My enquiry here concerns the way this proposition is inextricably bound up with the thinking and enactment of gender roles; does Bennett's critique of imperial and colonial modes of domination extend to their structural parallels in social, cultural, and psychological gendering? How do these gender representations, conceived during our contemporary "crisis of masculinity," relate to the book's concerns with international politics and colonial history, in whichever theatre that is played out? (2) Is there a homology or a contrast between Bennett's construction of gender relations and of black-white ones in Africa at the moment of decolonization?
33. Patricia J. Coughlan, "Does a Man Die at your Feet. . . . Gender, History, and Representation," in *The Catastrophist. (Critical Essay)* in *Irish University Review: A Journal of Irish Studies*; 9/22/2003.
34. The ranking was done by Machel, 2004, 71.

35. Norwegian Refugee Council and Global IDP Project, *Profile of Internal Displacement: Democratic Republic of the Congo, Global* IDP Project, Geneva, 2005, 7.
36. International Crisis Group, *The Congo Transition is Failing: Crisis in the Kivus,"* 30 March 2005
37. Integrated Regional Information Networks (IRIN), *Disarmament Launched in Ituri,* 3 September 2004; see also, Human Rights Watch (HRW), *The Curse of Gold: Democratic Republic of Congo,* 2 June 2005.
38. Amnesty International (AI), *Democratic Republic of Congo: Arming the East,* 5 July 2005.
39. Reuters, *DRC: Staging Congo Election, A Nightmare* 1 June 2005.
40. United Nations Security Council (UNSC), *Security Council Extends Mission in Democratic Republic Of Congo,* Resolution 1592 (2005), 30 March 2005.
41. Overseas Development Institute (ODI), Edward B. Rackely, *Predatory Governance in the DRC: Civilian Impact and Humanitarian Response,* Humanitarian Practice Network, 25 May 2005.
42. UNSC, *17th Report of the Secretary-General on the UN Mission in DR Congo*, 22 March 2005.
43. International Crisis Group (ICG), *The Congo Transition is Failing: Crisis in the Kivu,* 30 March 2005.
44. United State Agency for International Development (USAID), *DR Congo: Complex Emergency Situation Report,* No. 4, (FY 2004), 20 August 2004; see also, United Nations Organization Mission in the Democratic Republic of Congo (MONUC), "*RDC: La Situation humanitaire au Sud Kivu,"* 4 August 2004.
45. HRW, *DR Congo: War Crimes in Bukavu,* 12 June 2004.
46. HRW, *DR Congo: Fleeing Civilian Face Grave Risk,* 21 December 2004.
47. UN Office for the Coordination of Humanitarian Affairs (OCHA), *Consolidated Appeal Process (CAP): Mid-Year Review of Humanitarian Appeal for Great Lakes,* 23 June 2005.
48. OCHA, Monitoring de la Situation Humanitariare en RDC du 26 Mars au ler Avril 2005; see also, Agence France-Presse (AFP), DR Congo Militia Killed in Sweep, 19 April 2005.
49. OCHA, *UN Office Reports Disruption of Humanitarian Aid in DR Congo*, 8 June 2005; hereafter cited in text as OCHA UN Office Reports.
50. IRIN, *DRC: Insecurity Increases Food Shortages in Ituri,* 4 April 2005
51. IRIN, *DRC: Ituri Militia Take War to Civilian,* 23 March 2005.
52. IRIN, *DRC: Mayi-Mayi Attacks Displace 1, 700 in Katanga,* 8 June 2005.
53. OCHA, *Inter-Agency Internal Displacement Division (IDD) Mission to the Democratic Republic of Congo*, 7 June 2005.
54. MONUC, *RDC: La Situation humanitaire au Sud Kivu*, 13 June 2005.
55. UNSC, *Security Council, in Presidential Statement, Condemns Massacre of Women, Children in DR Congo*, 13 July 2005.

56. International Rescue Committee (IRC), *Mortality in Democratic Republic of Congo: Result from a Nationwide Survey,* 8 December 2004.
57. OCHA, *Inter-Agency Internal Displacement Division (IDD) Mission to the Democratic Republic of Congo,* 7 June 2005.
58. AI, *DR Congo: Addressing the Present and Building a Future,* 27 November 2003
59. AI, *Democratic Republic of Congo: Mass Rape- Time For Remedy,,* 26 October 2004
60. International Alert & al., *Women's Body as a Battleground: Sexual Violence against Women and Girls During War in the Democratic Republic of Congo South Kivu (1996–2003),* 2005.
61. IRIN, *DRC: Focus on Rampant Rape, despite end of War,* 8 March 2004.
62. OCHA, *Humanitarian Situation in DRC Monthly Update,* 31 July 2004.
63. OCHA, *DR Congo: OCHA Condemns Attacks on Civilian in Nindja,* 31 May 2005.
64. HRW, *Seeking Justice: The Prosecution of Sexual Violence in the Congo War,* 7 March 2005.
65. United Nations News Service, "Thousands of Women Assaulted; new fighting in Eastern DR of Congo," 4 November 2003.
66. UNSC, "17th Report," *22 March 2005, cited above.*
67. United Nations International Children Education Funds (UNICEF), Monthly Report of 7 May 2004.
68. Save the Children Fund (SCF-UK), *DRC: Has Burnia been taken over by Children?,* 9 June 2003.
69. Save the Children Alliance, *Forgotten Causalities of War: Girls in Armed Conflict,* 25 April 2005.
70. OCHA, *Monitoring de la situation humanitaire en RDC du 27 Decembre 2003 au Janvier,* 2004.
71. IRIN, *DRC: Suspected Plague Kills 58 in Ituri,* 29 July 2004
72. Reuters, *Two Dozen Die in Crowded Congo Camp Everyday,* 23 March 2005
73. IRIN, *DRC: Cholera Strikes IDP in Tche,* 22 April 2005
74. IRIN, *HIV/AIDS Prevalence 20 percent in Certain Region ,* 5 November 2003.
75. UNICEF, *UNICEF Humanitarian Action: Democratic Republic of Congo,* 7 May 2004.
76. Save the Children Alliance, *The True Face of War in DR Congo,* 27 April 2005.
77. UNICEF, *Conflict in Eastern DR Congo has Forced Millions to Flee Homes,* 16 December 2004.
78. OCHA, Email conversation with the Humanitarian Affairs Officer, DRC, 23 September 2004.
79. OCHA, *Inter-Agency Internal Displacement Division (IDD) Mission to the Democratic Republic of Congo,* 8 June 2005.
80. United Nations Secretary-General (UN SG), *Ross Mountain appointed Deputy Special Representative of Secretary General for Democratic Republic of Congo,* 18 November 2004.

81. OCHA, *Inter-Agency Internal Displacement Division (IDD) Mission to the Democratic Republic of Congo,* 8 June 2005.
82. IRIN, *Ituri: Militias take War to Civilians,* 23 May 2005.
83. Medair, *Repeated Violence against Humanitarian Organizations: Medair Protests by Reducing Its Activities in the Congo,* 17 June 2005.
84. Solidarites, *Solidarites: Tens of Thousands of People at Significant Risk in Gina, Dr Congo,* 19 July 2005.
85. OCHA, *Humanitarian Situation in DRC Monthly Update, 31* July 2004.
86. UNSC, *17th Report of the Secretary-General on the UN Mission in DR Congo,* 22 March 2005.
87. Tamuno N. Tekena, *Peace and Violence in Nigeria,* a Publication of the Panel on Nigeria Since Independence History Project, University of Ibadan, Nigeria, pp. xv-xvi.
88. British Broadcasting Corporations (BBC), News Bulleting *Nigerian Clashes: 50, 000 Killed,* 7 October 2004.
89. Peace and Development Projects and Friedrich Ebert Stiftung Foundation, *Annual Report on Violent Conflicts in Nigeria, 2003,* Sot Print Productions, Lagos, Nigeria, 2004.
90. Conflicts of this kind are commonplace in Nigeria. See also, Peace and Development Projects and Friedrich Ebert Stiftung Foundation, *Annual Report on Violent Conflicts in Nigeria, 2003,* Sot Print Productions, Lagos, Nigeria, 2004.
91. This position was canvassed by the cleric in an interview immediately after the Jos crisis on December 9, 2004.
92. BBC, News Bulleting, captioned *Muslims Seek Nigeria Clash Probe,* 5 May 2004
93. IRIN, *Nigeria: 30 Dead following Religious Riots in Kano,* 12 May 2004.
94. IRIN, *30, 000 Displaced by Religious Riots- Red Cross,* 28 November 2002.
95. HRW, *The O'Odua People's Congress: Fighting Violence with Violence,* February 2003.
96. International Committee of the Red Cross (ICRC), Email conversation of 18 March 2002
97. IRIN, *Nigeria: Over 100 Killed in month of Violence in Port Harcourt,* 10 September 2004.
98. AI, *Nigeria: Are Human Rights in the Pipeline?* 9 November 2004.
99. Poul Hartling, "The Un High Commission for Refugees and the Refugee Crisis in Africa: High Commissioner's Statement of Informal Meeting of Permanent Representatives of African States Accredited to the United Nations Office at Geneva, March 9, 1982," in *Issue: A Journal of Opinion,* Vol. 12 No. 1 / 2, African Refugee and Human Rights (Spring—Summer, 1982, 25–28.
100. Current estimate reveals that to 1 refugee, there exist about 3 or 4 IDPs. The total number of IDPs today, according the UNHCR and the Norwegian Global IDP Project, stands at between 35 and 45 million people.
101. The figure is based on the UNHCR and the Norwegian Global IDP Project's estimate.

102. The Norwegian Global IDP, *Internal Displacement: Global Overview of Trends and Development in 2004,* March 2005; hereafter cited in text as Internal Displacement.
103. Aderanti, The Refugee Situation, 31; See also, United Nations High Commissioner for Refugees (UNHCR), *Refugees, Geneva,* 1979, 64.
104. UNHCR, *News from the UNHCR,* No. 1. January/February 1981, 4.
105. Norwegian Refugee Council and Global IDP Project, *Profile of Internal Displacement: Democratic Republic of the Congo, Global* IDP Project, Geneva, 2005.
106. Norwegian Refugee Council and Global IDP Project, *Profile of Internal Displacement: Democratic Republic of the Congo, Global* IDP Project, Geneva, 2005.
107. B. A. Oyeniyi, "Problems of Inter-Group Relations in Nigeria: The Origin and Causes of Ife-Modakeke Conflicts," in Olayemi Akinwumi (ed.) *Inter-Group Relations in Nigeria in the 20th Century*, 2006.
108. B. A. Oyeniyi, *Group Memories and Conflict Resurgence in Africa: A Study of Crisis-Affected Youths in Nigeria 1900–2000,* Center for Historical Studies, Ibadan, Nigeria, Monograph 6, 2005.
109. Norwegian Refugee Council and Global IDP Project, *Profile of Internal Displacement: Democratic Republic of the Congo, Global* IDP Project, Geneva, 2005.
110. Akinjide Osuntokun, "The Independence Years," in Tamuno N. Tekena, *History of Nigeria*, Longman Nigeria, 1982.
111. The assertion was made on the National Television Authority during a media chat on *"The President Explains,"* 31 November 2005.
112. T. R. Cusak, "On the Theoretical Deficit in the Study of War: in The Process of War," In S. A. Bremer and T. R. Cusak (eds.); *Advancing the Scientific Study of War*, Gordon and Breach Publishers, Amsterdam, 1995, 191.
113. Forum on Early Warning and Early Response (FEWER), *Conflict Analysis and Response Definition* (Abridged version) Methodology, London, April 2001, 7.
114. Rwandans began fighting early in the year and the war lasted for many years, producing both the IDPs and the refugees at a rather large scale.
115. There are many works in this regards. Most of these works dwelt on different aspects of the Yoruba war. Ade-Ajayi, Robin Law, Smith, Oguntomisin, Falola, Ikime, Alagoa, etc and many more African and non-African scholars have worked extensively on different aspects of the war, its fall-out, and implications on the Yorubaland and Nigeria. One of the numerous implications is colonial rule.
116. Notable among such works are Norwegian Refugee Council and Global IDP Project, *Profile of Internal Displacement: Democratic Republic of the Congo, Global* IDP Project, Geneva, 2005; Norwegian Refugee Council and Global IDP Project, *Profile of Internal Displacement: Federal Republic of Nigeria, Global* IDP Project, Geneva, 2005; Jeremy Lind and Sturman Kathryn (eds.) *Scarcity and Surfeit: The Ecology of Africa's Conflict.* African Centre for Technology Studies and Institute for Security Studies, South

Africa, 2002; Collier, "Doing Well Out of War," 1999; B. A. Oyeniyi, "Problems of Inter-Group Relations in Nigeria: The Origin and Causes of Ife-Modakeke Conflicts," in Olayemi Akinwumi (ed.) *Inter-Group Relations in Nigeria in the 20th Century*, 2006.

117. Integrated Regional Information Network/ OCHA, *The Eight Plague: West African Locust Invasion.* The work is a documentary on how locust invasion in West Africa has led to widespread population dislocation and internal displacement of people searching for food and support.
118. Integrated Regional Information Network, *Bitter Sweet Harvest.* The work is a documentary on how drought has led to missed crop in the Horn of Africa and the Great Lake Region. This situation has also led to widespread population dislocation and internal displacement of people in search for food and support.
119. Australia is reported as at the time of writing this paper to be experiencing outbreaks of fire, which CNN claims has lasted the past five days. The fire is still raging and the number of the homeless and the dead are still undetermined.
120. The experience of the Asian Tsunami of 2004 is still fresh in the minds. The number of the IDPs is still unascertainable.
121. The number of causalities in hurricane Katrina and others in the US early in 2006 remains unascertainable also, as the government of the United State has not come out with any official figure to this effect.
122. Integrated Regional Information Network/ OCHA, "The Eight Plague: West African Locust Invasion," noted above.
123. F. D'Souza, *The Refugee Dilemma: International Recognition and Acceptance,* Report No. 43, Minority Rights Group, London, 1980.
124. UNHCR, *Refugees*, No. 4, July/ August, 1981, 3.
125. UNHCR, *UNCHR: The Last Ten Years,* Geneva, 1980, 2.
126. Marc Vincent, "Global IDP Survey: Involving the Beneficiaries," in Norwegian Refugee Council, Forced *Migration Review*, 1999, 45.
127. Norwegian Refugee Council and Global IDP Project, *Profile of Internal Displacement: Federal Republic of Nigeria, Global* IDP Project, Geneva, 2005, 6; hereafter cited in text as Norwegian Refugee Council.
128. Amy S. Patterson, "AIDS, Orphans, and the Future of Democracy in Africa," in Singhal Arvind and Howard W. Stephen, *The Children of Africa Confront AIDS*, Center for International Studies, Ohio University, USA, 2003, 12–39.
129. An unconfirmed report said that many Sudanese had to send their families to neighbouring countries to avoid the horrors of the war, while the husband stayed behind either to partake in the war or to watch-over their belongings. Many husband died in the process of going to these countries stealthily to check their families.
130. UNCHR, "*The Refugee Child,*" Geneva, 2002, 23.
131. UNCHR, "*Refugee,*" Vol. 223, No. 24, 1981, 2.
132. United Nations Development Programme (UNDP), (1994), Human Development Report, 1994. (New York, Oxford University Press).
133. See the analysis of David Baldwin (1997), "The Concept of Security," by Kanti Bajpai "Human Security: Concept and Measurement" Kroc Institute

Occasional Paper, No.19, OP.1, August 2000. Also UNDP (1994), "Redefining Security: The Human Dimension." Current History, vol. 94, 229–236.

134. Mahbub ul Haq has been closely associated with the idea of human security from the beginning. Much of his analysis appeared in "New Imperatives of Human Security," RGICS Paper No. 17, Rajiv Gandhi Institute for Contemporary Studies (RGICS), Rajiv Gandhi Foundation, New Delhi (1994).
135. IFPRI, *Assuring Food and Nutrition Security in Africa by 2020: Prioritizing Actions, Strengthening Actors, and Facilitating Partnerships*, International Food Policy Research Institute, Washington, DC, 2004.
136. See table next page.
137. M. De Onis, M. Blossner, E. Borghi, R. Morris, and E. A. Frongilla, "Methodology for Estimating Regional and Global Trends of Child Malnutrition," in *International Journal of Epidemiology;* Hunger Task Force, *Halving Hunger by 2015: A Framework For Action,* Interim Report of the Millennium Project (New York: United Nations Development Programme, 2003.)
138. Physician for Human Rights, *War Related Sexual Violence in Sierra Leone: A Population-Based Assessment* (Boston: Physician for Human Rights, 2002, 73)
139. The assertion was made at the monthly Presidential Media Chat: "The President Explains," 31 November 2005. The program is anchored monthly by the National Television Authority (NTA).
140. IRIN, "Our Bodies . . . Their Battleground," is a documentary produced and distributed by the Integrated Regional Information Networks, Kenya.
141. This was based on the testimony of combatants as reported by the IRIN in the above documentary. It is sad to note that, according to the judge, of about a hundred cases of gang-rape brought to the court only one soldier was found guilty so far.
142. Associates for Global Change; WHO, "HIV/AIDS in Sierra Leone: The Future at Stake," (Report by Associate for Global Change, December 2000.

Chapter Thirteen

Determinants of Ethiopian Refugee Flow in the Horn of Africa, 1970–2000

Solomon Addis Getahun

In the last decades of the twentieth century, Africa and Africans have suffered most from refugee crises. In those times, almost one in every three refugees in the world was African. Of the African refugees, many have been from Africa south of the Sahara. The majority of these have been from the Horn of Africa (Ethiopia, Eritrea, Somalia, Djibouti and Sudan), an area that has been in "permanent emergency" for decades. Of the countries of the Horn, Ethiopia accounted for the largest refugee population in Africa. While Ethiopia evolved as one of the main sources of refugees in Africa, Sudan became the main destination for Ethiopian refugees between the 1970s and 2000. This chapter's concern, however, is not why Ethiopia became the largest source of refugees in Africa—a subject matter which is fairly well-studied—but to explore why Sudan ended up being the favorite destination of Ethiopian refugees in the said period. Based upon interviews, U.S. Congressional archives and secondary sources, this chapter displays the role of geography, long-distance caravan trade, religion, Cold War politics and bilateral relations in shaping and reshaping, and determining refugee flows between the two African countries.

A BRIEF BACKGROUND TO THE REFUGEE CRISIS IN ETHIOPIA

The 1970s was a turning point era in Ethiopia's history. In 1974, the ancient regime that ruled the empire for centuries was overthrown in a popular revolution. Following this, a series of unprecedented events at local as well as regional levels took place. Somalia and Ethiopia, patronized and armed by the two super powers, Russia and the U.S. that were running a Could War sideshow in the Horn of Africa, switched allegiances. Ethiopia shifted its diplomatic and military ties from America and the Western world to the U.S.S.R and Eastern bloc countries. Siad Barre's Somalia, which had territorial claims over Ethiopia's Ogaden territory, abandoned its Soviet ties, thereby realigning itself with America and its allies. Egypt and Sudan, who were pro-Russian, also shifted gears and joined the "free world," and signed a mutual defense pact with unimaginable consequences for Ethiopia. These countries, who were arch supporters of Pan-Arabism and Pan-Islamism now also wore the mantle of anti-communism—one of their targets being "Communist" Ethiopia. They began fanning the already simmering Eritrean secessionist war and irredentist aspirations in Somalia. The latter declared war on Ethiopia in 1976 and occupied the Ogaden territory, eastern Ethiopia.[1]

Internally, the military junta (*Derg*) that hijacked power was confronted with a relentless protest from student-based political groupings such as the Ethiopian Peoples' Revolutionary Party (EPRP) and the All Ethiopian Socialist Movement (AESM). While the *Derg* was battling these parties who questioned its legitimacy, the Eritrean Liberation Front (ELF) and the Eritrean Peoples Liberation Front (EPLF) were almost on the verge of freeing Eritrea. The only territory that remained in the hands of the Ethiopian army was Asmara, the capital of Eritrea. The junta, using the nationalist slogan, "Revolutionary Mother Land or Death," rallied the masses behind it, though with devastating consequences for the country and its people. It mobilized almost half a million people for its army and sent it to battle Somali irredentism in the east, Eritrean secession in the north and political protest in the center.[2] The series of wars and political confrontations also involved mass arrest, torture and extra-judicial killings (interchangeably known as "Revolutionary Action" and "Red Terror"), and was coupled with economic dislocation, drought and famine to produce millions of Ethiopian refugees who sought sanctuary in neighboring countries, mainly Sudan.

THE DANGERS ASSOCIATED WITH FLEEING TO SOMALIA

Because of the 1976–77 Ethiopian-Somali war, otherwise known as the Ogaden War, the border between the two countries was not safe for Ethiopians to cross into Somalia. Both countries deployed a considerable number of their armed forces on the common border until the Djibouti accord of April 1988, in which both Ethiopia and Somalia agreed to pull out troops from the border.[3] Thus, not only was the border tightly monitored but it was also dangerous for refugees and political dissidents, especially for non-Somali speakers who might try to enter Somalia.

TABLE 13.1 Number of Ethiopian Refugees in Neighboring Countries, 1980-2000

Year	Country					Total
	Sudan	Kenya	Somalia	Djibouti	Ethiopia	Africa
1980	303,000	1,500	1,174,300	50,000	1,528,800	4,045,200
1981	490,000*	3,500*	1,540,000	42,000	1,967,000	3,589,340
1982	350,000	3,900*	700,000	30,000	1,083,900	2,251,600
1983	350,000	1,500	500,000	31,500	883,000	1,921,000
1984	484,000	2,000	700,000	23,000	1,209,000	2,633,000
1985	718,000	1,800	550,000	16,700	1,286,500	3,195,600
1986	656,000	1,850	550,000	17,000	1,229,850	3,112,950
1987	677,000	1,800	430,000	13,500	1,122,300	3,574,910
1988	660,000	2,200	365,000	2,000	1,101,200	4,088,260
1989	663,200	2,800	350,000	16,500	1,035,900	4,524,800
1990						
1991	700,000	3,000	355,000	6,400	1,066,300	5,443,450
1992	690,000	11,800	35,000	15,000	752,400	5,340,800
1993	730,000	80,000	10,000	11,000	834,800	5,698,450
1994	200,000	10,000	0	20,000	232,200	5,825,000
1995	160,000	10,000	0	20,000	190,750	5,880,000
1996	100,000	5,000	0	5,000	110,700	5,222,000
1997						
1998	40,000	5,000	0	2,000	48,000	2,944,000
1999	30,000	5,000	0	2,000	40,000	2,922,000
2000	30,000	20,000	0	2,000	50,000	3,147,000

Computed by the author from U.S. Committee for Refugees, World Refugee Survey (Washington DC)

It is also worth noting that the "Red Terror" and indiscriminate killings against political opponents were conducted mainly in the urban centers. Except in Tigray and Eritrea (the two northernmost provinces), many of the residents of these urban centers were Amharas, one of the largest ethnic groups in Ethiopia. While their primary residence is in the provinces of Gondar, Gojjam, Wallo and Shoa, they are also found in virtually all of the southern *ketmas* (towns), which initially were military garrisons, during

Emperor's Menelik's (r. 1889–1916) campaigns of territorial expansion in the late nineteenth century.[4] It was in the urban centers *(ketemas)* that the bloodiest battles between the *Derg* and its opponents were held. Thus, Amharas who were in the forefront against the ancien regime and the *Derg*, when persecuted, sought refuge either in the rural areas of the provinces or in the neighboring countries. However, while some of the Oromo elite and others considered the Amhara in Oromo lands (Wallega, Keffa, Bale, Arsi, Illubabor, and parts of Hara and Sedamo) as *neftegna* (colonizer/settler), neighboring states like Somalia associated the Ethiopian state with Amharas and detested the latter. Some Ethiopian highlanders who successfully trekked to Somalia were treated harshly.[5] For Amharas and others, who usually reside in the highland plateau, the Somali desert is unbearable. It is also difficult for Amharas to camouflage themselves as Somalis. Besides, many in the Somali government often suspected Ethiopian refugees of Amhara origin as spies of the Ethiopian government. Because of such circumstances, many Ethiopians seemed to prefer Sudan for refuge than Somalia.

Despite the aforesaid predicaments that they might have faced, there were a sizable number of Ethiopian refugees in Somalia on the immediate aftermath of the Ogaden War and until 1985. During this period, their number was much larger than those found in Sudan. However, as seen in Table 1, the number of Ethiopian refugees in Somalia contentiously dwindled after 1984 for reasons explained below. While the temporary hike in the number of Ethiopian refugees in Somalia could be partly ascribed to the drought and famine that swept Ethiopia in the early 1980s, ethnic affiliation could be another cause. The boundary between Ethiopia and Somalia is the result of colonial treaties that ignored the homogeneity and cultural ties of nationalities and ethnic groups in the region. As a consequence, we have Somalis who reside in borderlands straddling Ethiopia, Kenya and Djibouti. Hence, some of the Ethiopian refugees in Somalia could also be Somalis from Harar (the eastern province of Ethiopia that adjoins Somalia)[6] while others could be bilinguals who may have also understood and spoken Somali, in addition to Amharic, and thus eluded the ordeals associated with being an Amhara, *naftegna*.

THE DJIBOUTI OPTION

Djibouti (also known as French Somaliland until 1977 and Afar and Issa since then), compared to Ethiopia's three neighbors (Sudan, Kenya and Somalia), was less attractive to Ethiopian refugees. Aside from the ports of Massawa and Assab (now part of independent Eritrea since 1993), Djibouti served as one of the main outlets of Ethiopia's import-export trade. The completion of the Ethiopia-Djibouti railway in 1917 further enhanced the economic bond between the two countries. Annually, some 40 to 60 per cent of Ethiopia's import-export trade passes through Djibouti. The latter is, therefore, very dependant on Ethiopia for its foreign exchange. Ethiopia is also a major supplier of almost all agricultural goods including *kat* (a mild narcotic leaf that is chewed) to Djibouti.

Djibouti, like most of its neighbors, is a colonial creation and a multi-ethnic state. It is primarily composed of Somalis (Issas clan) and the Afar ethnic group that roughly constitute more than 50 and less than 40 per cent of the total population, respectively. While the Issa are affiliated with fellow Somalis in Somalia, the Afars are aligned with their co-ethnics in Ethiopia. Both ethnic groups are not enthusiastic about remaining Djiboutian—an identity and legacy of French colonialism. On the other hand, both Somalia and Ethiopia claimed Djibouti as theirs at one time or another. Until its independence in 1977, the French colonial presence in Djibouti deterred its giant neighbors form gobbling it up. Since its independence Djibouti has to walk a fine line—not antagonizing either of its neighbors.[7] Hence, the presence of Ethiopian refugees in Djibouti who might also be members of one of the many Ethiopian opposition political parties was unwelcome. Both the *Derg* and the current government in Ethiopia were reported to have kidnapped or killed political refugees who took shelter in Djibouti. For instance, in 1991, the Ethiopian government abducted and brought to justice some of the highly wanted *Derg* officials such as Major Melaku Tafera, the "butcher of Gondar," who took shelter in Djibouti.[8] Very recently (July 2005), in spite of international protest, Djibouti handed over Ethiopian air force pilots who sought refuge protesting the Ethiopian government's high-handed response to peaceful demonstrators in the capital, Addis Ababa, and some parts of the country.[9]

KENYA, AN EMERGING DESTINATION

Kenya, too, was not conducive for Ethiopian refugees at least until 1991. Because of the common threat of irredentism from Somalia, Kenya was always keen to work with Ethiopia. Somalia claimed Kenya's Northern Frontier District (NFD)—Somalis account for more than 60 per cent of the district's population. Both countries had concluded a mutual defense pact against Somalia in 1964. The pact was renewed in 1980 and 1987.

In 1991, many Ethiopian refugees, including hundreds of Addis Ababa University students, who fled to Kenya in the aftermath of Ethiopian Peoples' Revolutionary Democratic Forces' (EPRDF) victory in Ethiopia, had been repatriated to Ethiopia, willingly! Kenya, thus, did not want any troubles from Ethiopia because of refugees; and thus preferred to "repatriate" them anytime at the behest of the *Derg* or the current government in Ethiopia. In addition to official treaties, the Ethiopian government seemed to have a free hand in Kenya. By "infiltrating" refugee camps in Kenya, Ethiopian government agents were reported as threatening, kidnapping and killing political opponents who took sanctuary there.[10] Moreover, no international organization opposed this and similar *refoulements* by governments in the Horn of Africa.[11]

Since the mid-1990s, however, the Ethiopian refugee flight route has changed. Kenya is becoming one of the main destinations for Ethiopian refugees in the Horn of Africa. This shift is not accidental. It is a reflection of the changing politico-diplomatic realignment that is taking place among the countries of the Horn. Sudan, which served as the springboard for almost all anti-Ethiopian elements and hence became a haven for refugees, has ceased to provide the unconditional hospitality that it offered to Ethiopians since 1991. Its relationship with EPRDF has become very friendly for a number of reasons. One, its problems with Eritrea, which is also at loggerheads with Ethiopia, had compelled Sudan to seek friendly ties with the latter. The government in Addis Ababa, on its part, had refrained from supporting the Sudanese Peoples Liberation Army (SPLA) to which the *Derg*'s Ethiopia, for that matter Haile Sellassie's Ethiopia as well, were providing military training, weapons, and a safe heaven.[12] Second, unlike earlier times, north and northwestern Ethiopia—which used to be centers of political turmoil and hence major source of refugee flow to Sudan—are relatively calm. Meanwhile, south and southeastern Ethiopia, which had been relatively calm in earlier times, is not anymore. It is in these areas, including western Ethiopia, where one of the major opposition political party and national liberation movement such as the Oromo Liberation Front (OLF) is operating. As a consequence of this new political development in Ethiopia and due to the cultural ties that existed between some of the Oromo clans (Boren) in Ethiopia and Kenya, Ethiopians, mainly Oromo refugees, are entering Kenya in large numbers. Third, the dissolution of Somalia as a state—a state that posed a common threat due to its irredentist claims against Ethiopia and Kenya—seemed to have lessened the desire for Kenya and Ethiopia to watch each other's back; and hence Kenya's increased willingness to accept Ethiopian refugees, some of them members of Ethiopian opposition political groups with armed wings such as the OLF. Fourth, the statelessness in Somalia, a country which used to provide shelter to anti-Ethiopian parties, resulted in constant political turmoil in the country; hence no sane Ethiopian would want to go to Somalia seeking refuge. Those who dared, as Reuters reported, were hunted down by Ethiopian security operatives (with the help of Somali collaborators). The Ethiopian government was noted for establishing a clandestine security network throughout Somalia in guise of fighting "terrorism."[13] The absence of Somalia as a viable state increased Kenya's desirability for Ethiopians as a potential refugee center. Also, due to the global order of things, taking refuge in Somalia is dangerous. Fifth, there is also the potential of being associated with, or accused of terrorism—for Somalia is now widely believed to be the weakest link in the fight against international terrorism. Finally, an increased Ethiopian refugee presence in Kenya could also be attributed to changes in the global order of things. These days, contrary to the commonly held belief that Africans migrate to the Western World only, there is a radical shift in the migratory pattern of African professionals. They are remaining in Africa and Kenya is serving, like other countries in the continent, as a thoroughfare to favorite African refugee/immigrant destinations within the continent. Parts of Africa have developed to a degree of enticing fellow educated Africans to live and work in Africa, rather than leave the continent for the Western World. In this regard, the demise of apartheid in South Africa is one plausible factor for such development in southern Africa. African immigrant/refugee preferences to remain within the continent could also be the result of the contradictory nature of "globalization." The Western World that advocates the integration of world economies also tightly monitors its borders and more than often closes its doors against immigrants. As a result, many Ethiopians/Africans are using Kenya as a conduit (or a country of first asylum) to go to southern Africa—so much so, that there is even an illegal clandestine network that ferries illegal immigrants and refugees from Kenya to parts of Africa and beyond.[14] Therefore, because of the aforesaid developments (see also Table 1), there is an increasing shift in origin, ethnic composition and destination of Ethiopian refugees. Thus, when one looks at the overall figure of Ethiopian refugee destinations in the Horn of Africa, Sudan remains dominant. However, as of late, Kenya is increasingly emerging as a favorite destination for Ethiopians, especially since 2000 (see Table 2).

WHY SUDAN BECAME THE MAIN DESTINATION FOR ETHIOPIAN REFUGEES

There are a number of reasons why Ethiopians preferred Sudan as a point of initial refuge rather than other neighboring countries. Both Ethiopia and Sudan share the longest contiguous border in Africa—a border which also has lots of vents: There are many caravan trails and waterways that cut across the border. Some of these routes date from ancient times and continue to operate even today.[15] This is partly due to the North Central

TABLE 13.2 Total Number of Ethiiopian Refugees in the Neighboring Countries between 2001-2005

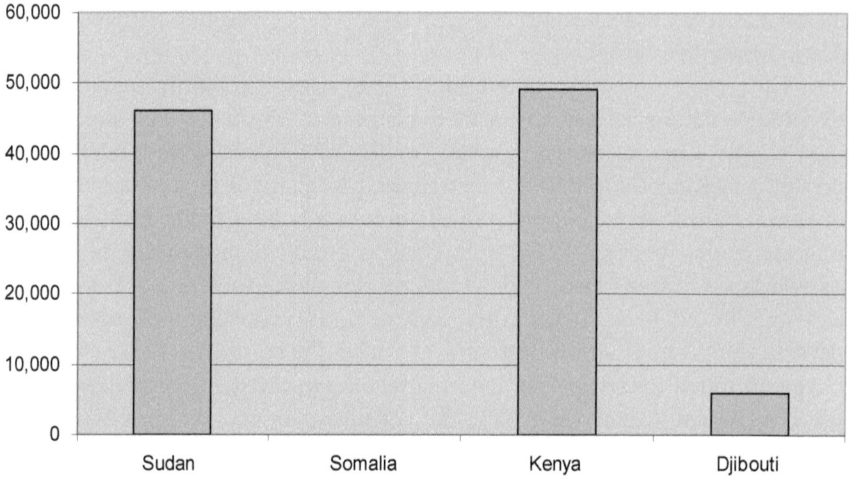

Massifs that made the caravan trails and some of the mountain passes attractive for traders.[16] Among such trade routes the Gondar, Matama and Basonda (in Sudan), and Gondar and Om Hagar (in present day Eritrea), then into Sudan, are some. These were a few of the main paths that connected the Ethiopian Empire with the historic Sudan (Nubia, Sinnar, Anglo-Egyptian Sudan) as well as modern-day Sudan for centuries, and continue to do so even today.[17] Many of the trade routes had their roots in the southern part of Ethiopia. In addition to this, the many trading posts which were established by colonial powers between Ethiopia and Sudan such as Gambella, (in Illubabor province of Ethiopia and on the Baro River), Kumiruk and Gizan (in Wallega Province) had further strengthened the relationship between the two neighbors. Gambella, for instance, accounted for 20 per cent of the Ethiopian export trade prior to the Italo-Ethiopian War of 1935.[18]

Traders continued to use some of these routes, despite the introduction of modern infrastructure. These traders often were contrabandists, encouraged by the scarcity of commodities especially during the reign of the *Derg*, whose command-economy principles had exacerbated such problems. Thus, notwithstanding the existence of stringent controls and the establishment of checkpoints (*kellas*), contraband trade between Ethiopia and Sudan flourished. Cattle from Ethiopia were exchanged for rifles, salt and other processed goods from Sudan.[19] Despite the ethno-nationalist war in Tigray (1977–1991), the Tigrian Peoples' Liberation Front (TPLF now EPRDF) was also involved in this illegal cross-border trade. It exported agricultural products to Sudan in exchange for items like salt, which it redistributed to the rest of Ethiopia.[20] However, most contraband traders were individuals drawn from the local peasants and farmer-traders, who reside along the Ethiopian-Sudanese border (Matemma and Humara localities) and there were also some traders from the highlands of Gondar.

It was also these traders who were increasingly involved in smuggling people across the border. In return for their daring service, they were paid handsomely, Eth$ 600 (Eth$1=$2.07 until 1991) and above, per person. It appears that a person who wanted to travel to Sudan during the rainy season was expected to pay more.[21] One rationale for the increase in guiding fee was the issue of rivers that usually overflow during the rainy season and, therefore, made travel difficult. Besides, it was during this time of year that peasants were engaged in farming. Thus, they did not want to risk the source of their main livelihood, farming, for a dangerous job that would not cover their annual income.

Almost throughout their modern history, Ethiopians seemed to have always looked towards Sudan as an abode in times of distress: During the reign of Yohanness IV (1871–1889), because of his religious policy, and during the Great Famine of 1889, people had migrated to Sudan.[22] In the years of Italian occupation (1935–1941), too, many Ethiopians had left for Sudan. It was also in Sudan that Emperor Haile Silassie and Orde Wingate planned the campaign against the Italians.[23] Sudan had other variables that bound it with Ethiopia, making it a favorite destination for Ethiopian refugees. One such factor is population movement within and outside of the politically delineated territories which is a common phenomenon in the African continent. Such movement could be triggered by natural calamities, population pressures or could be part of the survival mechanism of groups of people such as pastoralists. Accordingly, any cross border migration of Ethiopians into Sudan could also be the result of a combination of some or all of these factors. For instance, the Beni Amir and the Habab not only migrate to Sudan but also reside straddling the two countries.[24] For these two tribes and many others, Port Sudan, the largest city next to Khartoum, is the center of attraction. Kassala was another destination for Ethiopian migrants prior to the 1974 Ethiopian Revolution. It is only 40 kilometers away from the Eritrean town of Tessenei. So well-situated was the city that the Italians planned to construct a railway line that connected the Sudanese town of Kassla, and the Ethiopian town of Tessenei, and thence to Humera and Gondar.[25]

Aside from its geographic proximity, Kassala was also important as the spiritual capital for the Khatmiya Islamic sect, whose adherents reside on both sides of the Ethiopian-Sudanese border. The founder of the Khatmiya order, Al Sayed Al Hassan, was buried there. In addition, one of the founders of the Muslim League Party of Eritrea, Sayed Abu Baker al Mirghani, was a Khatmiya. As a result, Kassala became not only the spiritual center for the Eritrean Muslims, but also one of the very few places where the Eritrean Peoples Liberation Front (ELF) established branch offices in its early days.[26] Accordingly, it was natural for the first wave of Eritrean refugees to flee to Kassala in 1960s where they had no problem either identifying themselves as followers of the Khatmiya order or co-ethnics.

Capitalist penetration, such as the development of commercial farms in eastern Sudan in the 1960s added another dimension to the nature and pattern of cross border relations between Ethiopia and Sudan. The farming was capital intensive and mechanized. However, there was always a demand for farm labor, which now began to be supplied by Ethiopians, mainly from Eritrea. It was during this time that the secessionist struggle commenced in Eritrea; and thus people began to migrate to eastern Sudan. As a result, Tawawa, a small eastern Sudanese border town, evolved as one of the oldest refugee camps sheltering Ethiopians.[27]

In developed countries, governments maintain insurance programs that protect workers and their families from the risk of deteriorating economic conditions, injury in the work place, etc. But in poor countries like Ethiopia, there is no insurance against crop failure, unemployment, and disability. Thus, one safety valve against such disaster is to migrate in search of jobs that could help augment meager incomes.[28] Accordingly, the development of commercial farms in Sudan began to further attract laborers, mainly, but not exclusively from Tigray and Gondar. Among these laborers, some acquired their own farms while others evolved into tractor mechanics, drivers, and cross border traders. Some still continued to work in Sudan during off farming season in Ethiopia. These Ethiopians were sojourners. After the harvest season, they always returned to their home, Ethiopia, (Gondar, Tigray, Wollo and even Gojjam provinces).[29]

By the beginning of the 1970s, Ethiopia, too, had started commercial farms in the central and northwestern part of the country. The latter was in Gondar province, in the Matamma-Humera area, which adjoins the Sudanese border. With the help of the Extension and Project Implementation Department (EPID) of the Ministry of Agriculture, farmers were organized and established the Walqayt Satit-Humara Farmers Multipurpose Cooperative Society Ltd., in 1969. This enabled them to secure loans from the Agricultural and Industrial Development Bank (AIDB). Therefore, thousands of peasants from Gondar and Tigray moved to these farms. It is said that at the peak of the farming season the number of laborers in Matamma-Humara towns reached between 80,000 and 150,000 people.[30] In addition to the peasants, there were rural traders who were ferrying goods between these border towns and the nearby cities.[31]

However, the rise of the military junta to power, the nationalization of the rural and urban land and the prohibition of the use of hired farm labor changed the whole situation in the border towns. It virtually killed the commercial farms. As a result, it is said that thousands of peasants, most of them from Tigray, lost a good source of income, (Young, *Peasant Revolution*, 93–101). The destruction of the farms had other repercussions. The peasant-traders who used to trade between Humera-Matama and Gondar, and Humera-Matama and Tigray were negatively affected. The *Derg's* control of trade and the many checkpoints were discouraging, (Young, *Peasant Revolution*, 94; Clay and Holcomb, 53). Therefore, these people often had no choice except leaving the country for Sudan or to join one or the other guerilla movements operating in the region. The *Derg* tried to revive the commercial farms by changing them into state farms.[32] However, there was no labor force willing to work in these areas. Yet, to achieve success in the so-called Green Revolution, the *Derg* "began to capture and to forcefully transport vagrants and people considered undesirable from cities to work on these state farms," (Clay and Holcomb, 53). The working conditions were so harsh, and the laborers unskilled in the techniques of farming since most of them were drawn from the cities, that many fled to Sudan. It is worth remembering that the ghost of the Red Terror was still haunting people. Therefore, to be nearer to the Sudanese border was a blessing in disguise. By forcing the Ethiopians to work near the border, immediately following the Red Terror and mass killings, the *Derg* "helped" many Ethiopians, who wanted to leave the country, to avoid the danger of being caught on their way to Sudan.

The political crisis in Ethiopia in general, and the situation in the Humera-Matama area in particular, resulted in an influx of refugees into Sudan. The latter, which always faced a shortage of labor, seemed to have profited from the mayhem in Ethiopia. As Clay and Holcomb noted " . . . Most of the early refugees who arrived in Sudan from Gondar and Tigray were forced by the Sudanese to settle in refugee camps that became notorious for supplying cheap labor to neighboring agricultural schemes in eastern Sudan. They have consequently been widely referred as labor camps. Refugees in these camps were expected to work for nearby Sudanese farmers, and it was projected that they would become 'self-sufficient' from the wages they earned there," (Clay and Holcomb, 53). Thus, the temporary settlement sites in eastern Sudan, which initially have been designed as a labor pool for the country's commercial farms, were transformed into refugee camps, with of course the original purpose intact. Tawawa thus seems to have remained as the most favored refugee camp by the Sudanese government to which refugees from other sites were transferred. For instance, in 1979, some 20,000 refugees were forcefully brought to this camp from other sites.

The "tit-for-tat" policy of both Sudan and Ethiopia enabled antigovernment forces to operate in their respective territories. As a result, Sudan became the home of almost all Ethiopian opposition forces. It allowed them to function in its territory. For instance, Eritrean Liberation Front (ELF) had military training bases in Sudan.[33] Besides, when ELF finally lost the momentum against Eritrean Peoples Liberation Front (EPLF), and the *Derg's* Red Star Campaign, it retreated to Sudan, (Pool, "The Eritrean Liberation Front," 27). The latter disarmed some 3,000 ELF fighters who entered the country to repose and regroup.[34] Thus, ELF was able to survive and continued to be a viable factor on the issue of Eritrea by operating from Sudan. The same was true for the EPLF, which established its own aid organizations, the Eritrean Relief Association (ERA) in Sudan, and which ran many other branch organizations in Sudan. So much was the entrenchment of these fronts in Sudan, the EPLF leadership had openly threatened the Sudanese government if the latter tried to close the Ethiopian-Sudanese border in 1980. At that time, Col. Mengistu of Ethiopia and Gen. Numery of Sudan had reached an understanding to normalize their relationship and stop harboring and helping each other's enemies.[35]

The Sudanese government also accorded similar privileges and protection to the TPLF. The latter had its schools, health centers and aid organization, the Relief Society of Tigray (REST) in Sudan, (Dawit, 325). Besides, at the height of the 1984 famine during which the EPLF refused to let in relief supplies via Kassala, Sudan, into Tigray while millions of Tigrayans starved to death, the TPLF opened a new route to Sudan. The trail starts from Tambain, crosses western Tigray, passes through Wolqait (in North Gondar), and enters Sudan. Using this, the TPLF not only brought relief supplies from Sudan into Tigray, but also coordinated the migration of hundreds of thousands of peasant refugees from Tigray to the Wadi Hauli camp, near the Sudanese border, (Geday, 44–45).

Similarly, both the Ethiopian Peoples' Revolutionary Party (EPRP) and the Ethiopian Democratic Union (EDU) had used Sudan for various purposes. While the EDU in fact had a radio station in Omdurman and some of its prominent leaders and organizers had lived in Khartoum, EPRP often sent its severely wounded combatants to Sudan for treatment and recuperation. What is more, both EPRP and EDU, after the TPLF and the *Derg* kicked them out of Ethiopia, had taken shelter in Sudan.[36]

As a consequence of the aforementioned factors, the number of Ethiopians in Sudan, which was about 4000 in the early 1970s, reached hundreds of thousands by late 1970s and kept on growing. By March 1981, cities like Khartoum had 33,000; Gedarif 30,000; and Port Sudan 55,000 refugees. Moreover, the drought of 1984/1985 also drove hundreds of thousands more people into Sudan.[37] What is more, because of the secessionist movement in Eritrea, that province remained a steady and a major source of Ethiopian refugees in Sudan. It is said that as early as 1978, some 400,000 Eritrean refugees, who constituted 13 per cent of the Eritrean population, were in Sudan.[38]

By the 1980s, the political polarization between the central government and the secessionists had intensified. Severe drought and famine also struck the country. This, coupled with the hastily initiated resettlement program, pushed out around two million Ethiopians to neighboring countries, mainly Sudan, while making Ethiopia one of the major refugee-producing areas of the world.[39]

Since the seizure of power by the *Derg*, diplomatic relations between the U.S. and Ethiopia, mainly, and with other Western powers, generally, had cooled. Because of this and for ideological reasons, the *Derg* restricted permits to Ethiopians who were leaving the country for Western Europe and U.S. As a result, during the reign of the *Derg* many Ethiopians left the country on the pretext of business or visiting relatives residing abroad. The majority, however, took the arduous journey across the border illegally, (Koehn, *Refugees*, 79).

The *Derg* also denied access to overseas education for people who could afford to send their children. It also told academicians, even those who had successfully secured scholarships from the West, to pursue their education at home.[40] It was, therefore, only government officials and their relatives who could travel out of the country legally. Anyone who otherwise attempted was considered as a lackey of imperialism and thus reactionary. The way out was to go to Sudan or to some degree to Kenya. In fact, many well-off Ethiopians who had relatives in America and Europe, and those who had successfully resettled in the U.S. and other places, informed their families in Ethiopia to leave for Sudan. From there, it was relatively easy for Ethiopians residing in America to sponsor relatives from Ethiopia.[41] The presence of American and other refugee agencies in Sudan, such as the International Committee for Migration (ICM), the International Catholic Migration Committee (ICMC), International Rescue Committee (IRC), to name a few, whose main function was to facilitate the resettlement of Ethiopians in the U.S., further intensified the attraction of Ethiopians towards Sudan.[42]

Pan-Arabism also played a role in influencing Ethiopian refugee movements into neighboring countries, mainly Sudan. From the start, many Arab countries were opposed to Eritrea's union with Ethiopia. They viewed Eritreans as Arabs due to the presence of a sizable Muslim population in that province and because of their strategic interest in control over the Red Sea—Ethiopia was the only non-Arab country that had a share of the Red Sea coast. When the Eritrean secessionist struggle started in 1960s, Sudan and many Arab countries considered it as a struggle against Christian domination. The Eritrean secessionist movements, on their part, claimed Arab identity.[43] As Edward Morgan aptly noted, "although Eritrea supports a highly Islamicised population, whose cultural outlook is unquestionably oriented towards the Islamic world, the process of Arabisation does not permeate the character of Eritrea to the same extent as can be seen in Northern Sudan. However, the Islamic self-identity of the Eritreans has been consolidated, and perhaps to some extent exaggerated, as a reaction to both Christian Ethiopian attitudes as well as to external pressure applied by neighboring states." Morgan continued to indicate that Eritrean liberation fronts "had managed to attract considerable financial backing from Libya and other oil-rich Arab states . . . and enjoyed the full political support of the Arab League."[44]

Pan-Arabism coupled with Nile-water politics (Ethiopia is a source for 85 per cent of the Nile waters) on which Sudanese life depended, Sudan as well as other Arab countries such as Egypt were openly hostile to Ethiopia. Until very recently both Sudan and Egypt believed that a weaker Ethiopia that is incapable of using its natural resources, including the Nile River, is to their advantage. It guarantees them unlimited flow of the Nile waters. Hence, Sudan provided material support and served as a safe haven for Eritrean secessionists and partisan movements opposed to the Ethiopian government. Thus, they were most welcome in Sudan and the neighboring Arab countries.[45]

The TPLF was another beneficiary from Pan-Arab and Pan-Muslim governments in the Middle East and Africa. When established in 1977, TPLF's objective was the independence of Tigray from Ethiopian/Amhara domination. Because of its opposition to the unity of Ethiopia, countries like Sudan provided the TPLF with military bases, medical facilities and offices.[46] So much was the support from Sudan, the TPLF even organized the exodus of some 200,000 Tigrian peasants to Sudan in 1984–85. The refugees settled in the newly opened refugee camp, Wad Kauli. This camp was situated eleven km away from the Ethiopian border and 100 km from the Sudanese town of Gadarif.[47]

Apart from the TPLF-led peasant exodus, there were refugees, who fled resettlement sites in southwestern Ethiopia. These refugees trudged to Sudan from Matakel, Asosa, and Gambella areas. They began arriving in Sudan, the

Blue Nile and Upper Nile Administrative regions, sometime in 1985. Sudanese security officials and residents of the areas found some of these Ethiopians who were wandering in those regions without, however, being certain if they had crossed the Ethiopian border or not. They were picked up either by Sudanese security officials, people of the locality, or by one of the relief agencies such as Relief Society of Tigray (RST), the Oromo Relief Association (ORA), and Sudanese Commission of Refugees (COR). Upon arrival, they were collected at a holding center at Demazin. Many of these Ethiopians viewed their entry into Sudan as part of their journey back home, mainly Wallo Province of Ethiopia.[48]

At times Cold War politics also shaped the cross-border movement of people from Ethiopia into Sudan. [49] This was the case of the Beta Israel, pejoratively known as Flashas, migration to Sudan and thence to Israel. Until 1974, because of Ethiopia's amicable relationship with the West, no *aliya* (return) had been attempted. In fact, until 1975 the Israeli law of return did not include Ethiopian Jews. What the Israelis did in those days was to help some of the Beta Israel in Gondar. But since the days of the Revolution, all of a sudden the plight of the Beta Israel who were under Marxist rule became an issue.[50] Thus, Operation Moses, which smuggled thousands of Ethiopian Jews out of Ethiopia, was conducted in the early 1980s. The main center of operation was Sudan. Consequently, many Gondere (a person from Gondar) peasants and some from Tigray trudged to refugee camps in Sudan such as Gadarif and Tewawa either independently or through organizational channels.[51] Once in Gadarif, they were transferred to Port Sudan or Khartoum, mostly on trucks but sometimes by plane. From there, they were shipped or flown to Israel, mostly after detouring at a European or North American country so as not to risk suspicion. Beginning from the early 1980s, Israel was able to transplant around 7000 Beta Israel this way.[52]

The Beta Israel of Gondar also seemed to have benefited from the underground networks of EPRP and EDU, which the organizations charted between Gondar and Sudan. This happened either because some of the Beta Israel had been supporters and members of EPRP, or because of the proximity of some of the Beta Israel settlements to the city and the arterial roads. EPRP might have found it very important to include the Beta Israel in its urban and rural structures. In both cases, the Beta Israel communities were involved with EPRP and had benefited from its networks or the other way around, (Avraham and Kushner, *Treacherous Journey*, 51, 52, 55, 57, 70, 82, 86). Nevertheless, Operation Moses became an open secret and an embarrassment to both the Sudanese government and Ethiopia, who claimed to be avowed Arab and anti-Zionist, and anti-imperialist respectively.

CONCLUSION: PROSPECT AND RETROSPECT

Despite the glimmer of hope in parts of Africa on the aftermath of the Cold War, the Horn of Africa remained, as John Markakis indicated, "The Horn of Conflict."[53] While Somalia imploded, Sudan is confronted with another civil war, this time in Darfur and territories adjoining the newly independent Eritrea. So far, peace initiatives to solve the crisis in Somalia and Sudan have remained in vain. Djibouti, on its part, is still grappling with the Afar question. It has not come up with a mechanism that satisfies its Afar minority. In Ethiopia, despite the Ethiopian People's Revolutionary Democratic Front's (EPRDF) claims of ethnic federalism that brought together organizations like Oromo People's Democratic Organization (OPDO), Amhara National Democratic Movement (ANDM), Tigray People's Liberation Front (TPLF) and others, its critics are countering that EPRDF is no more than a façade used to cancel who the real rulers of Ethiopia are, the TPLF.[54] EPRDF's critics allege that the TPLF has monopolized power while its political nemeses blamed it for allowing the secession of Eritrea in 1993 and leaving Ethiopia without access to the sea. [55] The EPRDF government countered by condemning its opponents as *Timkitegna* (chauvinist) and *Neftegna* (colonizer) and began persecuting them. Disillusionment as the result of unfulfilled promises such as independence to the Oromos, the single largest ethnic group in the country, the realization that EPRDF is a hoax to cover the dominance of a single and yet a minority ethnic group, the Tigrayans (TPLF), (Leenco, 209–217 and Serra-Horguelin, 29–30) and the disbanding of the army (some 300,000) and its replacement with the TPLF's guerrillas force, further produced refugees, both economic as well as political, who continued to flee to Sudan and Kenya. The 1998–2000 Eritrean-Ethiopian war and the no peace/no war scenario following the boundary conflict, deportations of Eritrean and Ethiopian nationals from their respective countries, the sporadic student protest against the ethno-centrism of the EPRDF regime and allegations of election fraud, in addition to exposing EPRDF's undemocratic practices, has also continued producing refugees.

The new development, as seen in Table 2, is that Kenya is emerging as one of the favorite destinations for Ethiopian refugees. In fact, in 2005, which was one of the worst years of election-related political turmoil in Ethiopia, Kenya has, for the first time since the refugee crisis in Ethiopia began, surpassed Sudan as the main destination for Ethiopian refugees. Overall, however, Sudan has remained the main destination for Ethiopian refuges in the Horn of Africa.[56]

NOTES

1. John Markakis, "The Horn of Conflict," *Review of African Political Economy*, Vol. 97 (2003), 359–362; Steven David, "Realignment in the Horn of Africa: The Soviet Advantage," *International Security*, Vol. 4, No. 2 (Autumn, 1979), 69–90; Dan Connell, "Alignments in the Horn: Famine Reshuffles the Deck," *Middle East Report*, N0. 145 (Mar.-Apr., 1987), 29–30; "Israel and Ethiopia," *Journal of Palestine Studies*, Vol. 14. No. 4 (Summer, 1985), 194–196; Edward Morgan, "A Geographic Evaluation of the Ethiopia-Eritrea Conflict," *The Journal of Modern African Studies*, Vol. 15, No. 4 (Dec., 1977), 667–674.
2. On the revolution in Ethiopia and its consequences, see Andargachew Tiruneh, *The Ethiopian Revolution, 1974–1987: A Transformation from an Aristocratic to a Totalitarian Autocracy* (Cambridge: Cambridge University Press, 1993);Teferra Haile-Selassie, *The Ethiopian Revolution, 1974–1991: From a Monarchical Autocracy to a Military Oligarchy* (New York: Columbia University Press, 1997).
3. Lionel Cliffe, "Regional Dimensions of the Conflict in the Horn of Africa," in *Third World Quarterly*. Vol. 20, No 1, (1999), 91; Dawit Wolde Giorgis, *Red Tears: War, Famine, and Revolution in Ethiopia*, (Trenton: Red Sea Press, 1989), 309; see also David D. Latin and Said Samatar, *Somalia: Nation in Search of A State*, (Boulder: Westview Press, 1987)
4. Akalu Wolde Mikael, "Urban Development in Ethiopia in Time and Space Perspective," University of California, 1997. Ph. D dissertation; see also *idem*. "Some Thoughts on the Process of Urbanization in Pre-twentieth Century Ethiopia" *Ethiopian Geographical Journal*, Vol. 5, No., 2, (1967); also Harold G. Marcus, *A History of Ethiopia* (Berkeley: University Press, 1994), 105.
5. Ali Hassan, "*Yaetiyopiya sidategnoch basomaliya wusit 'baetiyopiyawiyan' eji ymifasamibachew gif*" [Ethiopian Refugees in Somalia: The Injustices they Suffered in 'Ethiopian' Hands] *Ethiopian Register*, Vol. I, No. 4, (May 1994), 89–92.
6. Mekuria Bulcha, "Conquest and Forced Migration: An Assessment of the Oromo Experience" (ed.) Seyoum Y. Hameso, Trevor Trueman, Temesgen M. Erena in *Ethiopia: Conquest and the Quest for Freedom and Democracy* (London: TSC Publication, 1997), 43–44.
7. Peter Schwab, "Col War on the Horn of Africa," *African Affairs*, Vol. 77, No. 306 (Jan., 1978), 6–20; Kassim Sheshim and James Searing, "Djibouti and the Question of Afar Nationalism," *African Affairs*, Vol. 79, No. 315 (Apr., 1980), 209–226; John Markakis, "Anatomy of a Conflict: Afar and Ise Ethiopia," *Review of African Political Economy*, No. 96 (2003), 445–453; Jeffery A. Lefebvre, " The United States, Ethiopia and the 1963 Somali-Soviet Arms Deal: Containment and the Balance of Power Dilemma in the Horn of Africa," *The Journal of Modern African Studies*, Vol. 36, No. 4 (Dec., 1998), 611–643; also on France's role in Africa in general and the Horn of Africa in particular, see Thomas A. Marks, "Djibouti: France's Strategic Toehold in Africa," *African Affairs*, Vol. 73, No. 290 (Jan., 1974),

95–104; Pierre Lellouche and Dominique Moisi, "French Policy in Africa: A Lonely Battle Against Destabilization," *International Security*, Vol. 3, No. 4 (Spring, 1979), 108–133.

8. Djibouti is country dominated by two major ethnic groups, the Afar and Issa, which in turn are subdivided into clans and sub clans. This ethnic fragmentation coupled with the absence of a democratic government in the country had made Djibouti a scene of ethnocentric conflict. The latter phenomena, in addition to weakening the central government, had created an opportunity for the neighboring countries such as Ethiopia and Somalia, and since 1993, Eritrea to muddle in the internal affairs of Djibouti. See Peter. J. Schraeder, "Ethnic Politics in Djibouti: From 'Eye of the Hurricane' to 'Boiling Cauldron," *African Affairs*, Vol.92, No. 367 (April 1993), 203–221.
9. UNHCR Briefing Notes, "Djibouti: AHC Morjane expresses UNHCR's 'deep preoccupation' over Ethiopians," July 15, 2005; UNHCR News Stories, "UNHCR Calls for Access to Three Ethiopian Defectors in Djibouti," July 15, 2005; Mohammed Adow, "Djibouti Deports Ethiopian Pilots," *BBC World Service*, July 19, 2005. http://news.bbc.co.uk/2/hi/africa/4696377.stm Accessed: January 31, 2006.
10. "UNHCR Scrapes Ethiopians Of Refugee Status," *Panafrican News Agency* (PANA), March 6, 2000; Stephen Muiruri, "186 Foreigners Deported," *The Daily Nation*, April 8, 2002; Nation Correspondent, "Ethiopian Refugees Stage Protest over Abduction," *The Daily Nation*, December 28, 2005.
11. Enocho O. Opondo, "Refugee Repatriation in the Horn of Africa: A Contextual Overview of Some Socio-Economic, Legal and Administrative Constraints," Tim Allen (ed.) *In Search of Cool Ground: War, Flight and Homecoming in Northeast Africa* (New Jersey: Africa World Press, Inc., 1996), 25.
12. Spencer, *Ethiopia at Bay*, 306, 321. Besides, Haile Sellassie had also promised Sudan that he will curtail the Ethio-Israeli support given to the southern Sudanese liberation movement, Anyana. In return, Sudan had agreed to limit its support to ELF. See Robert G. Patman, *The Soviet Union in the Horn of Africa: The Diplomacy of Intervention and Disengagement* (Cambridge: Cambridge University Press, 1990), 87–88.
13. Andrew Cawthorne, "Western Anti-terror Units Accused of Somalia Human Rights Abuse," Reuters, September 1, 2005. http://za.today.reuters.com/news/newsArticle.aspx?type=topNews&storyID=2005–09–01T115044Z_01_ALL142602_RTRIDST_0_OZATP-RIGHTS-SOMALIA-20050901.XML
14. Stephen Muiruri, "How Illegal Migrants Use Kenya's Airports," *The Daily Nation*, Feb 20, 2002.
15. Yuri M. Kobishchanov, *Axum*, J. W. Michaels (ed.) and Lorraine J. Kapilanoff (trans.), (London: The Pensylvania State University, 1979), 186.
16. F. J. Simoons, *Northwest Ethiopia: People and Economy*, (Madison: The University of Wisconsin Press, 1960), 205, Mesfin Wolde Mariam, *An Introductory Geography of Ethiopia*, (Addis Ababa, 1972), 37–38, 40.

17. See for the various trade routes that connected Ethiopia with Sudan and the other parts of the world C.F. Beckingham and G.W.B. Huntingford (trans, and eds.), *Some Records of Ethiopia 1593–1646*, (Nenden: Kraus Reprint Limited, 1967), 31, 39, 42, 191–192; James Bruce, *Travels to Discover the Source of the Nile in the years 1768, 1769, 1770, 1771, 1772 and 1773*, (Edinburgh: G.G.J. and J. Robinson, 1790), in five volumes. Volume III, 185, 490, 381; N. Pearce, *The Life and Adventure of Nationale Pearce*, J.J. Halls (ed.), (London: Heary Colburu and Richard Poentley, 1831), in two volumes Vol. II, 10; W. W. Plowden, *Travels in Abyssinia and the Galla Country with an Account of Mission to Ras Ali* (London: Gregg International Publishers Limited, 1972), 126–127; M. Abir, *Ethiopia: The Era of the Princes: The Challenge of Islam and the Reunification of the Christian Empire 1769–1855* (London: Longmans, 1968), 45, 51.
18. Margery Perham, *The Government of Ethiopia* (London: Faber and Faber Limited, 1969), 179; See also Eisei Kurimoto, "Trade Relations between Western Ethiopia and the Nile Valley during the Nineteenth Century," *Journal of Ethiopian Studies*, Vol. XXVIII, No 1, (1995), 53–63.
19. Shmuel Avraham and Arlene Kushner, *Treacherous Journey: My Escape from Ethiopia* (New York: Shapolsky Publishers, Inc, 1986), 135–136.
20. Alemsged Abbay, *Identity Jilted or Remaking Identity? The Divergent Paths of the Eritrean and Tigryan Nationalist Struggles* (New Jersey: Red Sea Press Inc, 1998), 120.
21. Tadele Seyoum Teshale With the Assistance of Virginia Lee Barnes, *The Life History of an Ethiopian Refugee (1984–1991): Sojourn in the Fourth World* (Lewiston: E. Mellen Press, 1991), 47.
22. Zewde Gebre-Sellassie, *Yohannes IV of Ethiopia: A Political Biography* (Oxford: At the Clarendon Press, 1975), 97, 170, 179.
23. Haile Sellassie I King of Kings of Ethiopia, *My Life and Ethiopia's Progress*, Vol. II, (ed.) Harold Marcus et al (East Lansing: Michigan State University, 1994), 109–140.
24. Ahmed Karadawi, "The Problem of Urban Refugee in Sudan," John R Rogge (ed), *Refugees: A Third World Dilemma* (New Jersey: Rowman & Littlefield Publishers, 1987), 117; See also J. Spencer Trimingham, *Islam in Ethiopia* (Oxford: Oxford University Press, 1952), 155–158.
25. E. Sylvia Pankhurst, *Eritrea on the Eve: The Past and the Future of Italy's 'First-born 'Colony, Ethiopia's Ancient Sea Province* (Essex: New Times and Ethiopian News Books, 1952), 16.
26. Karadawi, "The Problem of Urban Refugee in Sudan," 119; The Khatmyya order is also known as Mirghaniyya; see Trimingham, *Islam in Ethiopia*, 244–246.
27. Jerry L. Weaver, "Sojourners along the Nile: Ethiopian Refugees in Khartoum," *Journal of Modern African Studies*. Vol. 23, No. 1, 1985, 147; see also Jason W. Clay and Bonnie K. Holcomb, *Politics and the Ethiopian Famine, 1984–1985* (Cambridge: Cultural Survival Inc., 1986), 51.
28. Douglas Massey et al, "Theories of International Migration: A Review and Appraisal," *Population and Development Review*. Vol. 19, No. 3, (1993), 437.

29. Weaver, "Sojourners along the Nile," 147; Clay and Holcomb, *Politics and the Ethiopian Famine*, 51. Because of the proximity of Gojjam to Wallega, one of the major coffee producing areas in Ethiopia, many Gojjames migrate to Wallega during the coffee harvesting seasons (approximately between December and May). As a result of this, all daily laborers in Wallega are referred "Goje," meaning "a man from Gojjam." However, these seasonal labor migrants also include people from Gondar, especially a locality called Iste, in southern Gondar and from Wollo. Thus, seasonal labor migration to areas of cash crop from the northern half of the country is not unknown among Ethiopians, during pre and post-revolution days.
30. Solomon A Getahun, *History of the City of Gondar* (Trenton, NJ: The Red Sea Press, 2006), 232, 233.
31. See for the establishment and impact of commercial farming on the peasants in the central part of the country Bulcha, "Conquest and Forced Migration," 38–41; for earlier periods of agricultural development, labor migration to northwestern part of Ethiopia, and cross-boarder trade between Ethiopia (Humera), Sudan and Italian Eritrea see James C McCann, "A Dura Revolution and Frontier Agriculture in Northwest Ethiopia, 1898–1920" *The Journal of African History*, Vol. 31, No. 1 (1990), 121–134.
32. Addis Zemen, 38th year, No. 60, Friday Hidar 13; and No. 105, Wednesday, Ginbot 5, 1972 EC.
33. Cliffe, "Regional Dimensions," 92, 93, 107. The Ethiopian government, on its part, had allowed Sudanese People Liberation Army (SPLA), to use Gambella. See Dawit, 310.
34. *Africa Confidential*, Vol. 22, No. 25, December 9, 1981.
35. *Africa Confidential*, Vol. 21, No. 8, April 9; No. 24, Nov. 26, 1980.
36. Young, "The Tigray People's Liberation Front," in Christopher Clapham (ed.), *African Guerrillas* (Oxford: James Currey, 1998), 39–40; *Africa Confidential*. Vol. 19, No. 31, January 6, 1978; Vol. 21, No. 16, July 30, 1980; Vol. 24, No. 19, September 21, 1983.
37. Karadawi, "The Problem of Urban Refugee in Sudan," 115; Tina Wallace, "Briefing: Refugee and hunger in Western Sudan," *Review of African Political Economy*. No 33, (August 1985), 64.
38. Peter H. Koehn, *Refugee from the Revolution: US Policy and Third-World Migration* (Boulder: Westview Press, 1991), 83.
39. Getachew Metaferia and Maigenet Shifferraw, *The Ethiopian Revolution of 1974 and the Exodus of Ethiopia's Trained Human Resources* (Lewiston: E. Mellen Press, 1991), 2.
40. It seems that one of the intentions of the *Derg* in establishing the Graduate Program of the Addis Ababa University in 1979 was to limit the Western trained intellectuals of Ethiopia any chance of escape to the West. If there was anything that the country's university could not teach, students were sent to Eastern Bloc countries, where escape to western countries was difficult if not impossible.
41. Informant: Shakespeare. He is the son of one of the well to do families in Ethiopia. Because his family was unable to send him to the U.S., they sent him to Kenya, and told him to stay until he got a visa to America. During

all these times, his family covered his expenses. Interview: Seattle, WA, May 27, 1997.

42. From Powell A. More, Assistant Secretary for Congressional Relations to the Honorable Clarence D. Long, Chairman, Subcommittee on Foreign Operations, Committee on Appropriations House of Representatives. Washington D.C., May 12, 1982. See also Karadawi, "The Problem of Urban Refugees," 128.
43. Alemsged Abbay, *Identity Jilted or Remaking Identity? The Divergent Paths of the Eritrean and Tigryan Nationalist Struggles* (New Jersey: Red Sea Press Inc, 1998), 113; See also Ruth Iyob, *The Eritrean Struggle for Independence: Domination, Resistance, Nationalism, 1941–1993* (Cambridge: Cambridge University Press, 1995)108–120.
44. Edward Morgan, "A Geographic Evaluation of the Ethiopia-Eritrea Conflict," *The Journal of Modern African Studies*, Vol. 15, No. 4 (Dec. 1977), 669–670.
45. Ethiopia, too, was not averse to such machinations. It had, at one time or another, conspired and allied with the U.S. and Israel in destabilizing Sudan. Besides providing a safe-haven for the Sudan Peoples' Liberation Army (SPLA), it served as a conduit for weapons destined to the front and as a listening post for Israeli and American agents against the surrounding Arab countries and communist states. For Nile-water politics and Israeli-Ethiopian co-operation, see Jutta Brunnee and Stephen J. Toope, "The Changing Nile Basin Regime: Does Law Matter?" *Harvard International Law Journal*, Vol. 43, No. 1 (Winter 2002), 105–159; Views from Abroad, "Israel and Ethiopia," *Journal of Palestine Studies*, Vol. 14, No. 4 (Summer, 1985), 194–196; Dan Connell, "Alignment in the Horn: Famine Reshuffles the Deck," *Middle East Report, No. 145 (Mar.—Apr., 1987), 29–30; Daniel Kendie, The Five Dimensions of the Eritrean Conflict, 1941–2004: Deciphering the Ggeo-political Puzzle* (Signature Book, 2005).
46. Young, *Peasant Revolution*, 80–117, 167–168; Vestal, *Ethiopia*, 183–192; Assefa, *The Pillage of Ethiopia*, 79–83.
47. Young, *Peasant Revolution*, 131; Dawit, *Red Tears*, 133, 314; Clay & Holcomb, *Politics and the Ethiopian Famine*, 53, 65–57, 70–71; Young, *Peasant Revolution*, 133; Alemseged, *Identity Jilted*, 129, 132; Barbara Hendrie, "Assisting Refugees in the Context of Warfare," Tim Allen (ed.) in *In Search of Cool Ground: War, Flight and Homecoming in Northeast Africa* (New Jersey: Africa World Press, Inc, 1996), 35.
48. Clay and Holcomb, *Politics and the Ethiopian Famine*, 77–78, Young, *Peasant Revolution*, 133, Dawit, *Red Tears*, 325.
49. Judith Bentley, *Refugees: Search for a Heaven* (New York: Julian Messner, 1986), 53.
50. The former Prime Minster of Israel, Ariel Sharon, who visited Ethiopia in the early 1970s, and who met some of the Beta Israel in Gondar, noted that the Beta Israel were surprised to find out that there were Jews in other parts of the world. See Ariel Sharon with David Chanoff, *Warrior: The Autobiography of Ariel Sharon* (New York: Simon & Schstor, 2001), 172–174, 419–420; Ian Blank and Benny Morris, *Israel's Secret Wars: A History*

of Israel's Intelligence Services (New York: Grove Press, 1991), 185–187, 427; Dawit, *Red Tears*, 244–250, and his view of Operation Mosses, 317–320; See also Mitchell Bard and Howard Lenhoff, "The Humanitarian Side of the Reagan Administration, The Rescue of Ethiopian Jews: Who Would Believe that the CIA and the Reagan Administration had Worked Covertly in a Foreign country for a Humanitarian Goal?," *The Humanist*, Vol.47 (November/December, 1987), 25–26; Ahmed Karadawi, "The Smuggling of the Ethiopian Falasha to Israel Through Sudan," *African Affairs*, Vol. 90, No. 358 (January 1991), 23–49; Avrham and Kushner, *Treacherous Journey*, 47.

51. Ahmed Karadawi, "The Smuggling of the Ethiopian Falasha to Israel Through Sudan," *African Affairs*, Vol. 90, No. 358 (January 1991), 23–49; *Newsweek*, January 14, 1985; Dawit, *Red Tears*, 113–119.
52. Tadele, *The Life History of an Ethiopian Refugee*, 2; See also *Newsweek*, January 14, 1985; Dawit, 317–318; Also Ahmed Karadawi, "The Smuggling of the Ethiopian Falasha to Israel Through Sudan," *African Affairs*, Vol. 90, No. 358 (Jan., 1991), 23–49. For a detailed account of the Beta Israel exodus, see Tudor Parfitt, *Operation Moses: The Untold Story of the Exodus of the Falasha Jew From Ethiopia* (London: Weidenfeld and Nicholson, 1985).
53. John Markakis, "The Horn of Conflict," *Review of African Political Economy*, No. 97 (2003), 359–362.
54. Kidane Mengisteab, "Ethiopia's Ethnic Based Federalism: 10 Years After," *African Issues*, Vol. 29, No.1/2 (2001), 20–25; Arnault Serra-Horguelin, *The Federal Experiment in Ethiopia: A Socio-Political Analysis* (Bordeaux IV: Institut D'Etudes Politiques De Bordeaux, 1999); Assefa Negash, *The Pillage of Ethiopia by Eritreans and their Tigrean Surrogates* (Los Angeles: Adey Publishing Company, 1996); Aaron Tesfaye, *Political Power and Ethnic Federalism: The Struggle for Democracy in Ethiopia* (Lanham: University Press of America, 2002); Leenco Lata, *The Ethiopian State at the Crossroads: Decolonization and Democratization or Disintegration* (Lawernceville: The Red Sea Press, Inc, 1999); Theodore M. Vestal, *Ethiopia: A Post-Cold War African State* (Westport:Praeger, 1999).
55. Of the 500 or so seats in the Ethiopian parliament, *shengo*, the TPLF occupies 34. However, almost all key government positions such as prime minister, foreign affairs, internal affairs (security) and defense are in the hands of TPLF. In terms of budgetary allocation, Tigray's share is much larger in relation to its population. The country's businesses are also directly in the hands of the TPLF or under one of its affiliates. See, Siegfried Pausewang, Kjetil Trovnvoll and Lovise Aalen, "Democracy Unfulfilled?" in Siegfried Pausewang, Kjetil Trovnvoll and Lovise Aalen (eds.), *Ethiopia Since the Derg: A Decade of Democratic Pretensions and Performances* (London: Zed Books, 2002), 230–244; Assefa, *The Pillage of Ethiopia.*

Conclusion

"Unknown Immigrant:" The Persistence of Migration Blues

Toyin Falola and Niyi Afolabi

> "We cannot ignore the real policy difficulties posed by migration, but neither should we lose sight of its immense potential to benefit migrants, the countries they leave and those to which they migrate." Kofi Annan, UN Secretary-General

According to two recent reports by *The Guardian* of September 8, 2006, and the French Press Agency [*Agence France Presse* (AFP)] of September 29, barely three weeks apart, international migration continues to be in a persistent state of crisis and flux. While these two articles focus on the death toll of African migrants who regularly risk their lives to cross into the European Union in nightmarish journeys across the Mediterranean, the lessons of opportunity cost on the part of the migrants on the one hand, are balanced on the other by the supply-demand or push-pull dynamics that compel migrants to brave the odds by seeing some light at the end of the tunnel. This paradoxical light often turns out to be imaginary in the end, and may well be an invitation to darkness. Be that as it may, the persistence of migration blues notwithstanding, African migrants continue undeterred in their quest for greener pastures across the globe.

The first article, captioned "The D-Day Package from Senegal to Spain," captures the objectifying and dehumanizing nature of migration. The urgency evoked in "D-Day," a term used to refer to the fishing boat or *pirogue* is equally telling, as the report narrates that 3,000 illegal immigrants from Senegal have risked their lives to make a "nightmarish sea journey from West Africa." Portraying the risk-taking migrants as some alien bunch in the midst of British tourists and sunbathers on the beach, one gets the sense of horror and nightmare as the narrative details an unending saga of boats "carrying men in various states of desperation," that is, migrants who have not had much to eat or drink for five days of a tortuous journey. A local doctor who examined them is quoted as reporting "a mixture of burns from the sea salt and the petrol from the boat's engine," and even more serious still, in some cases, some unlucky ones have had their limbs amputated when their cases are severe. Other horror tales include the exorbitant economic cost: a boat with 60 passengers charges £400 per person. It was also reported that a quarter of such passengers do not make it since most do not know how to swim, receive sores on their backs and shoulders—all in the spirit of migration fantasies and blues. The dreams and aspirations are vividly captured by Mamadou Gueye, a seventeen year old, who just arrived, "I'm the oldest of four, I had to come here to help my parents . . . It's just a normal part of life. At home, everyone knows someone who has left by boat. I came in a pirogue with 140 people, none of whom I knew. We sailed for a week, eating rice. When the waves got high, the others said 'Don't worry as soon as we got to Spanish waters, our suffering will be over." This optimism is the key to success, since the migrants have to look at the legacies of those who achieved and not those who failed.

The reaction of Spaniards to this wave of African migrants is mixed, however. From those who worry about the security of their jobs and the probability of the education of their children being indirectly devalued, since attention must be paid to Africans learning Spanish in order to integrate within the new community, to those who actually sympathized with the ordeal of the immigrants, recalling their own historical emigration of the 1940s and 1950s when some locals, "leftists" as they were called, were obliged to risk their own lives on "rickety boats" to reach Venezuela in search of a new life, the reality is that these African migrants are seen as unfortunate intruders, whose graves, when they die on land are marked "unknown immigrant" and if they die at sea, serve as a haunting metaphor for the blue expanse of the island, now occasionally referred to as the "watery graves of Africa." Despite these horrific migration "tales from the Crypt," African migrants remain undaunted.

Captioned "Deaths Highlight EU Immigration Troubles," the second report focuses, ironically, on the question of human rights for migrants. The International Organization for Migration (IOM), in their 2003 report, estimate that the illegal immigration business across Turkey into Europe alone, is estimated at half a billion dollars (415 million) per year with each migrant paying an average of $2,500 to traffickers. The deaths of five people, following a clash of hundreds of would-be immigrants who stormed the fence on the Spanish-Moroccan border was the primary trigger for the revisitation of the problems of illegal immigration into the European Union. According to the toll compiled by Agence France Presse, between the years 2000 and 2004, some 387, 000 illegal immigrants and about 5,000 suspected traffickers were detained. In addition, the International Organization for Migration estimates the annual number of illegal immigrants using Turkey as transit into Europe at about 200,000. Italy is quoted, however, as expelling a number of illegal immigrants to Libya under an undisclosed bilateral agreement. The fact that it usually takes some tragedy to get the attention of the world on the persistent problem of global migration is indeed an ample proof that the tendency is to be indifferent about the issue, since there is some mutual understanding of the push-pull dynamics promoting voluntary migration.

As these two episodes clearly indicate, the issue of African migration continues to be a topical one—one that is not going away any time soon. We may well return to the wisdom of the diplomatic solution proposed by Kofi Annan, the UN Secretary-General, quoted above. Ultimately, the solution to the economic tensions, political controversies, and human costs involved in African migrations, lies in inviting a spirit of collaboration and partnership between beneficiaries and benefactors.

Contributors

JAMAINE M. ABIDOGUN holds a Ph.D. in Curriculum and Instruction in Secondary Education with a minor in African and African-American studies from the University of Kansas. She is currently the Program Coordinator for Missouri State University's BSED Secondary Social Studies Program in the Department of History at Springfield, Missouri. Her academic background incorporates cultural and education studies. She most recently received a Fulbright Scholar Award to conduct research on education and gender issues in Nsukka, Nigeria for the 2004–2005 academic year. Her work, "Yoruba Cultural Influence on Junior and Senior Secondary Curriculum," appeared in *The Yoruba in Transition,* edited by Toyin Falola and Ann Genova (2006). Moreover, her article, "Ghana: Educational and Cultural Transformation," was published in the *International Journal of Diversity in Organizations, Communities, and Nations*(2003). She has served as Vice President of the National Association for Multicultural Education, Region VII and has taught in both secondary and higher education.

CHARLES ADEYANJU holds a Ph.D. in Sociology from McMaster University, Canada. He is currently an assistant professor of Sociology at the University of Victoria, British Columbia, Canada. His primary areas of research are social inequality, racial and ethnic group relations, transnational migration (especially Africa), and media and society. Dr. Adeyanju's current research focuses on news discourse and ethno-racial representation in the Canadian press.

NIYI AFOLABI, PhD, is co-editor of *The Human Cost of African Migrations*. He teaches African and African Diaspora studies at the W.E.B. Du Bois Department of Afro-American Studies at the University of Massachusetts at Amherst. He is the author of *The Golden Cage: Regeneration in Lusophone African Literature and Culture* and editor of *Marvels of the African World.*

OBIJIOFOR AGINAM is Professor of Law at Carleton University, Ottawa, Canada. Born in Nigeria, he holds a Ph.D. in Law from the University of British Columbia, Canada. Since 1993, Dr. Aginam has been an Attorney & Research Associate, *Olisa Agbakoba* & Associates (a leading Nigerian law firm), and legal consultant to numerous governmental and civil society organizations. He was Global Health Leadership Officer, World Health Organization, Geneva, Switzerland 1999–2001, and a Fellow of the Social Science Research Council (SSRC) of New York on Global Security and Co-operation 2003–2004. He has published numerous articles in leading international journals; he is also co-editor of *Humanizing Our Global Order: Essays in Honour of Ivan Head* (University of Toronto Press, 2003), and author of *Global Health Governance: International Law and Public Health in a Divided World* (University of Toronto Press, 2005). He has served as an international law consultant for the World Health Organization, and as a visiting professor at the International University of Peoples' Institutions for Peace (IUPIP), Rovereto, Italy, and most recently at the UN-affiliated University for Peace, Costa Rica (2005). He is an active member of the Academic Council on the United Nations System (ACUNS), and the Canadian Council on International Law. He is currently a recipient of the Canadian Social Sciences and Humanities Research Council (SSHRC) 3-year research grant (2005–2008), to study aspects of AIDS and Human Security in Nigeria and South Africa.

ENYI ANOSIKE graduated from the College of Medicine, University of Nigeria, in 1998. He is currently working as a community psychiatrist in East Anglia, United Kingdom, and pursuing a master's degree in public health at the University of Cambridge.

IKE ANYA graduated from the College of Medicine, University of Nigeria, in 1995. He is currently a Specialist Registrar in Public Health Medicine on the South West Regional Training Programme in Bristol, England, and teaches at the London School of Hygiene and Tropical Medicine and the University of the West of England.

TOYIN FALOLA, Ph.D., is a University Distinguished Teaching Professor, University of Texas at Austin. He has held numerous appointments and received various awards, most recently the 2006 Cheickh Anta Diop Award for Exemplary Scholarship in African Studies. Author of various books, including the edited collection, The *Yoruba in the Atlantic World*, Professor Falola is also a poet.

SOLOMON ADDIS GETAHUN, Ph.D., is an Assistant Professor of African History at Central Michigan University, Mount Pleasant, Michigan. His book, *The History of the City of Gondar, 1927–1966 EC*, is forthcoming from Africa World Press. He has also published the following articles and chapters that deal with Ethiopia: "The Evolution and Development of the Public Health College and Training Center in Gondar: Che-Che-La from an Italian Consular Office to a Medical College, 1910s–1970s" (2005); "The History of Addis Alam" (2003); "Brain Drain and Its Effect on Ethiopia's Institutions of Higher Learning, 1970s–1990s" (2002); "Health and Sanitation in Gondar: The History of the Public Health College and Training Center, PHC and TC, 1950s–1990s" (2001); and "Addis Alem: The Nucleus of Gondar, 1630s–1970s" (1997). Currently, he is working on the history of the post-1960s Ethiopian / African immigrants in the United States.

CHIKWE IHEKWEAZU graduated from the College of Medicine, University of Nigeria, in 1996. He is currently a Specialist Registrar in Public Health Medicine with the Health Protection Agency London, England.

KATHRYN H. JACOBSEN earned an M.P.H. in International Health and a Ph.D. in Epidemiology from the University of Michigan. She is currently an Assistant Professor of Epidemiology in the Department of Global and Community Health at George Mason University in Fairfax, Virginia.

MYRA MABOYA is principal and history teacher at Sukani Primary School in Giyani town, Mopani District in Limpopo Province, South Africa. She has recently developed an interest in academic writing and research. Her main areas of interests are school governance and school migration / student mobility in South African rural areas.

SIFISO MXOLISI NDLOVU is a Senior Researcher at the South African Democracy Education Trust (SADET), gained his MA in history from the University of Natal and his Ph.D. from the University of the Witwatersrand. He is the author of the *Soweto Uprisings: Counter Memories of 16 June 1976* and co-editor of *Soweto '76: Reflections on the Liberation Struggles*. His other main research field is the pre-colonial history of South Africa, and he has published academic articles in this field including a journal article, "Johannes Nkosi and the Communist Party of South Africa: Images of 'Blood River' and King Dingane in the late 1920s-1930s," published in *History and Theory* 39 (2000).

BUKOLA ADEYEMI OYENIYI is currently Head of the Department of History and Strategic Studies at Redeemer's University (RUN) and a doctoral candidate at the University of Ibadan, Department of History. His teaching and research interests are in African history and diplomatic history. He recently compiled a documentary sourcebook, *Conflict in Nigeria: 1900–1960*. Another of his works on conflict resolution and peace building is forthcoming: *Peace-Building in Composite Communities: The Ife-Modakeke Example, Book Builders*. He is currently a member of the Committee of Ife-Modakeke Conflict Resolution Group, constituted of eminent Yoruba leaders of thought in Nigeria. He has authored more than twenty scholarly papers on African history, including diplomatic and strategic issues. He has been a Research Fellow of the Center for Historical Studies since 2003.

VICTOR NNAMDI OPARA holds an LL.M. from New York University School of Law, and another LL.M. from the University of Toronto Law School, Canada. He is a Member of the Bars of Ontario (Canada) and Nigeria. He was a Shell Nigeria University Scholar for Academic Excellence 1993–1998, a University of Toronto Graduate Fellow 2001–2002, and a Graduate Editor of the *New York University Journal of International Law and Politics*. He was also the recipient of the Rotaract Club of University of Benin Best Dressed Male Award in 1997. Victor Opara has a variety of interests, including Executive Modeling, Academics, and Law Practice. He has an Executive Modeling Portfolio (High Fashion) with two top Canadian modeling agencies. He is well published in various fields of law. His representative publications include "Re-Characterizing Abortion in Nigeria: An Appraisal of the Necessity Test" (2004) 11 *ILSA Journal of Internationall & Comparative Law* 143–171; "Sovereign & Diplomatic Immunity as Customary International Law: Beyond R. v. Bow Street Metropolitan Stipendiary Magistrates and Others, Ex Parte Pinochet Ugarte" (2003) 21 *Wisconsin International Law Journal* 255–297; "Police Right of Audience in Nigerian Courts: Olusemo v. The Commissioner of Police Revisited" (2000) 4 *Nigerian Law & Practice Journal* 92–105; "Emerging Issues in Nigerian Abortion Jurisprudence," in Toyin Falola & Matthew H. Heaton, eds., *Endangered Bodies: Women, Children and Health in Africa* (Trenton, New Jersey: Africa World Press, 2006) 19–74; as well as a chapter he authored in a book project commissioned by the Canadian Safe Boating Council: "Legal Issues on Mandatory Lifejackets / PFD Wear in Canada," in Philip Groff & Jen Ghadiali, eds., *Will It Float? Mandatory PFD Wear Legislation in Canada* (Toronto, Ontario: SMARTRISK, 2003) 241–286. He has worked for the Attorney General of Ontario (Canada), where he contributed to several cutting-edge and high profile issues in legislation, policy, comparative Canada-US constitutional analysis, autism, gender reassignment surgery, and employment discrimination, among others. He is presently practicing law ina Bay Street law firm in Toronto, Canada where he concentrates in Corporate & Commercial Law, Labor & Employment Law, Intellectual Property, Immigration, Torts, and Criminal Law.

ELINAMI VERAELI SWAI received her D.Ed in Adult Education from The Pennsylvania State University, United States. She also holds B.Ed (Honors) and M. Ed degrees from the University of Dar-es-Salaam, Tanzania. She taught at the Institute of Adult Education, Dar-es-Salaam, and the University of Dar-es-Salaam between 1997 and 2000. She is currently teaching Women's Studies at Central Washington University, and has made several presentations at national and international conferences. Elinami has written and contributed chapters in books such as Moses Oketch and Maurice Amutabi (Eds.). *The Distance Future: Perspectives on Lifelong Learning in Africa* (Forthcoming, London: Kluwer, 2007); Fassil Demissie, (Ed.).*Colonial Architecture and Urbanism: Intertwined and Contested* (Forthcoming from Pretoria: University of South Africa Press, 2007); Toyin Falola and Matthew Heaton, (Eds.). *Endangered Bodies: Women, Children and Health in Africa* (Trenton: Africa World Press, 2006).

Index

For Product Safety Concerns and Information please contact our EU representative GPSR@taylorandfrancis.com
Taylor & Francis Verlag GmbH, Kaufingerstraße 24, 80331 München, Germany

www.ingramcontent.com/pod-product-compliance
Ingram Content Group UK Ltd.
Pitfield, Milton Keynes, MK11 3LW, UK
UKHW040855180926
475701UK00001B/17
9780415802390